Drug Discovery

**Science and Development
in a Changing Society**

Drug Discovery
Science and Development
in a Changing Society

Two symposia sponsored by
the Division of Medicinal
Chemistry at the 160th
Meeting of the American
Chemical Society, Chicago,
Ill., Sept. 15-16, 1970.

Barry Bloom and Glenn E. Ullyot,

Symposia Chairmen

ADVANCES IN CHEMISTRY SERIES **108**

AMERICAN CHEMICAL SOCIETY
WASHINGTON, D. C.   1971

Coden: ADCSAj

Copyright © 1971

American Chemical Society

All Rights Reserved

Library of Congress Catalog Card 70-184206

ISBN 8412-0136-6

Advances in Chemistry Series

Robert F. Gould, *Editor*

FOREWORD

ADVANCES IN CHEMISTRY SERIES was founded in 1949 by the American Chemical Society as an outlet for symposia and collections of data in special areas of topical interest that could not be accommodated in the Society's journals. It provides a medium for symposia that would otherwise be fragmented, their papers distributed among several journals or not published at all. Papers are refereed critically according to ACS editorial standards and receive the careful attention and processing characteristic of ACS publications. Papers published in ADVANCES IN CHEMISTRY SERIES are original contributions not published elsewhere in whole or major part and include reports of research as well as reviews since symposia may embrace both types of presentation.

CONTENTS

PREFACE

"The world is a scene of changes, and to be constant in nature were inconstancy." No one takes issue with this expression from the pen of Abraham Cowley, but too often we fail to recognize the direction of change and adjust our way of life to accommodate it. Thus we become trapped and bogged down in outmoded institutions, obsolescent methods, and unproductive traditions.

Several years ago, the Public Affairs Committee of the ACS Division of Medicinal Chemistry began to reflect upon the profound changes taking place in the world about us. How were these changes going to affect the coalition of industry, universities, and government involved in the drug discovery process? This was the concern.

Many of the changes were taking place in the science of drug discovery itself. We had witnessed the beginning of the application of computer technology to the synthesis of chemical compounds. Chromatographic devices and spectroscopic instruments had begun to revolutionize the art of structure determination. The probing of biological processes at the molecular level was beginning to unravel some of the mysteries of disease states. These developments, among many others, were already affecting the drug discovery process. Even more significant changes could be expected in the future.

Society itself was also in the throes of fundamental changes, and the effect was certain to influence the system for drug discovery and development. It had become national policy that health care is the right of everyone. Drugs are an important part of the care system, and although they represent only 20% of the total health care cost, their price had come under heavy attack and criticism. The movement toward increased government regulation of the drug industry was another facet of the kaleidoscopic environment. Altogether such factors were fast becoming determinants in the economics of drug discovery. Indeed, had the research and development process reached the point where it was no longer paying for itself?

The Public Affairs Committee concluded that a critical look at the process of change and the influence of such change on future drug development would be constructive. From this nebula arose the two symposia "The Science of Drug Discovery" and "Drug Discovery and Development in a Changing Society," which were organized under the able leadership of Barry Bloom and Glenn Ullyot, respectively. The papers from these symposia comprise the substance of this volume.

Abbott Laboratories   WARREN J. CLOSE
North Chicago, Ill.
August 1971

Drugs from Natural Products—Plant Sources

S. MORRIS KUPCHAN

University of Virginia, Charlottesville, Va. 22901

The plant kingdom has served as one of man's oldest sources of useful drugs. The history of classic plant-derived medicinals, such as morphine and quinine, illustrates the origin of the older medicinals as major and relatively easily isolated constituents of folk remedies. More recently discovered agents, such as reserpine and vincaleukoblastine, have been minor constituents of complex mixtures, whose isolation was guided by pharmacological assay. A model for future searches for plant derived medicinals is illustrated by the isolation and characterization of the tumor inhibitors vernolepin and jatrophone. Screening of many hundreds of crude extracts yielded a significant number of active extracts, and fractionations guided by biological assays have yielded a fascinating array of novel biologically active plant products.

The use in medicine of drugs derived from plants goes back to antiquity. When one considers the therapeutic impact of morphine, quinine, digitalis, ergot, atropine, cocaine, reserpine, and vincaleukoblastine, to name but a few, it is evident how great is the debt of medicine to plant-derived drugs even today. If one adds the synthetic derivatives and variants of plant-derived products, the role of natural products from plant sources has been most impressive.

The most important plant-derived drugs were developed between 1800 and 1950. The past few decades have witnessed an unquestionable diminution in the number of such compounds introduced into medicine. These facts have led to suggestions that the intensive investigations of the past century have nearly exhausted the plant kingdom as a potential source for new drugs and that future work in this area is unlikely to be rewarding. I address myself to the contrary thesis—*viz.*, that the plant kingdom continues to offer a rich and virtually inexhaustible supply of new potential drugs. However, the success in tapping this source will depend upon the extent to which newer approaches to the study of biologically-active plant constituents are used.

1

The Past: Morphine and Quinine

As we look to the past, morphine and quinine represent classic examples of early plant-derived medicinals. Opium, the sun-dried latex of the unripe fruit of *Papaver somniferum*, is believed to have been used before history was recorded. The first undisputed reference to poppy juice is found in the writings of Theophrastus in the third century B. C. Dioscorides in the first century A. D. was fully acquainted with the method for collecting and preparing opium, and his directions for preparing syrup of poppy are essentially unchanged in modern pharmacopeias. Arabian physicians were well versed in the uses of opium. This drug was introduced to the Orient and China by Arabian traders. The spread of the opium habit throughout China did not occur until the latter part of the eighteenth century when the Portuguese and later the English started to exploit the natives in this regard. The war against opium has continued in the Orient and elsewhere ever since.

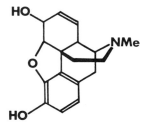

Figure 1.   Morphine

From the sixteenth century and well into the nineteenth century the uses of opium for its analgesic and hypnotic properties were fairly well understood in Europe. In 1805 a young German pharmacist in Hanover named Sertürner isolated and described morphine. This epochal finding went unnoticed until his later publication in 1816. Sertürner almost lost his life by experimenting with morphine on himself. The discovery of other alkaloids in opium quickly followed that of morphine, and the use of pure alkaloids rather than crude preparations soon spread throughout the medical world. Extensive structural studies led to elucidation of morphine's structure by Gulland and Robinson in 1925 (*1*), and total syntheses by Gates and Tschudi (*2*) and by Elad and Ginsburg (*3*) confirmed completely the structure and stereochemistry of the molecule (Figure 1). It is noteworthy that morphine is the major alkaloid of opium; in a good grade of opium it averages 10%, although samples containing over 20% have been reported.

Quinine is the chief alkaloid of cinchona, the bark of the cinchona tree indigenous to certain regions of South America. The first written record of the use of cinchona occurs in a religious book written in 1633 and published in Spain in 1639. A variety of colorful and fanciful versions of the discovery of the fever bark exist. A popular and persistent version is that the bark was used in 1638 to treat Countess Anna del Chinchon, wife of the viceroy to Peru, and that her miraculous cure resulted in the introduction of cinchona into Spain in 1639 for the treatment of ague. By 1640, the drug was being used for fevers in Europe. The term "cinchona" was chosen by Linné (who accidentally misspelled it) for the species of plants yielding the drug. Jesuit priests were the main importers and distributors of cinchona in Europe, and the name "Jesuit bark" soon became attached to the drug.

For almost two centuries, the bark was used in medicine as a powder, extract, or infusion. In 1820 Pelletier and Caventou isolated quinine and cinchonine from cinchona, and the use of the alkaloids as such gained favor rapidly. Extensive and classic studies led to elucidation of the structure of quinine (Figure 2) (4) and to its total synthesis in 1944 (5). Cinchona contains 25 closely related alkaloids, of which the most important are quinine, quinidine, cinchonine, and cinchonidine. The average yield of alkaloid is about 6–7%, of which one-half to two-thirds is quinine. It has been said that quinine owes its dominant position in the treatment of malaria only to the fact that it was the first alkaloid isolated from cinchona, and that there is little among the four major alkaloids to choose from in treating this disease (6).

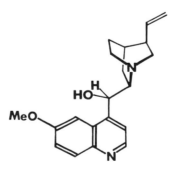

Figure 2.   Quinine

The history of morphine and quinine, like that of most classic plant-derived medicinals, reveals that the compounds represented major and relatively easily isolated plant constituents. The ready accessibility of the compounds played a major role in their characterization as the active principles of the plants.

The Present: Reserpine and Vincaleukoblastine

Reserpine and vincaleukoblastine represent the most important plant-derived medicinals introduced into medicine by our generation, and it is instructive to compare their history with those of morphine and quinine. Descriptions of the use of extracts of plants resembling *Rauwolfia* may be traced back to ancient Hindu ayurvedic writings. They were used in primitive Hindu medicine for a variety of diseases, including snake bite, hypertension, insomnia, and insanity. The early remedies were used for various other purposes, but it seems clear now that our present day application of *Rauwolfia* alkaloids in treating hypertension and mental disease was foreshadowed in the folk medicine of the Eastern peoples.

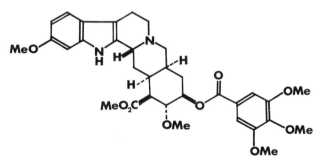

Figure 3. Reserpine

Although *Rauwolfia* was investigated in the nineteenth century and the presence of alkaloids indicated, a systematic investigation of *Rauwolfia* was only started by Siddiqui and Siddiqui in 1931 (*7*). Five alkaloids were isolated at that time, and despite the fact that one alkaloid (serpentine) had a blood-pressure reducing effect, none of the five showed the characteristics which were later called "reserpinelike" (*8*). Chopra and others concluded that additional pharmacologically active material must be present in the whole root for which the crystalline alkaloids available at the time could not account (*9, 10*). The *Rauwolfia* problem received a great stimulus from the 1949 paper by Vakil in the *British Heart Journal* on the antihypertensive effects of *Rauwolfia* extracts in man (*11*). In the newer studies, systematic fractionation and isolation were coupled with pharmacological evaluation, and it became apparent that the hypotensive and alkaloidal material was concentrated into the "oleoresin" fraction. Reserpine, the most important *Rauwolfia* alkaloid, was isolated from the "oleoresin" fraction in 1952 (*12*), and shortly afterward it was shown to be responsible for most of the tranquilizing and hypotensive effects of *Rauwolfia* extracts. The elucidation of its structure (Figure 3) (*13*) and an elegant total synthesis (*14, 15*) constituted major achievements in alkaloid chemistry. Reserpine is one of over 50 alkaloids isolated from various *Rauwolfia* species.

The beneficial properties of the periwinkle plant, *Vinca rosea* Linn., have been described in medicinal folklore for many years in various parts of the world. An alleged activity as an oral hypoglycemic agent prompted its phytochemical examination in two different laboratories independently. While neither group could substantiate this reported activity in either normal or experimentally-induced hyperglycemic rabbits, the Canadian group of Noble, Beer, and Cutts observed a peripheral granulocytopenia and bone marrow depression in rats associated with certain fractions (*16*). These effects guided the extraction and purification of an active alkaloid, termed vincaleukoblastine. The Lilly group, which included Johnson, Svoboda, and others, demonstrated that certain alkaloidal fractions inhibited the growth of an acute lymphocytic leukemia in mice. Fractionation, followed by assay in the leukemic mice, yielded vincaleukoblastine, vincristine, and two other active dimeric alkaloids (*17*, *18*). Vincaleukoblastine and vincristine are now among the most important drugs for the treatment of acute leukemia of childhood and other neoplasms (*19*). The molecular structures of vincaleukoblastine and vincristine were determined by chemical studies in 1964 (Figure 4) (*20*), and the complete stereochemistry and absolute configuration were elucidated by x-ray crystallographic analysis in 1965 (*21*). Vincaleukoblastine is one of more than 50 alkaloids isolated from *Vinca rosea*.

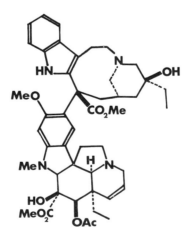

Figure 4.   Vincaleukoblastine

The review of the history of reserpine and vincaleukoblastine reveals that each alkaloid was a minor constituent of a complex mixture and that its isolation from the mixture was guided in each case by assay for characteristic pharmacological properties. It is likely that, had the investigations of *Rauwolfia serpentina* and *Vinca rosea* proceeded along classical phytochemical lines, without pharmacological guidance, the discovery of reserpine and of vincaleukoblastine would have been postponed by many years.

The Future: Vernolepin and Jatrophone

The past and present states of any field are far simpler to comment upon than the future. On the other hand, the absence of clear-cut guidelines provides the writer considerable latitude in discussing the future.

Below I outline briefly some recent findings in my laboratory in a program directed at tumor inhibitors of plant origin. This program, which has already led to the isolation of the active principles of more than 80 tumor-inhibitory extracts, has been the subject of two recent reviews (22). For this discussion of the future of plant-derived drugs, the stories of vernolepin and jatrophone will exemplify one important approach.

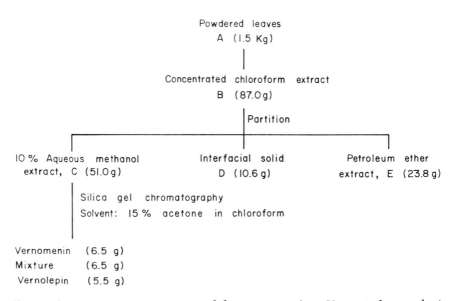

Figure 5.   Fractionation of tumor-inhibitory extract from Vernonia hymenolepis

In our program, the fractionation and isolation studies are guided at every stage by biological assays. The systematic fractionation has made possible the isolation of important minor constituents which would most probably have been missed in the classical approach. During the screening program sponsored by the Cancer Chemotherapy National Service Center, an extract of *Vernonia hymenolepis, A. rich,* was found to show significant and reproducible cytotoxicity against the KB tissue culture of human carcinoma of the nasopharynx. Figure 5 summarizes the fractionation procedure that led to the isolation of the cytotoxic principles, vernolepin, and vernomenin. Although the compounds were concentrated and isolated solely on the basis of *in vitro* cytotoxicity, vernolepin was subsequently found to show significant *in vivo* tumor inhibitory activity against the Walker 256 carcinosarcoma in the rat. Vernolepin and its isomer, vernomenin, were interrelated by conversion to a common methanol adduct. A combination of degradative, spectral, and x-ray crystallographic studies resulted in assignment of the biogenetically novel, elemanolide dilactone structures shown in Figure 6 (*23, 24*).

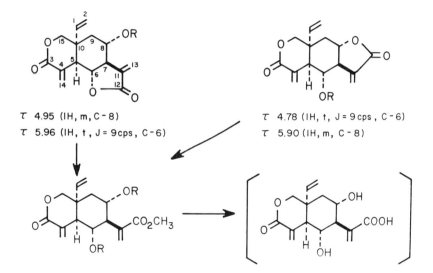

τ 4.95 (IH, m, C-8)
τ 5.96 (IH, t, J = 9cps, C-6)

τ 4.78 (IH, t, J = 9cps, C-6)
τ 5.90 (IH, m, C-8)

Figure 6. Structures of vernolepin (upper left, R=H) and vernomenin (upper right, R=H)

Several recent observations have focused attention on the importance of the conjugated α-methylene lactone function for the biological activity of vernolepin and other sesquiterpene lactones. Furthermore, the results support the view that the α-methylene lactones may exert their effects on cells by interacting with sulfhydryl enzymes that regulate cellular growth. For instance, vernolepin is a potent inhibitor of the extension growth of wheat coleoptile sections (*25*); this inhibitory effect is blocked completely by adding sulfhydryl compounds such as mercaptoethanol to the medium. Second, vernolepin and other sesquiterpene lactones can inhibit phosphofructokinase by reacting with the enzyme's sulfhydryl groups (*26*). Third, as shown in Figure 7, the cytotoxicity of vernolepin derivatives appears to be related directly to the presence of free conjugated α-methylene lactone functions. Thus, selective reduction of the ethylidene

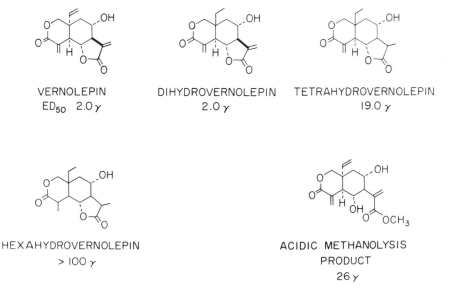

Figure 7.   Cytotoxicity of vernolepin derivatives

double bond does not appear to affect the cytotoxicity. However, modification of the α-methylene-γ-lactone (by trans-esterification to the methanol adduct or by hydrogenation) results in a 10-fold diminution in cytotoxicity. Modification of both α-methylene lactone systems, as in hexahydrovernolepin, leads to a derivative which is essentially inactive. [The synthesis of dihydrovernolepin exemplifies a new blocking sequence for the protection of the highly reactive conjugated α-methylene groups of lactones (Figure 8). Vernolepin was treated with excess n-propylthiol at pH 9.2 to give a bisthiol adduct. Hydrogenation of the bisthiol adduct (with one mole equivalent of hydrogen), followed by methyl iodide methylation and sodium bicarbonate-catalyzed elimination, gave dihydrovernolepin (27).] Recently we studied the reactions of several conjugated α-methylene lactones with model biological nucleophiles, such as cysteine, lysine, and guanine (28). Thiols such as cysteine were the most reactive, and the rate of reaction was of the same order as that of cysteine with iodoacetate, a commonly used sulfhydryl reagent (Figure 9). The biscysteine adducts, in accord with expectations, were essentially inactive.

Extracts of *Jatropha gossypiifolia* L. and related species have been used for many years in Costa Rica to treat cancerous growths. An alcoholic extract of the roots of *Jatropha gossypiifolia* (supplied by J. A. Saenz Renauld of the University of Costa Rica) was found by CCNSC to show inhibitory activity against four standard animal tumor systems (sarcoma 180, Lewis lung carcinoma, and lymphocytic leukemia P-388 in the mouse, and the Walker 256 intramuscular carcinosarcoma in the rat) and *in vitro* against cells derived from human carcinoma of the nasopharynx (KB). Figure 10 summarizes the fractionation procedure that led to the isolation of the cytotoxic principle, jatrophone. After isolation on the basis of fractionation guided by assay against KB cell culture, jatrophone showed reproducible inhibitory activity against the P-388 lymphocytic

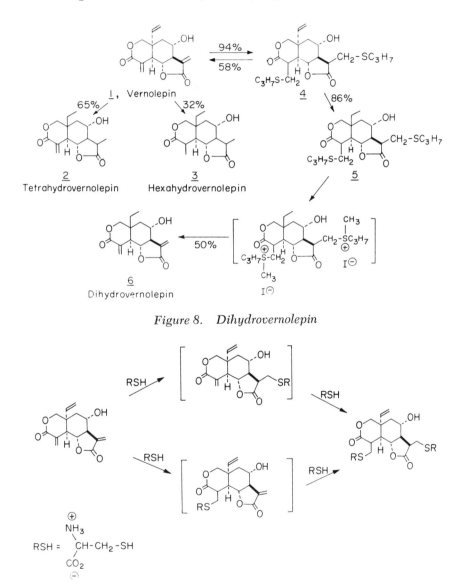

Figure 8. Dihydrovernolepin

Figure 9. Reaction of vernolepin with L-cysteine at 25°C, pH 7.4. Initial reaction rate: $k_2 = 12,000$ liters/mole/min.

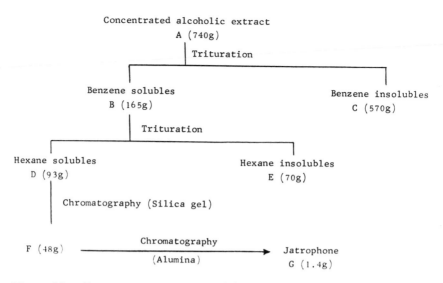

Concentrated alcoholic extract
A (740g)

Trituration

Benzene solubles
B (165g)

Benzene insolubles
C (570g)

Trituration

Hexane solubles
D (93g)

Hexane insolubles
E (70g)

Chromatography (Silica gel)

F (48g) ————— Chromatography —————→ Jatrophone
(Alumina)   G (1.4g)

Figure 10. Fractionation of tumor-inhibitory extract from Jatropha gossypiifolia *L.*

leukemia as well. The novel macrocyclic diterpenoid structure shown in
Figure 11 was assigned on the basis of spectral studies of jatrophone and
several derivatives, as well as x-ray crystallographic analysis of jatrophone
dihydrobromide (29). Hydrobromination of jatrophone in glacial acetic
acid gives the unique dihydrobromide adduct; stirring a chloroform solution of the dihydrobromide with a suspension of neutral alumina regen-
erates jatrophone. The ready formation of the dihydrobromide adduct
is envisioned as a result of two novel transannular conjugate addition
reactions, and the stereochemical representation of these conjugate additions is shown in Figure 12. Thiols attack jatrophone with great ease,
and studies of the interaction of sulfhydryl enzymes with jatrophone are
currently underway. These and other experiments are designed to eval-

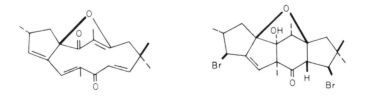

JATROPHONE   JATROPHONE DIHYDROBROMIDE

Figure 11. Antileukemic principle of Jatropha gossypiifolia

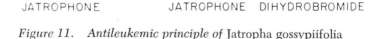

uate whether jatrophone and other plant-derived tumor inhibitors may act by selective alkylation of sulfhydryl enzymes that regulate cellular growth.

This discussion of vernolepin and jatrophone illustrates our approach to the isolation from plants of new, novel, and biologically active natural products. Both examples involved biological assays for growth-inhibitory activity, but any other satisfactory biological assay could be used in a search for other types of compounds. To the investigator who will undertake such a systematic approach to biologically active natural products,

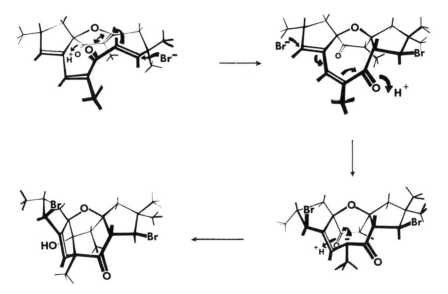

Figure 12.   Transannular conjugate additions of HBr

the plant kingdom represents a virtually untapped resource. Our botanist colleagues estimate that approximately 500,000 species of plants occur, and that perhaps 10% have been investigated phytochemically. Of the small minority which have received chemical attention, only a tiny proportion have ever been attacked with a systematic approach involving any type of biological assay. Different bioassays will provide "handles" for isolating new compounds from those few plants which have already been examined with the guidance of one assay system. Indeed, we have already witnessed the effectiveness of this approach in the plant tumor-inhibitor program. Periodic reexamination of plant recollections with new screening systems continues to yield new actives. As one looks to the future, plant sources may prove to be inexhaustible since periodic reexamination of extracts of the same plant will be desirable as new and sensitive bioassay procedures for different types of activity are discovered.

One important question remains: where will the new leads come from? So many of the older plant-derived medicinals have sprung from folk remedies that many readers assume that only plants reported to be therapeutically useful should be examined for pharmacological properties. Selected individual folk remedies whose reported pharmacological properties are detectable in objective assays will continue to provide some leads. However, logistic considerations will require that the majority of future leads in this area will emerge from large scale random screening of plant extracts. It is significant that of the first 40,000 crude extracts prepared from plants collected by the CCNSC randomly from around the world approximately 3% showed reproducible activity in one or another of the tumor systems used (30). The demonstrated effectiveness of random screening of plant extracts in uncovering significant leads for systematic isolation of growth-inhibitory compounds supports confidence in this approach to new compounds with other desired pharmacological properties.

Our small incursion into the search for plant-derived tumor inhibitors during the past decade has yielded a fascinating array of novel biologically active natural products. The plant kingdom will continue to yield novel drugs to those who will use biological assay as a "divining rod" in their highly significant and challenging explorations.

Literature Cited

(1) Gulland, J. M., Robinson, R., *Mem. Proc. Manchester Lit. Phil. Soc.* (1925) **69**, 79.
(2) Gates, M., Tschudi, G., *J. Am. Chem. Soc.* (1952) **74**, 1109; (1956) **78**, 1380.
(3) Elad, D., Ginsburg, D., *J. Chem. Soc.* (1954) 3052.
(4) Turner, R. B., Woodward, R. B., *The Alkaloids* (1953) **3**, 1.
(5) Woodward, R. B., von E. Doering, W., *J. Am. Chem. Soc.* (1944) **66**, 849; (1945) **67**, 860.
(6) Russell, P. B., in "Medicinal Chemistry," A. Burger, Ed., p. 821, 2nd ed., Interscience, New York, 1960.
(7) Siddiqui, S., Siddiqui, R. H., *J. Indian Chem. Soc.* (1931) **8**, 667; (1932) **9**, 539; (1935) **12**, 37.
(8) Woodson, R. E., Jr., Youngken, H. W., Schlittler, E., Schneider, J. A., "Rauwolfia," Little, Brown, & Co., Boston, 1957.
(9) Chopra, R. N., Chakravarti, M., *Indian J. M. Res.* (1941) **29**, 763.
(10) Chopra, R. N., Gupta, J. C., Bose, B. C., Chopra, I., *Indian J. M. Res.* (1943) **31**, 71.
(11) Vakil, R. J., *British Heart J.* (1949) **11**, 350.
(12) Mueller, J. M., Schlittler, E., Bein, H. J., *Experientia* (1952) **8**, 338.
(13) Dorfman, L. A. *et al.*, *Helv. Chim. Acta* (1954) **37**, 59.
(14) Woodward, R. B., Bader, F. E., Bickel, H., Frey, A. J., Kierstad, R. W., *J. Am. Chem. Soc.* (1956) **78**, 2023, 2657.
(15) Woodward, R. B., Bader, F. E., Bickel, H., Frey, A. J., Kierstad, R. W., *Tetrahedron* (1958) **2**, 1.

(16) Noble, R. L., Beer, C. T., Cutts, J. H., *Biochem. Pharmacol.* (1958) **1**, 347.
(17) Johnson, I. S., Wright, H. F., Svoboda, G. H., *J. Lab. Clin. Med.* (1959) **54**, 830.
(18) Svoboda, G. H., Johnson, I. S., Gorman, M., Neuss, N., *J. Pharm. Sci.* (1962) **51**, 707.
(19) National Advisory Cancer Council Report, "Progress Against Cancer, 1969," U. S. Department of Health, Education, and Welfare, Washington, D. C.
(20) Neuss, N., Gorman, M., Hargrove, W., Cone, N. J., Biemann, K., Buchi, G., Manning, R. E., *J. Am. Chem. Soc.* (1964) **86**, 1440.
(21) Moncrief, J. W., Lipscomb, W. N., *J. Am. Chem. Soc.* (1965) **87**, 4963.
(22) Kupchan, S. M., *Trans. N.Y. Acad. Sci.* (1970) **32**, 85; *Pure Appl. Chem.* (1970) **21**, 277.
(23) Kupchan, S. M., Hemingway, R. J., Werner, D., Karim, A., *J. Org. Chem.* (1969) **34**, 3903.
(24) Kupchan, S. M., Hemingway, R. J., Werner, D., Karim, A., McPhail, A. T., Sim, G. A., *J. Am. Chem. Soc.* (1968) **90**, 3596.
(25) Sequeira, L., Hemingway, R. J., Kupchan, S. M., *Science* (1968) **161**, 789.
(26) Hanson, R. L., Lardy, H. A., Kupchan, S. M., *Science* (1970) **168**, 378.
(27) Kupchan, S. M., Giacobbe, T. J., Krull, I. S., *Tetrahedron Letters* (1970) 2859.
(28) Kupchan, S. M., Fessler, D. C., Eakin, M. A., Giacobbe, T. J., *Science* (1970) **168**, 376.
(29) Kupchan, S. M., Sigel, C. W., Matz, M. J., Saenz Renauld, J. A., Haltiwanger, R. C., Bryan, R. F., *J. Am. Chem. Soc.* (1970) **92**, 4476.
(30) Hartwell, J. L., Abbott, B. J., *Advan. Pharmacol. Chemother.* (1969) **7**, 117.

RECEIVED November 5, 1970.

2

Drugs from Natural Products—Animal Sources

J. A. HOGG

The Upjohn Co., Kalamazoo, Mich. 49001

Comparative analysis of the timetables depicting break-through events in the development of the steroid hormone and the prostaglandin fields, when viewed in relation to certain developments in the field of science as a whole, reveals some of the factors which most influenced their genesis. The most prominent factor in regulating the pace of progress was the emergence of new supporting technology in other fields of science. The breakthrough event itself often served to stimulate the pace. Despite numerous similarities between the two fields the pattern of the prostaglandin effort has not been a duplication of the steroid developments, but the influence of advances in the science of drug discovery in general is recognizable. The potential for drug discovery from animal sources remains high as judged by the promise of numerous emerging new fields.

An analysis and evaluation of the scientific aspects of drug discovery from animal origin should provide some enlightenment on the future of this drug source. Most of the major classifications of drug candidate substances known to be produced by the various animal categories (Table I) are still under active investigation today. However, since this entire field is so vast, only two categories are discussed: the steroid hormone field and the prostaglandins. The former is older in vintage and more mature in its development while the latter is a field in which there are as yet no products in therapeutic use. Neither category is limited in origin to mammalians and in the case of steroids not even to animals. These two exciting fields of drug research are analyzed by using timetables for each which depict breakthrough events. Perhaps some of the lessons learned from the steroid experience may be used in developing the prostaglandins.

14

Table I.   Drugs from Animal Sources

Animal Category	Drug (Candidate) Substances
Vertebrates	steroid hormones
aquatic	peptide hormones
terrestrial	vitamins
	enzymes
Invertebrates	vaccines
aquatic	prostaglandins
terrestrial (e.g., insects)	miscellaneous
	pheromones
	predator–prey defense
	parasite–host defense

Steroid Hormones

Figure 1 shows the basic carbon structures for these two classes of substances. All steroids contain the perhydrocyclopentanophenanthrene ring system while the carbon skeleton basic to all prostaglandins has been called prostanoic acid. The steroid hormones are discussed first.

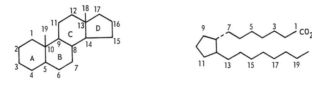

PERHYDROCYCLOPENTANOPHENANTHRENE   PROSTANOIC ACID

Figure 1.   Basic carbon skeletons of steroids and prosta-glandins

The sequence of events which normally occurs in the discovery of a naturally occurring substance is usually initiated by some biological event which signals the possibility of drug potential. This "biodetection" endpoint may or may not reveal a specific area of medicinal interest for the unknown substance. In some instances the initial biological activity can be developed into a quantitative assay method, which can then be used to guide the isolation of active substance. Most hormonal substances are present in tiny amounts so that isolation cannot be achieved without the help of such an assay.

This is especially true for the primary steroid hormones shown in Table II. The isolation of estrone would have been much delayed had Zondek not discovered that the urine of pregnant women is a much richer source than ovarian extract, where its presence had first been detected.

The magnitude of the task involved in one of these isolations can be appreciated from the fact that Butenandt was able to isolate only 20 mg of pure progesterone from 625 kg of ovaries obtained from 50,000 sows. The large scale extractions were carried out by Schering AG laboratories.

The first testicular hormone isolated was androsterone, a metabolite of testosterone. This also was achieved by Butenandt starting with an extract from 15,000 liters of urine supplied by Schering from which he obtained only 15 mg of pure crystals. Four years later, Laquer isolated 10 mg of the primary male sex hormone, testosterone, from 100 kg of steer testis. In all cases on this table the key to isolation was the quantitative bioassay as listed.

Table II.   Source Concentrations of Steroid Hormones

Hormone	Source	Concentration	Assay
Estrone	human pregnancy urine	1 mg/liter	Allen-Doisy (1)
	pregnant mare urine	10 mg/liter	
	palm kernel	18 mg/50 kg	
Progesterone	sow ovaries	625 kg yielded 20 mg	Corner-Allen (2)
Testosterone	urine	1 mg/liter (15,000 liters yielded 15 mg (3)	Coxcomb test
Hydrocortisone	beef adrenal	37 mg/1000 lb	Ingle work test (4)

The dates of these isolations and others of the primary steroid hormone group are recorded in Table III. This overall timetable of events also shows other key stages in the discovery and development of drugs from natural sources. Most of these stages normally occur but not always in the order listed.

The members of this group of naturally occurring hormones are similar in structure. In their biochemical evolution nature has used a common raw material—namely, cholesterol, yet their physiological roles are vastly different. It would seem that nature is the original practitioner of molecular modification.

The most striking fact revealed on this chart is that the isolation, structure, and partial synthesis of all of the primary hormones in each class, excepting aldosterone, were achieved concurrently within the 1930's, a ten-year period. It would be tempting to assume from this table that structure determination and synthesis are routine consequences of the isolation. The isolations of this entire group, excepting aldosterone, occurred rather close together. However, the reasons which explain the

Table III.   Steroid Hormones—Discovery and
Development (Timetable)[a]

	1930	34	38	42	46	50	54	58	62
Female Hormones Equilenin		(1)	(2)	(3)					
Estrone	(1)	(2,6) (5)	(3)		(4)				
Progesterone		(1,2,3) (5,6)					(4)		
Male Hormones Testosterone		(1,2,3,6)					(4)		
Adrenal Steroids (30) Cortisone		(1) (2)	(3)			(5)	(4) (6)		
DOC		(2,3) (1)					(4)		
Aldosterone						(1,2)	(4)		

[a] Legend: (1) isolation, (2) structure, (3) partial synthesis, (4) total synthesis, (5) therapeutic use, (6) analogs.

rapid breakthroughs in structure and synthesis seen here relate to preceding events and are of considerable importance to the process of natural product drug discovery. These reasons are discussed below.

The total synthesis of these substances lagged another dozen years and then broke across the board. Gifted scientists in both industry and universities were responsible for developing the necessary technology. Scientists in both environments were motivated by the challenge and importance of the goals set up by the successes of the steroid hormone decade. The risk for the industrial scientist to become involved at this early stage is greater since he is also accountable for the practicality of his results.

The therapeutic utilization of steroids did not reach significant proportions until the early 1950's, following the cortisone breakthrough in 1949. Merck and Co. assumed the primary risk for developing methodology and preparing large quantities of cortisone for clinical evaluation. Hench, at the Mayo Clinic, then discovered the clinical efficacy of cortisone in relieving the symptoms of arthritis. One immediately obvious consequence of this breakthrough, now well known, was a world-wide, upward surge of steroid research in general and adrenal steroid research in particular.

In addition to the competition to exploit the medical markets so long sought for, other technical factors contributed to the research buildup through the 1950's. The now readily available steroid substances were ideal models to study stereochemistry, reaction mechanisms and rates, conformational analysis, and the application of new instruments to structure characterization. All of these studies, although not necessarily aimed at drug discovery, were nonetheless contributory. Scientific breakthrough continued to add fuel to the fire. The microbiological 11-oxygenation of Peterson and Murray (5) in 1952 greatly expanded the technical capability to produce steroids. The synthesis of the highly active 9-fluoro analog of hydrocortisone in 1954 by Fried (6) was the forerunner of a vast adrenal steroid analog program. However, the concept of molecular modification (i.e., analogs) was not new to the steroid field. Diethylstilbestrol was synthesized by Cook (7) at about the time the estrone structure was elucidated, presumably not by design but in connection with studies on the structure of estrone. Probably few analog programs can match the scope of the modified estrogen program that followed. Methyltestosterone was synthesized in the same year that saw the birth of testosterone itself. Steroids are still being chemically modified today.

Some indication of the magnitude of the steroid effort is noted by Fieser and Fieser (8), who observed that even as early as 1936 publications were appearing at the rate of 300 per year. Applezweig (9) notes that in 1960 there were 1,123 reported analogs emulating the natural hormones.

Table IV provides a quick visual impression of some 50 or 60 separate drug entities, excluding derivatives and formulations, available for therapeutic use in the United States today. Progress in population control and family planning was certainly enhanced by the development of the steroid-based pill, which contains progestins and estrogens. However, the entire steroid hormone development would have been delayed markedly had it not been for preceding developments, outlined in Table V.

The highlights in the long history of research that preceded the steroid hormone era of the 1930's are shown here. This timetable records the discovery and characterization of a select few from literally hundreds of naturally occurring steroid substances, which were later to become important as raw materials in man's preoccupation with steroid synthesis. During this period it was learned that cholesterol, first discovered (10) in 1812 and characterized structurally in 1932, is actually the biogenetic raw material for all of the steroid hormones; in turn, it is preceded biogenetically by the isoprenoid—squalene—a fact which was suggested as a possibility long before the structure of cholesterol became known. Except for cholesterol and the bile acids these substances are of plant origin, so that the subject of drug discovery from animal sources cannot be divorced entirely from plant sources. Of the main steroid classifications only the cardiac glycosides are not represented. Although medically important, the latter are of plant origin and have not become meaningful to steroid hormone research. All of the steroid substances shown in this table have been or now are important raw materials used to manufacture steroid hormones.

Table IV.   Available Drug Entities

Corticosteroids

Betamethasone
Cortisone
Desoxycorticosterone
Dexamethasone
Fludrocortisone
Fluprednisolone
Hydrocortisone
Methylprednisolone
Paramethasone
Prednisolone
Prednisone
Triamcinolone

Progestins

Dydrogesterone
  (Duphaston)
Ethisterone (Pranone)
Hydroxyprogesterone
  (Prodox)
Medroxyprogesterone
  (Provera)
Norethindrone (Norlutin)
Progesterone

Contraceptives

Chlormadinone + mestranol
  (C-Quens)
Dimethisterone + ethinyl
  estradiol (Oracon)
Ethynodiol + mestranol
  (Ovulen)
Medroxyprogesterone +
  ethinyl estradiol (Provest)
Norethindrone + ethinyl
  estradiol (Norlestrin)
Norethindrone + mestranol
  (Ortho-Novum)
Norethynodrel + mestranol
  (Enovid-E)

Topical A.I.F. Agents

Dichlorisone
  (Diloderm)
Flurandrenolide
  (Cordran)
Fluocinolone
  (Synalar)
Fluorometholone
  (Oxylone)
Hydrocortamate
  (Magnacort)

Anabolic Agents

Ethylestrenol
  (Maxibolen)
Methandrostenolone
  (Dianabol)
Nandrolone
  (Durabolin)
Norethandrolone
  (Nilevar)
Oxandrolone
  (Anavar)
Oxymetholone
  (Adroyd)
Stanazolol
  (Winstrol)

Androgenic Agents

Fluoxymesterone (Halotestin)
Methyltestosterone
Stanolone (Neodrol)
Testosterone

Estrogens

Estradiol
Estriol
Estrone
Ethinyl estradiol

Miscellaneous

Dehydrocholic acid (choleretic)
Digitalis (cardiotonic (mixture of steroid glycosides))
Dihydrotachysterol (treatment of hypoparathyroidism)
Dromostanolone (2α-methylandrostan-17β-ol-3-one, 17-propionate (anabolic–androgenic, for cancer only)
Hydroxydione (Viadril) (anesthetic)
Pregnenolone (listed in Modell, use unknown)
Medrysone (ophthalmic)
Sitosterols (antihypercholesterolemic)
Vitamin D (Calciferol) (vitamin)

The 120-year-long investigation on the structure of cholesterol, marked especially by the brilliant research of Windaus and Wieland in the early 1900's, succeeded in 1932. This knowledge was the key to the structures of all steroid classes under investigation, including the steroid hormones, which quickly fell in place. Whereas the birth of the steroid hormone era has been attributed to the 1930–40 period, we see that this period marks instead the maturation of the steroid field as a whole. Consideration of the events before 1930, therefore, can not be excluded in searching for significant factors in understanding the process of drug discovery from natural sources and in particular steroid hormones.

There is some merit in thinking of the pre-steroid hormone era as the subconscious phase of steroid hormone research, the results of which later provided goals clearly relating to drug potential. Early research in the separate steroid categories in Table V were conducted without knowledge of the structural similarity that existed between their members. However, throughout these widely separated studies numerous inter-relationships were established. For example, in 1919 the conversion of cholesterol to cholanic acid showed for the first time that these two major categories are both steroidal. The established facts of each series accumulated over a century now became applicable to the other.

The long periods of time required for these early developments have no relation to the availability of the natural steroid substances because they were abundantly available for research purposes. This is in sharp contrast to the availability of steroid hormone substances discussed earlier. However, the entire science of organic chemistry was emerging during this period so that the rate of progress in steroid reseach kept pace with the developing general methodology.

Table V.   Precursors of Steroid Hormones (Timetable of Discovery)

	1800	15	30	45	60	75	90	1905	20	35	50
Sterols (hundreds) Cholesterol			(1)						(2)		(3)
Ergosterol							(1)		(2)		
Stigmasterol								(1)			
Bile Acids (20)									(2)		
Cholic acid				(1)					(2)		
Sapogenins (40 ±) Diosgenin						(isolation of gitogenin)				(1) (2)	

Steroid Hormone Era (↓ at 20)   Cortisone Era (↓ at 35, ↓ at 50)

ᵃ Legend: (1) isolation, (2) structure, (3) configuration.

**Table VI.   Instrumental and Analytical Techniques Applied to
Steroid Research (Timetable)**

Instrument	Application to Steroids	Comment
Ultraviolet absorption	1930	Beckman DU available 1940
Paper chromatography	1949	by Zaffaroni
Infrared spectrometry	early 1950's	
Rotatory dispersion	1955	Commercial instrument same year
Nuclear magnetic resonance	1958	Commercial instrument in 1955–56
X-ray diffraction	late 1950's	—
Mass spectrometry	1958–59	—
Gas chromatography	1959–60	Instrumentation in 1951–52

The entire period, especially as we approach the steroid hormone era, is marked by the confluence of numerous other lines of endeavor, both chemical and biological, which cumulatively resulted in the rapid progress from 1930 to 1940. However, the goals of the individual researchers of the time were usually technical in nature. Söderbaum reflects this on the occasion of the Nobel lectures of 1928 by Windaus and Wieland when he said that the investigations on steroids "were all designed to explain the internal structure of organic materials, their relationship with one another and their transitions into one another." He continues: "for this reason they are of fundamental importance for our knowledge of a number of processes occurring in both the healthy and diseased organism, and therefore of greatest significance, not only for the chemistry as such, but also for the sister sciences, physiology and medicine" (*11*). From this it is clear that the scientific community, on the eve of the steroid hormone era, had clearly sensed the potential importance of the developing field. It has also been said that Windaus held this view long before.

The spread of steroid research on a world-wide basis is typical of a phenomenon in research in which trends develop spontaneously, resulting in global research teams and remarkably well balanced but competitive programs. Equally spontaneous is the assumption of leadership in guiding such trends; usually one can identify a few pioneers who were responsible for shaping the course of the overall effort even though it is widespread.

It would seem that the early steroid work now stands as a model of basic research which in its entirety provides evidence that basic research relating to natural products need not be without purposeful direction, and that private and public funds, properly administered in support of similar

research, can bring rich rewards. It is of interest that at least 10 research
pioneers have received Nobel prizes for their research in or related to
the steroid field.

Before leaving the steroids to take up the prostaglandins, it is important to assess the impact of modern instrumental and analytical techniques
on steroid hormone research. Table VI shows that the general use of
these techniques in steroid research began during the 1950's, too late to
assist in the steroid hormone era. The cortisone era through the 1950's

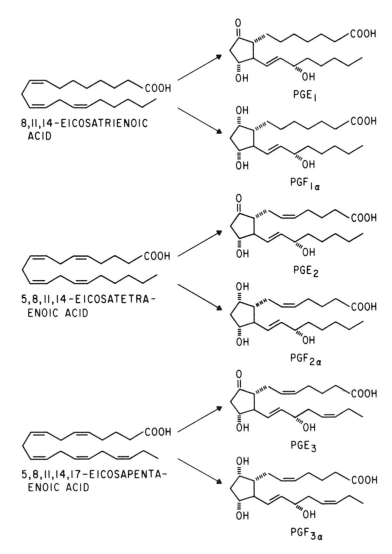

Figure 2.   The naturally occurring

benefitted increasingly as judged by the timetable of application to
steroids shown here. However, as we shift now to the emerging field of
prostaglandin research, we see that several of these developing techniques
provided the key to opening up this field.

Prostaglandins

Biodetection of the substances now known as the prostaglandins
was first reported in 1930 by Kurzrok and Lieb (*12*), who demonstrated

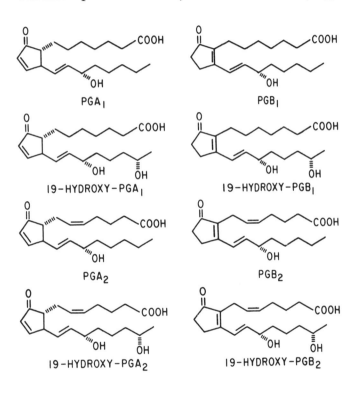

prostaglandins and their precursors

that fresh human semen could cause strong contractions or relexation when applied to strips of the human uterus. Note that this date coincides with the beginning of the steroid hormone era. It is a curious coincidence that in the August 1935 issue of *Klinische Wochenschrift* there appeared on consecutive pages the assignment of the name prostaglandin to this new substance by von Euler (*13*) and the assignment of the term progesterone to the newly isolated steroidal corpus luteum hormone by Butenandt (*14*). That both substances should eventually promise means of population control is even more intriguing.

Figure 2 shows structures for the entire prostaglandin family. The second column shows the six primary prostaglandins, so designated because in their biogenesis none are precursors of the other. The prostaglandins may be defined as lipid-like, local hormones, present in numerous mammalian tissues. Amusing but superficial analogies to the steroids are the cyclopentane ring, the 20 carbon atoms, and the presence or absence of an hydroxyl group at position 11. More meaningful is their formation biogenetically from the essential polyunsaturated acids by enzyme catalyzed cyclization as shown in this figure (*15*), a striking analogy to squalene as precursor to cholesterol. The fatty acid precursors of the prostaglandins are counterparts of the steroids of the pre-hormone era, but the vast fatty acid technology did not match the steroid counterpart in contributing later to the rapid development of prostaglandins, excepting their use as biosynthetic raw material.

Table VII shows a partial list of demonstrated occurrences in mammalian tissues for the six primary prostaglandins. In the early years the facts that the prostaglandins are ubiquitous in their distribution, are rapidly metabolized, are not circulating hormones, and elicit multiple biological responses led some to argue that they would never have useful medicinal properties. Others interpreted these facts in just the opposite way.

Table VIII shows that the concentration of PGE_1 equivalents in several sources is very small, a fact which accounts greatly for the delayed development of the prostaglandins. The special problem of collecting large quantities of some of these substances richest in prostaglandins is obvious. Sheep vesicular glands eventually proved to be the most practical source. The prostaglandin discovery and development timetable shown in Table IX, when compared with the steroid timetables, reveals some of the differences as well as similarities between these developments.

The prostaglandin era began with its biodetection by Kurzrok (*12*) in 1930 in human semen, which was shown to contract or relax strips of human uterus. For the next 29 years prostaglandin research moved at a slow pace, averaging one publication per year, while steroid hormone

Table VII.   Occurrence of Prostaglandins

Source	PGE_1	PGE_2	PGE_3	$PGF_{1\alpha}$	$PGF_{2\alpha}$	$PGF_{3\alpha}$
Vesicular gland, sheep	+	+	+	+		
Seminal plasma, human	+	+	+	+	+	
sheep	+					
Menstrual fluid		+			+	
Lungs, sheep		+			+	
pig					+	
bovine					+	+
guinea pig					+	
monkey					+	
man					+	
Iris, sheep					+	
Brain, bovine					+	
cat						
Thymus, calf	+					
Pancreas, bovine		+			+	
Adrenal, cat				+		
Fat, rat	+					
Kidney, rabbit		+				
Intestine, frog	+			+		
Spinal cord, frog	+			+		

Table VIII.   Concentration of Prostaglandins

Tissue	PGE_1 Equivalent
Sheep vesicular gland	10–500 μgram/gram
Human semen	25–780 μgram/ml
Cat thymus	0.8 μgram/gram
Dog spinal cord	104 μgram/gram

	$PGF_{2\alpha}$
Sheep lung	0.5 μgram/gram
Human lung	0.02 μgram/gram

research matured and reached its peak during the same period of time. These early publications emanated largely from a few laboratories: von Euler in Sweden, Goldblatt in England, and Bergström in Sweden. This is in sharp contrast to the effort on steroid hormone and pre-hormone steroids, which occurred in many laboratories around the world. Even though Windaus has been called the father of steroids, many other pioneers are recognized.

Probably the most significant factor in the slow pace during the early years (1930–1956) was the scarcity of the naturally occurring materials which contained only low levels of the active substances. When Bergström of the Karolinska Institute, who likes to "isolate things," came back to the problem in 1956–57, he brought with him a vast experience with nature's acidic substances, the bile acids, and essential fatty acids, fields in which he was already prominent. This background was an important adjunct to the task at hand and probably enhanced the fascination for isolating this unknown acidic lipid-like substance called prostaglandin.

Two important differential technological factors contrasted the real beginning of the prostaglandin era in 1956 and the steroid hormone era of the 1930's. One of these is the maturation of modern instrumental

Table IX.   The Prostaglandins—Discovery

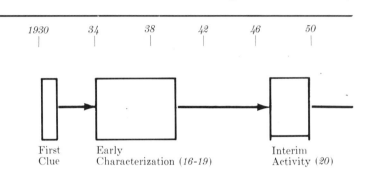

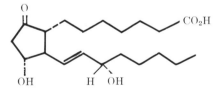

Prostaglandin E₁

and analytical techniques, which arrived too late to help in the steroid hormone breakthroughs. Gas chromatography, mass spectrometry, and ultramicroanalytical techniques were applied in a series of brilliant investigations from which the structure (23, 24) of PGE$_1$ (1962) as well as the whole family of new prostaglandin substances emerged (by 1966). Isolation was guided by the smooth muscle strip assay. These achievements stand as the classic example of the first structure elucidation of a

and Development (Timetable)

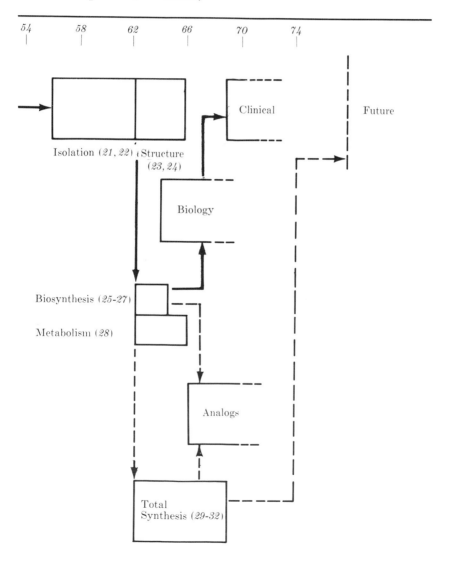

family of new and important natural products utilizing advanced instrumentation, especially mass spectrometry.

The other important difference from the steroid hormones is the
complete absence of awareness of tie-in with investigations along other
lines of natural product research prior to the structure determinations,
which were therefore essentially *de novo*. However, after the structures
became known, three different laboratories (*25–27*) independently recognized the possibility of the C_{20} unsaturated fatty acids as biosynthetic
precursors (Figure 2). Thus the essential fatty acid technology became
useful to the prostaglandin effort but at a later point on the timetable—
namely as readily available starting material for enzymatic conversion
in tissue homogenates to the prostaglandins. With prostaglandins produced in this manner the biological phase of prostaglandins became
possible. The Upjohn Co. which holds a basic U.S. patent to this process
(*27*), provided hundreds of laboratories with research quantities of the
prostaglandins.

Industrial collaboration with academic institutions was characteristic
during the steroid developments. The same is also true for the prostaglandins. Prior to the Karolinska assault on the prostaglandin structure,

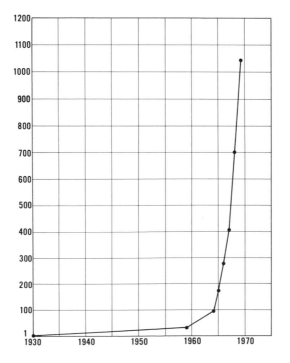

*Figure 3.   Accumulated publications on pros-
taglandins*

David Weisblat arranged for The Upjohn Co. to assist the project through support for collecting large quantities of sheep seminal vesicular glands; this collaboration, involving an exchange of materials and technology, has continued.

Table X. Areas of Potentials Use for Prostaglandins

Multiple smooth muscle properties
Intermediary metabolism
Physiology of the central nervous system
Gastrointestinal physiology
Cardiovascular physiology
Reproductive physiology

With the prostaglandin structures known, the goal for total synthesis was established. Such studies began in several laboratories long before clear evidence of therapeutic potential was established. The first synthesis of a prostanoic acid, one of the metabolites of prostaglandin E_1, was reported (29) in 1966. Since then the total synthesis of all of the primary prostaglandins has been reported (30–32). These developments, coupled with the biosynthetic techniques, provided technology for analog synthesis, an activity which also preceded established therapeutic potential. Several analogs prepared by the biosynthetic route have been reported. In our laboratories several hundred analogs and isomers have been synthesized, an endeavor based on the conviction that the prostaglandins would eventually play an important role in therapy.

The upsurge of interest in prostaglandin research is dramatically revealed in Figure 3 which shows the number of publications against time. The asymptotic increase in publications from 1965 to 1970 reflects the renewed interest in biology made possible by the aforementioned generous distribution of biosynthetic prostaglandins for biological research.

The clinical phase of prostaglandin research is now well advanced in the United States and abroad. Table X summarizes some of the areas of biological and medical interest. The clinical efficacy of PGE_2 and $PGF_{2\alpha}$ in abortion and labor induction has been established. Clinical studies in cardiovascular disease and as gastric antisecretory agents are also in progress. The alleviation of the symptoms of asthma in humans with the E prostaglandins has been reported (34).

The geneses of drug developments, illustrated specifically by the steroid hormones and prostaglandins, are nurtured by the developments in the basic sciences and are often extensions of research aimed at other goals. Probably the greatest single factor in pacing the rate of discovery and development of new fields is the availability of adequate technology.

Patterns of drug development are obvious for both fields discussed. These patterns are variations of the order in which the key stages on the timetable occur. Not obvious is the formula for initiative. Whereas integrated worldwide trends involving global research teams evolve as general awareness in any given field increases, the breakthroughs into truly virgin territory come from those very few leaders with intuition and insight.

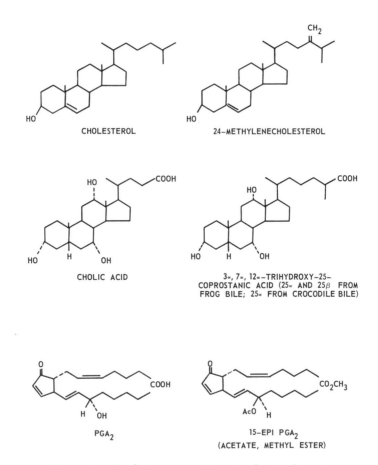

CHOLESTEROL

24—METHYLENECHOLESTEROL

CHOLIC ACID

3ᵅ, 7ᵅ, 12ᵅ—TRIHYDROXY—25—
COPROSTANIC ACID (25ᵅ AND 25β FROM
FROG BILE; 25ᵅ FROM CROCODILE BILE)

PGA₂

15—EPI PGA₂
(ACETATE, METHYL ESTER)

Figure 4.   Evolutionary variation in chemical species

The record of the past and the high promise in currently emerging new fields of natural products of animal origin attest to the potential for the future in this field. The probability for future discovery of entirely new classes of substances of animal origin cannot be guessed. Even without breakthroughs into new areas, several active fields of today promise contemporary breakthroughs which will become the historical accounts of tomorrow's success stories—*e.g.*, the peptide hormone field wherein progress has kept pace with emerging technology.

However, substances of animal origin which serve to regulate body function have unique potential for therapeutic usefulness relative to other substances of natural origin. Bergmann in his review (35) of the evolutionary aspects of sterols observed that cholesterol, the dominant sterol produced in higher forms of animal life, had numerous chemically related companions in lower forms of life, one of which is 2,4-methylene cholesterol. Even the bile acids appear in different structural modifications in lower forms of life such as the frog and crocodile. Bergmann defines the emergence of cholesterol as the dominant sterol in higher animals as a "phenomenon of bio-chemical evolution" and concludes that "It would appear that in cholesterol we witness the survival of the fittest sterol." Already in the new field of prostaglandins we have an example in *P. Homomalla*, a gorgonian of the coral reefs and a lower form of animal life, which produces a prostaglandin substance (36). This prostaglandin differs from PGA$_2$ only in the stereochemistry at carbon-15. (Figure 4)

It is reasonable to conclude that the perpetuation of regulatory chemical species or their precursors as products of mammalian biochemistry is a result of the survival value they have contributed to the organism they serve, and therefore such substances will in some way directly or indirectly be found to play a role in human medicine.

Literature Cited

(1) Allen, E., Doisy, E. A., *J. Amer. Med. Assoc.* (1923) **81**, 819.
(2) Corner, G. W., Allen, W. M., *Amer. J. Physiol.* (1928) **86**, 74.
(3) Fieser, L. F., Fieser, M., "Steroids," p. 503, Reinhold, New York, 1959.
(4) Ingle, D. J., *Amer. J. Physiol.* (1936) 622.
(5) Fieser, L. F., Fieser, M., *op. cit.*, p. 673.
(6) Fried, J., Sabo, Emily F., *J. Amer. Chem. Soc.* (1954) **76**, 1455.
(7) Cook, J. W., Dodds, E. C., Hewett, C. L., *Nature* (1937) **131**, 56.
(8) Feiser, L. F., Fieser, M., *op. cit.*, p. iii.
(9) Applezweig, Norman, "Steroid Drugs," p. 88, McGraw-Hill, New York, 1962.
(10) Fieser, L. F., Fieser, M., *op. cit.*, p. 3.
(11) Söderbaum, H. G., presentation of Nobel prize in chemistry to Wieland and Windaus, in "Nobel Lectures in Chemistry, 1922–1941," p. 89, Elsevier, Amsterdam, 1966.
(12) Kurzrok, R., Lieb, C. C., *Proc. Soc. Exptl. Biol. Med.* (1930) **28**, 268.
(13) von Euler, U. S., *Klin. Wochenschr.* (1935) **14**, 1182.
(14) Allen, W. M., Butenandt, A., Corner, G. W., Slotta, K. H., *Ibid.*
(15) Bergström, S., Carlson, L. A., Weeks, J. R., "The Prostaglandins, a Family of Biologically Active Lipids," *Pharmacol. Rev.* (1968) **20** (1), 1–48.
(16) Goldblatt, M. W., *Chem. Ind. (London)* (1933) **52**, 1056.
(17) Goldblatt, M. W., *J. Physiol. (London)* (1935) **84**, 208.
(18) von Euler, U. S., *Arch. Exp. Pathol. Pharmakol.* (1934) **175**, 78.
(19) von Euler, U. S., *J. Physiol. (London)* (1937) **88**, 213.
(20) Bergström, S., *Nord. Med.* (1949) **42**, 1465.

(21) Bergström, S., Sjövall, J., *Acta Chem. Scand.* (1957) **11**, 1086.
(22) *Ibid.*, (1960) **14**, 1693, 1701.
(23) Bergström, S., Ryhage, R., Samuelsson, B., Sjövall, J., *Acta Chem. Scand.* (1962) **16**, 501.
(24) Bergström, S., Ryhage, R., Samuelsson, B., Sjövall, J., *J. Biol. Chem.* (1963) **238**, 3555.
(25) Bergström, S., Danielsson, H., Samuelsson, B., *Biophys. Acta* (1964) **90**, 207.
(26) van Dorp, D. A., Beerthuis, R. K., Nugteren, D. H., Vonkeman, H., *Biochim. Biophys. Acta* (1964) **90**, 204.
(27) Beal, P. F. III, Fonken, G. S., Pike, J. E., U.S. Patent **3,296,091** (Jan. 3, 1967).
(28) Bergström, S. *et al.*, *Pharmacol. Rev.* (1968) **20** (1), 4, 30.
(29) Beal, P. F. III, Babcock, J. C., Lincoln, F. H., *J. Amer. Chem. Soc.* (1966) **88**, 3131.
(30) Axen, U. F., Lincoln, F. H., Thompson, J. L., *Chem. Commun.* (1969) 303.
(31) Just, G., Simonovitch, C., Lincoln, F. H., Schneider, W. P., Axen, U. F., Spero, G. B., Pike, J. E., *J. Amer. Chem. Soc.* (1969) **91**, 5364.
(32) Corey, E. J., Andersen, N. H., Carlson, R. M., Paust, J., Vedejs, E., Vlattas, I., Winter, R. E. K., *J. Amer. Chem. Soc.* (1968) **90**, 3245.
(33) Struijk, C. B., Beerthuis, R. K., van Dorp, D. A., Nobel Symposium 2, "Prostaglandins," p. 51, S. Bergström, B. Samuelsson, Eds., Almqvist and Wiksell, Stockholm, 1967.
(34) Cuthbert, M. F., *Brit. Med. J.* (1969) **4**, 723.
(35) Bergmann, W., in "Cholesterol," R. P. Cook, Ed., Chap. 12, Academic, New York, 1958.
(36) Weinheimer, A. J., Spraggins, R. L., *Tetrahedron Letters* (1969) **59**, 5185.

RECEIVED November 5, 1970.

3

Discovery of Drugs from Microbiological Sources

LLOYD H. CONOVER

Pfizer Medical Research Laboratories, Groton, Conn. 06340

Demonstration of the safety and therapeutic value of penicillin coupled with the discoveries of tyrothricin, actinomycin, and streptothricin initiated the halcyon era of antibiotic discovery (1940–1959). During this period, the prototypes of virtually all families of antibacterial antibiotics now important in medicine were discovered. After 1959, discovery of medically useful new drugs from microbiological sources dropped sharply while partial synthesis of new antibiotics (notably β-lactams and tetracyclines) having improved biological properties increased sharply. A landmark discovery was the first preparation of semisynthetic penicillins by Sheehan (1958). Guided by increased understanding of action and resistance mechanisms, chemical synthesis of new congeners will provide important antibiotic discoveries in the future. Examination of previously little studied genera of microorganisms for antibiotic elaboration, use of new culturing and detection techniques, and testing for more diverse types of biological activity will also provide significant new discoveries.

The mycelia of the fungus *Calviceps purpurea* which infects flowering rye was used for centuries by the practitioners of European folk medicine. A book published in 1582 recorded the use of sclerotia from *Secale cornutum* to control postpartum hemorrhage. In 1918 Stoll crystallized the alkaloid ergotamine, small doses of which elicited rapid and long lasting uterine contractions. The medicinal use of materials of microbiological origin is thus very old. In contrast, significant use of the presently most important drugs of microbiological origin—the antibiotics—extends back a scant 30 years.

It seems at first glance that with the isolation of tyrothricin by Dubos (*1*), actinomycin, streptothricin, and streptomycin by Waksman *et al.* (*2, 3, 4*) and penicillin by Florey, Chain *et al.* (*5*), the era of antibiotic discoveries was fully launched with little scientific precedent save Fleming's now celebrated chance observation (*6*). In reality these were the culminating discoveries that transformed investigation of microbial antagonism and antibiotic substances from an obscure erratically pursued academic endeavor to a highly organized applied science. The discovery of antibiotics widely useful in medicine was in fact presaged by many pregnant observations. Fascinating reviews of these early findings have

Table I.   Some Early Observations of Antimicrobial

Substance or Preparation	Microbial Source	Organism(s) Inhibited or Killed
"Cuxum"	fungus of roasted green corn	bacteria
Muscus ex cranio humano	fungus	bacteria
Moldy bread	*Penicillia*	bacteria
Liquid culture	*Penicillium species*	bacteria
Mycophenolic acid (crystalline)	*Penicillium brevicompactum*	*Bacillus anthracis*
Liquid culture	*Penicillium glaucum*	fowl plague
Kojic acid	*Aspergillus oryzae*	bacteria, fungi
Mycelial extract	*Aspergillus fumigatus*	*Mycobacterium tuberculosis*
Penicillic acid (crystalline)	*Penicillium puberulum*	*Escherichia coli*
Agar culture medium	actinomycete	*Bacillus mycoides* *Bacillus vulgatus*
Agar culture medium	actinomycete	bacteria
Sparassol (crystalline)	*Sparassis ramosa*	fungi
Liquid culture medium	actinomycetes	gram-positive, gram-negative bacteria
Gliotoxin	*Trichoderma lignorum*	fungi
Actinomycetin (protein precipitate)	*Streptomyces albus*	bacteria

[a] The work of Welsch with actinomycetin was a continuation of the investigations of Gratia.

been written by Waksman (7) and the Oxford group (8). A representative selection of these observations is summarized in Tables I and II.

The following are worthy of special mention: (1) use of molds to combat superficial infections was a part of European and Mayan folk medicine; (2) Gratia and Dath (1926) consciously undertook to isolate actinomycete and fungal cultures that produced substances antagonistic to bacteria; their sources were mud, tap water, and air; (3) Louis Pasteur was one of the first to record (1877) the phenomenon of microbial antagonism; (4) the basic methodology now used to detect antibiotics both in liquid and solid growth media was evolved by a number of early

Activity Produced by Fungi, Molds, and Actinomycetes

Therapeutic or Other Application	Discoverer or Recorder of Antimicrobial Action	Year
infections of skin and intestines	Mayan Indians	Pre-Columbian period
wounds	J. Parkinson	1640
wounds	European peasants, etc.	—
—	Tyndall	1876
—	Gosio	1896
—	Tartakovski	1904
—	Saito	1907
human tuberculosis	Vaudremer	1913
—	Alsberg & Black	1913
—	Grieg-Smith	1917
—	Lieske	1921
—	Falck	1923
immunization with bacterial lysates	Gratia & Dath	1926
plant fungus infections	Weindling & Emerson	1936
immunization with bacterial lysates	Welsch[a]	1937

Table II.   Some Early Observations of

Substance or Preparation	Microbial Source	Organism(s) Inhibited or Killed
Liquid culture	aerobic bacteria	*Bacillus anthracis*
Liquid culture medium	bacteria	bacteria
Gelatin culture medium	*Staphylococci*	*Bacillus anthracis*
Gelatin culture medium (containing diffusable secretory products)	*Bacillus fluorescens*	*Staphylococcus aureus*
Gelatin or agar culture medium (zones of inhibition)	cocci	*Bacillus anthracis*
"Pyocyanase" (crude precipitate)	*Pseudomonas aeruginosa*	bacteria
Agar and liquid culture medium (containing diffusable inhibitory material)	*Micrococcus tetragenus*	*Bacillus anthracis* *Staphylococcus aureus*
Agar and liquid culture media	bacteria	bacteria
Liquid culture medium	*Bacillus subtilis*	bacteria
Liquid culture medium	*Bacilli*	*Mycobacterium tuberculosis*
Liquid and agar culture medium	*Bacillus mesentericus*	*Proteus, Meningococcus, Corynebacterium diphtheriae*
"Sentocym" (bacterial lysates)	bacteria	bacteria
Liquid culture medium	*Bacillus scaber*	*Bacillus anthracis, Vibrio cholcrae*

Antimicrobial Activity Produced by Bacteria

Therapeutic or Other Application	Discoverer or Recorder of Antimicrobial Action	Year
—	Pasteur & Joubert	1877
—	Soyka	1885
—	Babès	1885
—	Garré	1887
—	Doehle	1889
human meningitis, diphtheria, grippe, local infections (commercially produced 1901-1935)	Emmerich & Low	1899
(not therapeutic in animals)	Lode	1903
—	Frost	1904
—	Nicolle	1907
guinea pig tuberculosis	Rappin	1912
human upper respiratory infections (local application)	Pringsheim	1920
human dysentary, typhoid fever, urinary tract infections	Much	1925
—	Rosenthal	1926

Table II.

Substance or Preparation	Microbial Source	Organism(s) Inhibited or Killed
Pyocyanine (crystalline)	Pseudomonas aeruginosa	bacteria
Prodigiosin	Serratia marcescens	trypanosomes, fungi
Hemopyocyanine (crystalline)	Pseudomonas aeruginosa	bacteria, fungi
Iodinin	Chromobacterium iodinum	bacteria

investigators, among whom Frost (1904) was notable; (5) "Pyocyanase" must be considered the first commercial antibiotic product; it was produced in Germany between 1901 and 1935, and when properly prepared, it had a therapeutic effect against bacterial infections in man and animals. In retrospect, it seems that the discovery and broad application of antibiotics in medicine was overdue when it came to pass. In the preceding decades scientists primarily interested in controlling infectious diseases were engrossed in the immunological approach, had been disillusioned with chemotherapy by the failure of disinfectants to control systemic infections and finally were encouraged by the success of the sulfonamides to seek additional synthetic antimetabolites.

The "Golden Era" of Antibacterial Microbial Metabolite Discoveries, 1940–1959

One of the remarkable aspects of the era that followed the discoveries of Dubos, Florey, Chain, and Waksman was the rapidity with which major drugs were discovered and put to practical use. The long induction period which preceded exploitation of microbial sources of antibacterial drugs permitted this exploitation to be rapid, once begun. By 1940, basic knowledge and experimental techniques were in hand which permitted: (1) facile collection, isolation, and growth of cultures of fungi, molds, bacteria, and actinomycetes; (2) detection, biological assay, purification, isolation, and structure proof of complex, unstable metabolites having antimicrobial activity; (3) evaluation of the chemotherapeutic efficacy and safety of antibacterial drugs in laboratory animals and man; (4) artificial mutation of antibiotic-producing microorganisms with selection of mutants having improved productivity; and (5) development of industrial-scale submerged, aerated fermentations, and of recovery proc-

Continued

| | *Discoverer or Recorder of* | |
Therapeutic or Other Application	Antimicrobial Action	Year
human diphtheria carriers (upper respiratory disinfection)	Hettche	1932 (isolated in 1860)
trypanosomiasis of mice	Masera, Fischl	1934–1935
—	Kramer	1935 (possibly isolated in 1863)
—	McIlwain	1941

esses for the antibiotics produced thereby. The requisite knowledge, methods, and techniques were drawn from mycology, bacteriology, plant, and soil microbiology, microbial genetics, chromatography, experimental chemotherapy, chemical engineering, and industrial fermentation technology.

A coincidence of key technical developments and external influences accelerated developments in the field, once its potentialities were recognized. Thus, the development of practical manufacturing processes for the new antibiotics discovered after 1944 was greatly facilitated by the existence of the basic technology perfected in the wartime "crash" effort devoted to penicillin production. The discovery of paper chromatography in 1944 was exceptionally timely (9). This technique, by providing a simple and sensitive analytical method for associating a specific chemical entity with *in vitro* antimicrobial activity, made possible the screening of large numbers of microbial cultures for small concentrations of new, active entities.

The years between 1940 and 1959 have been justly called the golden era of antibiotic discovery. During this period every important class of antibacterial antibiotic now known was recognized (Table III). Indeed, many specific drugs (*e.g.*, benzylpenicillin, streptomycin, oxytetracycline, chloramphenicol, neomycin, and erythromycin) which presently occupy major places in therapeutic practice were discovered during that period.

The Decline in Antibacterial Microbial Metabolite Discoveries, 1960–1970

Since 1959 relatively few newly discovered microbial metabolites have reached general use in human or veterinary medicine (Table IV); most of the major discoveries (the penicillinase-resistant penicillins, the

Table III.   Year of Discovery of Structural Classes
of Antibacterial Antibiotics

Year of First Literature Report	Class	First Discovered Member	First Generally Useful Member
1939	cyclic peptide	tyrothricin	Polymyxin
1940	penicillin	penicillin F, G, etc.	penicillin G
1943	steroid	helvolic acid	fusidic acid (1962)[a]
1944	aminoglycoside	streptomycin	streptomycin
1947	chloramphenicol	chloramphenicol	chloramphenicol[a]
1948	tetracycline	chlortetracycline	chlortetracycline
1950	macrolide	picromycin	erythromycin (1952)
1953	virginiamycin	streptogramin[b]	virginiamycin (1955)
1955	lincomycin	celesticetin	lincomycin (1962)
	cycloserine	cycloserine	cycloserine[a]
1956	novobiocin	novobiocin	novobiocin[a]
	cephalosporin	cephalosporin C	cephalothin, cephaloridine (1962)[c]
	vancomycin	vancomycin	vancomycin[a]
1957	ansamacrolide	streptovaricins	rifamycin SV (1961)[c]

[a] Only useful member to date.
[b] PA-114 was the first member to be recognized as a synergistic mixture (*119*).
[c] Semisynthetic.

broad-spectrum penicillins, doxycycline, the new cephalosporins, and rifampicin) have been made by chemical modification of existing antibiotics. This shift with time in the source of major discoveries is shown graphically in Figure 1. The relationships of lincomycin (*10, 11, 12, 13*), fusidic acid (*14, 15, 16, 17, 18, 19, 20, 21*), gentamicin (*22, 23, 24, 25*), and capreomycin (*26, 27, 28, 29*) (which were discovered after 1959) to their structural antecedents are shown in Figure 2.

Clearly, the felicitous combination of technical factors which facilitated the initial burst of microbial metabolite drug discoveries no longer operates with the same effect. This has led to a judgment on the part of some that no important new antibacterial drugs or drug classes will be derived directly from microbiological sources in the future.

The validity of this judgment obviously will not be known until a number of years have passed. Those presently seeking to discover superior new antibacterial drugs must, however, make an assessment based upon available evidence. Any rational attempt to make this assessment brings to mind a complex of subsidiary questions—*e.g.*, can the causes for the decrease in microbial metabolite drug discoveries depicted in Figure 2 be identified? Do these suggest possibilities for increasing the discovery rate? These and other questions concerning the future course and nature of drug discoveries from microbiological sources were incor-

Table IV. Timing and Source of Significant Antibacterial
Antibiotic Discoveries 1939–1969

Year of First Literature Report	From Structural Modification	From Structural Modification by Bio- or Chemical Synthesis
1939	tyrothricin [tyrocidin, gramicidin][a]	
1940	penicillin,[b] actinomycins[a]	
1944	streptomycin	
1945	bacitracin	
1946		dihydrostreptomycin
1947	chloramphenicol, polymyxins	
1948	chlortetracycline	phenoxymethylpenicillin[c]
1949	neomycin	
1950	oxytetracycline	
1951	viomycin	
1952	erythromycin	chloramphenicol palmitate
1953	leucomycins	tetracycline
1954	oleandomycin	
1955	spiramycin, virginiamycin,[d] cycloserine, cephalosporin C[a]	
1956	novobiocin, vancomycin, mikamycins[d]	
1957	kanamycins, 6-demethyltetracycline	triacetyloleandomycin
1958		proprionylerythromycin, pyrrolidinomethyltetracycline
1959	rifamycins, paromomycin, tylosin[d]	phenethicillin, propicillin
1960		methicillin
1961		ampicillin, nafcillin, oxacillin, methacycline, rifamycin SV
1962	lincomycin, fusidic acid	cephalothin, cephaloridine, doxycycline, cloxacillin, lysinomethyltetracycline, phenbenicillin
1963	gentamicin, capreomycin	
1965		rifamide, dicloxacillin, cephaloglycine
1967		cephalexin, rifampicin, carbenicillin
1968		clindamycin
1970[e]		

[a] Historically important; not used or not now important as an antibacterial drug.
[b] Report on therapeutic efficacy of crude penicillin.
[c] Produced by "biosynthetic" methods; not utilized until 1953.
[d] Used primarily or exclusively in animals.
[e] Newer discoveries whose utility has not yet been established have been omitted.

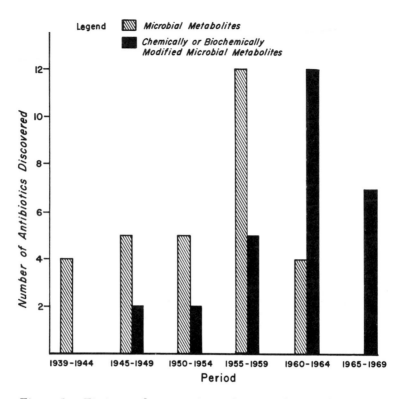

Figure 1.   Timing and source of significant antibacterial antibiotic discoveries, 1939–1969

porated into a questionnaire sent to some 120 scientists in industrial, academic, and government laboratories; completed questionnaires were received from 70 individuals. The panel of respondents includes men responsible both for past antibiotic discoveries and for present-day microbial metabolite and antibacterial drug research. The questionnaire sought to obtain the same global judgments, synthesis of views, and definition of problems and opportunities that would have emerged had first-hand discussions been possible with all of the respondents. Much of the remainder of this paper is devoted to a summary and interpretation of the responses to the questionnaire.

The first section of the questionnaire probed the causes for the drop in the discovery rate of useful new antibacterial microbial metabolites, then sought judgments as to whether, and if so how, this trend could be reversed. Finally it asked the respondents to rate the potentialities of five discovery approaches for providing useful new antibacterial drugs over the next decade.

The Nature and Causes of the Decline in Discovery Rate of Antibacterial Microbial Metabolites. The panel does not support the hypothesis that virtually all of the potentially useful structural classes of antibacterial antibiotics have been discovered. The thrust of the majority opinion (83% agreement) is that the search for antibacterial microbial metabolites, massive and prolonged as it has been, has not drawn upon the total reservoir of antibiotic-producing organisms and their secondary metabolites; the same sector of the total microbial population has been repeatedly sampled and examined for antibiotic elaboration by techniques which have changed little in 30 years. Potentially valuable new antibiotics have been missed because the producing organism was not isolated, did not grow, or did not produce a sufficient quantity of antibiotic to be detected under the conditions employed. Some respondents reported that changes in media and fermentation conditions on the one hand and/or application of new, more sensitive detection methods on the other have been responsible for discoveries in their own laboratories. The composition or temperature of the culture medium or the duration of the fermentation may determine whether an antibiotic is detected or, in some cases, what antibiotic is detected. Antibiotics produced in minor amounts, especially in the presence of other easily detected antibiotics, have undoubtedly been overlooked in the past. (Conversely, some such antibiotics owe their discovery to the fact that they were present in broths which were being investigated intensively because of other components present. Cephalosporin C, for example, is so weakly active that had it not been accompanied by penicillin N and cephalosporin P, it might easily have been overlooked.)

There are genera and species of antibiotic-producing microorganisms that, relatively speaking, have been neglected for the past 20 years. From about 1950 onward, *Streptomyces* species obtained from soil have received by far the greatest study (*30*). In the early years, there was good reason for this: they could be obtained easily in seemingly endless variety, and they were a rich source of new antibiotics. In more recent years known metabolites of *Streptomyces* have been rediscovered repeatedly. The discoveries of phosphonomycin, negamycin, sparsomycin, actinonin, showdomycin, and kasugamycin (Figure 3) were cited by respondents as evidence that even so, *Streptomyces* species are still capable of providing antibacterial antibiotics of novel structure.

The majority of respondents (69%) feel that the spectacular successes achieved by chemical modification of existing antibiotics in the late 1950's and early 1960's caused a shift of research effort away from soil sample screening and that this was in part responsible for the smaller number of significant fermentation-antibiotic discoveries. A substantial minority (23%) hold, however, that in absolute terms the effort applied to discovery of microbial metabolites has not decreased; only the proportion of the total discovery effort so applied has decreased as the semisynthetic efforts have grown quite large. Published statistics which reflect the level of fermentation-antibiotic discovery effort over the years do suggest that there has been no real curtailment of this activity. Berdy and Magyar's tabulation (*30*) of antibiotic discoveries (Table V) shows an absolute increase in the number of new antibiotics reported over each successive five-year period from 1940 through 1965. Perlman's analysis (*31*) of year-by-year totals (1940–1968) shows a steady increase until 1961, then a leveling off at a rate well above the average for the previous two decades.

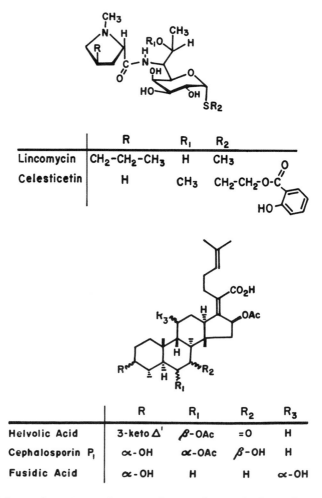

	R	R_1	R_2
Lincomycin	$CH_2-CH_2-CH_3$	H	CH_3
Celesticetin	H	CH_3	CH_2-CH_2-O-C

	R	R_1	R_2	R_3
Helvolic Acid	3-keto Δ^1	β-OAc	=O	H
Cephalosporin P_1	α-OH	α-OAc	β-OH	H
Fusidic Acid	α-OH	H	H	α-OH

*Figure 2. Relationship of significant antibacterial microbial metabo-
chemistry shown for the*

These statistics point up a fact that may not be generally appreciated: while the discovery rate for antibacterial microbial metabolites reaching general use in human or veterinary medicine has indeed dropped sharply, the total number of antibiotics discovered annually has not decreased.

Unquestionably, many of the new antibiotics isolated in the period 1960–1969 would have constituted significant discoveries in the 1940's when antibiotics were filling a virtual chemotherapeutic vacuum. Standards for medical and commercial acceptance have risen continuously as have requirements for regulatory approval of new antibiotics. In the past decade these influences properly discouraged the development and commercialization of new antibiotics not possessing significant advantages

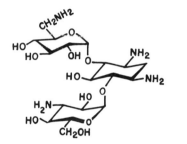

Kanamycin A

Gentamicins	R	R_1
C_1	CH_3	CH_3
C_{1A}	H	H
C_2	CH_3	H

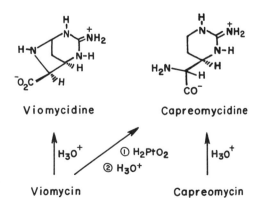

Viomycidine   Capreomycidine

Viomycin   Capreomycin

lite discoveries 1959–1970, to structural antecedents. The stereo-gentamicins is tentative (140).

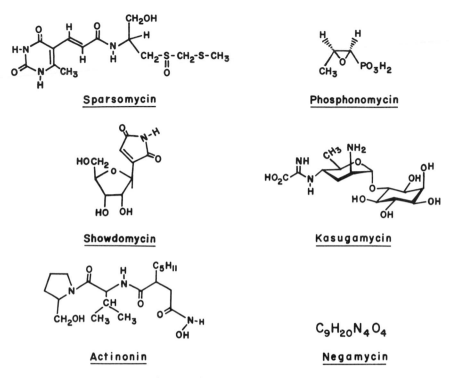

Figure 3.   Recent antibacterial antibiotic discoveries of novel structure

over existing drugs. One can be quite sure, however, that some new antibiotics have been rejected without benefit of the extensive comparisons
with existing drugs that would have revealed unique superiorities. A
great investment in time and resources is usually required to obtain the
quantities of a purified newly discovered antibiotic needed for a definitive
assessment. While in most cases this investment proves fruitless, valuable
properties can only be discovered if they are tested for.

Table V.   Cumulative Totals of New Antibiotics from
Three Major Sources 1940–1965

| | Schizomycetes | | Other Classes | | Five-Year |
Year	Actinomycetales	Eubacteriales	of Fungi[a]	Totals	Increase
1940	6	14	19	39	
1945	14	26	52	92	53
1950	82	100	143	325	233
1955	363	141	220	724	399
1960	812	187	282	1281	557
1965	1266	222	374	1862	581

[a] Fungi imperfecti, basidiomycetes, ascomycetes, phycomycetes.

Proposals Designed to Increase the Discovery Rate of Antibacterial Microbial Metabolites. The questionnnaire cited five specific approaches that have been advocated as means of increasing the rate at which discoveries of significant new antibacterial antibiotics are made. The panel was asked to evaluate the validity of each approach separately, then to rank these five approaches "in order of their practical potentiality for increasing the rate of discovery . . . over the next decade." Table VI lists these approaches and summarizes the responses. The two approaches

Table VI. Ranking of Approaches to Increased Antibacterial Microbial Metabolite Discovery 1970–1979

Approach	Rank[a]	Percent Judging Approach Fruitful[b]
Application of new techniques for collecting, storing, and processing soil samples, for isolating and growing potential antibiotic-producing microorganisms, and for detecting new antibiotics	1	67
Examination of genera of microorganisms that have received relatively little attention thus far in the search for antibiotics	2	58
Examination of marine microorganisms	3	53
Examination of terrestrial microorganisms that grow under unusual or extreme environmental conditions	3	42
Examination of microorganisms that grow in the presence of pathogens	4	33

[a] The over-all rank was derived from individual rankings by use of a weighted scoring system.

[b] Respondents were asked whether a given discovery approach could be expected to be fruitful for the discovery of useful new antibacterial antibiotics in the next decade.

given strongest support (application of new techniques and examination of neglected genera of microorganisms) were forecast by the analysis of the causes of the historical decline in discovery rate. Marine microorganisms are not expected to provide a cornucopia of new antibiotics; they constitute one category of little studied organisms which deserves study but which may pose special problems in terms of collection, isolation, and growth. The questionnaire reconfirmed the generally accepted conclusion that antibiotics do not play an ecological role, and thus there is no reason to expect a higher proportion of antibiotic producers in an environment where pathogens abound.

I should like to consider in some detail the basis for the expectation that structurally novel antibiotics will be discovered if efforts are concentrated upon species within "neglected" genera of microorganisms. First, this expectation is supported by past experience; secondly, it rests upon the proposition that the structures of microbial secondary metabolites are an expression of the genetic individuality of the elaborating species. To the extent that classical taxonomy reflects the magnitude of genetic difference between microorganisms, taxonomically widely separated organisms should elaborate antibiotics which differ widely in structure while closely related organisms may produce the same or closely related antibiotics.

Figure 4 shows in simplified form the taxonomic locations of microbial classes, orders, and families which produce the known structural classes of useful antibacterial antibiotics. None of the useful structural classes originally discovered as products of Schizomycetes has been isolated from a species of the *Fungi imperfecti;* there is but one preliminary report (32) that a *Streptomyces* species has been isolated which produces penicillin N, otherwise known exclusively as a product of *Fungi imperfecti.* Even elaboration of the same antibiotic by organisms belonging to different orders of the same class is rare. Cycloserine which is synthesized by several *Streptomyces* species and by *Pseudomonas fluorescens* (33) constitutes one of the few known examples.

The most common finding is the elaboration of the same or very closely related substances by different strains of the same species or

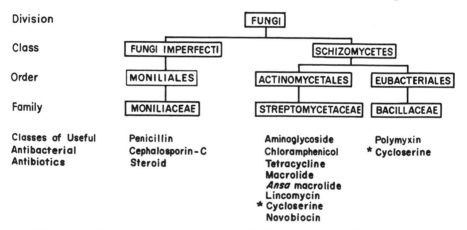

Figure 4. Taxonomic location of microbial orders and families producing useful antibacterial antibiotics. Other classes of fungi known to produce antibiotics are basidiomycetes, ascomycetes, and phycomycetes. For simplicity, the older classification of Schizomycetes as a class of fungi has been used. Schizomycetes and blue-green algae are generally now placed in a kingdom distinct from that of fungi. This classification in no way alters the argument that Fungi imperfecti and schizomycetes, being very widely separated taxonomically, may be expected to produce structurally distinct secondary metabolites.

different species of the same genus. Species belonging to different genera of the same family may produce the same antibiotic, but in notable instances they produce structurally distinctive analogs. Figure 5 illustrates this point with the β-lactams and some of the aminoglycosides and macrolides. Penicillin N is elaborated by several species of *Cephalosporium*, and a *Paecilomyces* species (and perhaps by some *Aspergillus* and *Trichophyton* species—all members of the Moniliaceae family). The other "natural" penicillins are only produced by *Penicillia* while cephalosporin C, a structural relative of penicillin N, has not been found as a metabolite of a *Penicillium*. (Penicillin N and cephalosporin C have also been isolated from the species *Emericellopsis terricola* which falls in the class Ascomycetes. Since these organisms are the perfect stage of a *Cephalosporium*, the taxonomic separation is not considered pertinent to the present discussion.)

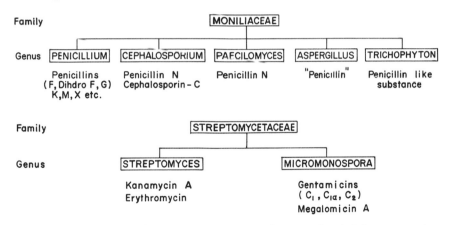

Figure 5. Taxonomic location of genera-producing related β-lactam, aminoglycoside, and macrolide antibiotics

Among the aminoglycosides, the gentamicin C family has thus far only been obtained from *Micromonospora* while the kanamycins are elaborated only by *Streptomyces* species. Megalomicin A (34) produced by a *Micromonospora* species represents a novel analog of erythromycin C, a product of *Streptomyces* species (Figure 6).

A detailed consideration of the neglected genera is beyond the scope of this discussion. This subject has received attention from Waksman (35) and other authors. It does appear that structurally novel congeners of a given antibiotic may be found by examining organisms falling in a genus closely related to that of the known producer. This would suggest examination of genera of Streptomycetaceae other than *Streptomyces*, and of Moniliaceae other than *Penicillium*. The fact that through 1955 more antibiotics had been reported from the *Fungi imperfecti*, basidio-

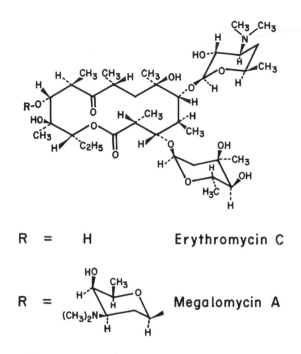

R = H   Erythromycin C

R =   Megalomycin A

Figure 6.   Erythromycin and megalomycin A

mycetes, ascomycetes, and phycomycetes than from the schizomycete order actinomycetales, suggests that classes of fungi other than schizomycetes should be examined more thoroughly (*see* Table V and Figure 7). Just as all drug research is becoming more difficult and time consuming, some of the neglected genera will prove more difficult to collect, isolate, and grow than the *Streptomyces,* and the proportion of active cultures they provide may be lower. The chance that their secondary metabolites, once detected, will be new should be greater, however.

Evaluation of Proposed Approaches to Antibacterial Drug Discovery, 1970–1980

It is germane to consider not only means by which discoveries of useful antibacterial microbial metabolites might be increased in the future but also to weigh the relative potentialities of all approaches to antibacterial drug discovery. Perhaps the reward for effort expended would be greater elsewhere. The questionnaire requested a ranking of the following five approaches in terms of their "practical potentiality for providing useful new antibacterial drugs over the next decade": (1) isolation of new microbial metabolites; (2) preparation of structural analogs of existing useful antibiotics by chemical or other means; (3) preparation of structural analogs of existing toxic or poorly efficacious antibiotics by chemical or other means; (4) empirical screening of organic compounds unrelated to existing antibiotics; (5) directed synthesis of organic compounds based upon a biochemical rationale.

The successes achieved in the past decade with chemically modified penicillins, tetracyclines, and lincomycin, undoubtedly influenced the judgment of the panel that preparation of structural analogs of useful antibiotics by chemical or other means should be ranked as one of the two most promising discovery approaches for the next decade. Before proceeding further with the evaluation made by the respondents of the five approaches (Table VII), some aspects of the history and nature of the structural modification approach are examined.

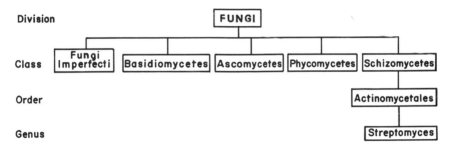

Figure 7.   Classes of fungi

Structural Modification of Antibiotics. HISTORICAL REVIEW. Writing in 1945, Waksman (7) set forth in prophetic terms the role that the medicinal chemist was to play in the antibiotic field.

. . . the discovery of new chemical agents possessing antibacterial or antifungal properties offers the chemist many new models to draw upon for varied types of syntheses.

Although only very few antibiotic agents have so far been isolated, and even fewer crystallized, it is already well established that we are dealing here with a great variety of chemical compounds. . . . Many a chemist is awaiting the solution of the problem of the chemical nature of penicillin before beginning new syntheses.

Doubtless most of the compounds that prove to be useful as chemotherapeutic agents will sooner or later be synthesized. The contribution of the bacteriologist may be all but forgotten in the light of forthcoming chemical developments, but even the bacteriologist will be grateful for new tools to help combat disease-producing agents. . . .

It is fitting that Waksman's own discovery, streptomycin, provided the vehicle for making the first useful semisynthetic antibiotic—dihydrostreptomycin (36, 37). It is interesting that dihydrostreptomycin was subsequently found as a microbial metabolite (38).

The massive wartime British-American investigation of penicillin chemistry included attempts to ". . . modify penicillin chemically in the hope of obtaining new compounds which might differ qualitatively or quantitatively in their biological activity, stability or rate of excretion . . . there was always the hope that a chemical modification of the molecule might so alter the specificity of the drug as to greatly broaden its field of application" (*39*). The thiazolidine carboxyl of benzylpenicillin and the activated ortho positions of *p*-hydroxybenzylpenicillin (Figure 8) proved amenable to chemical modification, but no new penicillins superior in chemical stability or chemotherapeutic action were identified in this work. Most of the chemical reactions of penicillins observed in early studies destroyed or reduced biological activity.

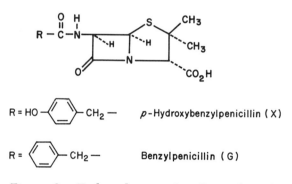

*Figure 8. Early substrates for chemical modi-
fication of penicillins*

From the point of view of importance and chemical feasibility, chloramphenicol (Figure 9) presented an excellent subject for structural modification. It was the first truly broad-spectrum antibiotic isolated, and its structure and total synthesis were both reported two years after the discovery was announced (*40, 41, 42*). The synthesis of chloramphenicol analogs proved to be one of the great disappointments of early chemical research in the antibiotic field. Hundreds of analogs were synthesized, but none was found superior to the parent drug in terms either of antimicrobial activity or therapeutic index (*43*). The palmitate and hemisuccinate esters have provided superior dosage forms for oral and parenteral use. One synthetic analog, thiamphenicol (*44*) has achieved limited use in human and veterinary medicine.

Because early experience with the penicillins, streptomycin, and chloramphenicol did not fulfill Waksman's optimistic prediction, there followed a period of skepticism regarding the potential value of chemical modification of antibacterial substances derived from microbiological sources; it was argued in some quarters that antibiotics represented the

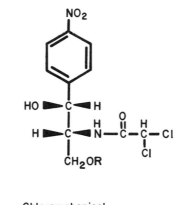

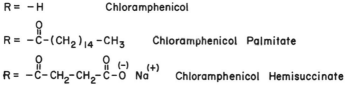

R = −H   Chloramphenicol

R = −C−(CH₂)₁₄−CH₃   Chloramphenicol Palmitate

R = −C−CH₂−CH₂−C−O Na   Chloramphenicol Hemisuccinate

Figure 9.   Chemical modification of chloramphenicol

culmination of an evolutionary process designed to give the elaborating organism the optimum chemical weapon in the competition for survival.

Robinson expressed this skepticism (*45*) when he wrote in 1953: ". . . indeed one of the disappointments in antibiotic work is that it seems impossible to modify the molecule without reducing or eliminating its antimicrobial activity . . ." The discoveries early in the 1950's of tetracycline and phenoxymethylpenicillin established beyond doubt, however, that modification of antibiotics by chemical or biosynthetic means could yield superior drugs.

SEMISYNTHETIC TETRACYCLINES. Tetracycline (Figure 10, Table IV) (*46, 47, 48*) was the first major semisynthetic antibiotic discovered. This product was discovered independently in my laboratory and that of Boothe at Lederle after the structures of oxytetracycline and chlortetracycline had been determined by the Pfizer group in collaboration with Woodward (*49, 50, 51, 52*). It was formed by the catalytic hydrogenolysis of chlortetracycline. Tetracycline was found to be a potent broad-spectrum antibiotic which was more stable and better tolerated than its fermentation-produced progenitor. In a few years it almost completely displaced chlortetracycline from medical practice. Interestingly, as happened in the case of dihydrostreptomycin, tetracycline was found as a microbial metabolite after its chemical synthesis had been accomplished (*53*). Further selective transformations of tetracycline antibiotics affording useful new drugs were slow in coming. It was to be 10 years before

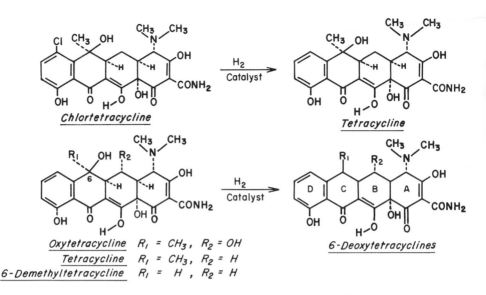

Figure 10.   Tetracycline and 6-deoxytetracyclines

Stephens, von Wittenau, Blackwood, and co-workers of Pfizer reported the discoveries of methacycline and doxycycline (54, 55). Woodward has characterized the molecule of oxytetracycline as a "diabolical concatenation of reactive groupings" (56). Indeed, the complexity and lability of the parent tetracyclines proved to be a great obstacle to drug discovery. At the outset the tetracyclines, like a number of other antibiotic classes (β-lactams, macrolides, aminoglycosides), were not amenable to facile molecular modification for exploring relationships between structure and biological properties. The most reactive functionalities proved, in general, to be required for biological activity. In the end, control of the chemistry of the C6 hydroxyl function provided the key to new drug discovery.

In 1958, the Pfizer group reported the successful hydrogenolysis of the C6 hydroxyl of oxytetracycline, tetracycline, and 6-demethyltetracycline (Figure 10) (57). Similar work was reported later by McCormick et al. of Lederle (58). The reaction products were of interest in that they were biologically active and also because they were stable to the conditions of electrophilic aromatic substitution reactions. It was now possible to prepare a large variety of D ring-substituted tetracyclines for biological study. From such studies came the discovery of minocycline by Martell and Boothe of Lederle (59). This compound is unique in its *in vivo* efficacy against some infections caused by tetracycline-resistant pathogens.

Insights were sought at Pfizer by which molecular structure and shape, electronic properties, acid strength, chelating ability, and lipophilicity might be related to potency or range of antibacterial activity. These studies were complicated by the fact that large differences observed *in vitro* were often reduced or completely nullified *in vivo*. Such observations focused attention upon the interplay of structural and pharmacokinetic properties of tetracyclines.

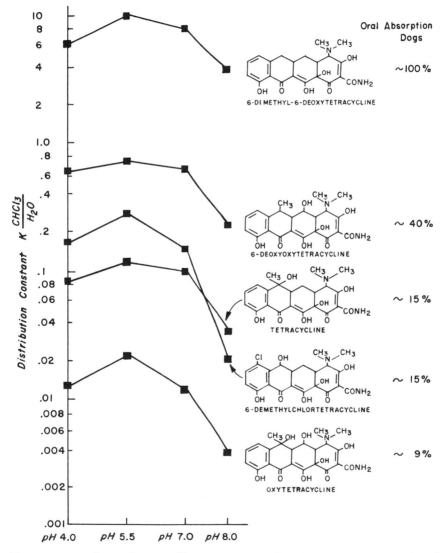

Figure 11. Relationship of chloroform–water distribution constants and oral absorption in dogs for some tetracyclines

Studies by von Wittenau and co-workers demonstrated that for most tetracycline antibiotics studied, *in vivo* behavior (such as completeness of oral absorption, degree of serum protein-binding, tissue affinity, rate of urinary excretion, and biological half-life) important to drug efficacy could be related to drug lipophilicity as reflected by chloroform-buffer distribution constants (*60, 61, 62, 63*). The principles which emerged based on studies in dogs proved applicable in man. Figure 11 indicates the relationship between oral absorption in dogs and chloroform–water distribution constants for a group of tetracyclines.

The 6-deoxytetracyclines provided a series in which the biological consequences of removing the 6-hydroxyl group, of modulating lipophilicity, and of altering configuration at C6 could be studied. Studies with 6-demethyl-6-deoxytetracycline indicated that although this analog retains essentially the same *in vitro* spectrum as tetracycline, is chemotherapeutically effective, is efficiently absorbed and affords a long serum half-life, its great tissue affinity is reflected in increased toxicity. While the *in vitro* potency of this compound against gram-positive organisms is generally enhanced compared with its parent, catalytic hydrogenolysis of oxytetracycline gives a 6-deoxy compound having lower *in vitro* potency. The explanation for this anomaly lies in the fact that during the hydrogenolysis of oxytetracycline inversion occurs at C6, presumably because the α face of the molecule is less hindered (Figure 12).

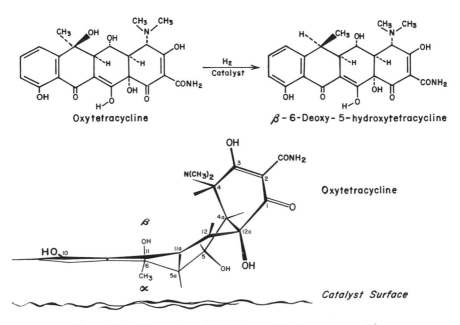

Figure 12.   Formation of β-6-deoxy-5-hydroxytetracycline

6-Deoxy-5-hydroxytetracycline having the normal α-methyl configuration at C6 had been sought in chemical studies starting as early as 1952. Discovery and development of this compound (which proved to have somewhat enhanced *in vitro* antibacterial activity, lower affinity for calcium, a lower effect on the gastrointestinal flora, and near ideal pharmacokinetic properties) was made possible by the mastery of further new chemistry at C6. In the end, two stereoselective routes to the elusive compound were discovered (*54, 55*). The key reactions are shown in Figure 13. Note that success in the direct hydrogenation route required reversal of the usual preference for catalytic hydrogenation to occur at the least hindered face of a molecule.

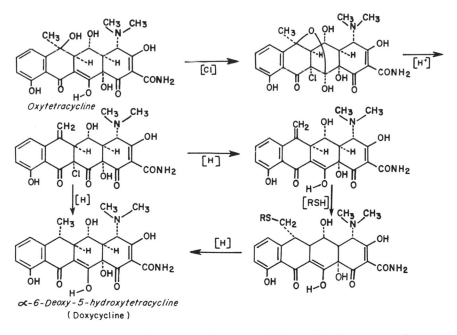

Figure 13. Stereoselective synthesis of α-6-deoxy-5-hydroxytetracycline

SEMISYNTHETIC PENICILLINS. Just as the independent lines of inquiry of Dubos, Waksman, and the Oxford group converged to open the antibiotic era, the period of semisynthetic penicillin discoveries was initiated by a similar convergence. As an outgrowth of the early observation that the chemical nature of the penicillins produced by fermentation was influenced by the composition of the growth medium, the preparation of "biosynthetic" penicillins was accomplished by adding substituted phenylacetic acid derivatives (and related structures) to penicillin fermentations. By this method Behrens and co-workers at the Eli Lilly Co. had by 1948 prepared some 30 penicillins modified in the acyl moiety (*64*).

In principle, only the limitations in substrate structure imposed by the specificities of the enzyme or enzymes involved in the activation and coupling reactions prevented this and other biosynthetic investigations from anticipating the major discoveries made a decade and more later by the semisynthetic approach. As it was, it appeared initially that the only useful advantage possessed by a biosynthetic penicillin was lower allergenicity. This property which was attributed to penicillin O (allylmercaptomethylpenicillin) (Figure 14) proved illusory.

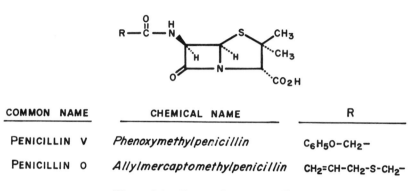

COMMON NAME	CHEMICAL NAME	R
PENICILLIN V	*Phenoxymethylpenicillin*	$C_6H_5O-CH_2-$
PENICILLIN O	*Allylmercaptomethylpenicillin*	$CH_2=CH-CH_2-S-CH_2-$

Figure 14.   Biosynthetic penicillins

In 1954, however, Brandl and Margreiter (65) reported that biosynthetic phenoxymethylpenicillin (penicillin V) was superior to benzylpenicillin in terms of acid stability. Since this compound retains good activity against penicillin-sensitive gram-positive bacteria penicillin V quickly gained acceptance as the only reliable penicillin for oral administration.

The fledgling Beecham penicillin research team was stimulated by the advent of phenoxymethylpenicillin to seek additional superior penicillins modified in the acyl moiety (66). The general approach envisioned was the conversion of one penicillin bearing a reactive functionality to a variety of new modified penicillins; specifically biosynthetic p-aminobenzylpenicillin was selected for modification via acylation of the amine function (Figure 15).

During the same period, Sheehan was working toward a total synthesis of penicillins. In 1958, he announced the synthesis of 6-aminopenicillanic acid (6-APA) and its utility for the preparation of new penicillins by acylation (67, 68). (Almost 10 years earlier, this substance had been postulated to be an intermediate in the biosynthesis of penicillins (69, 70). Prior Japanese literature also contained clear suggestions that it had been formed by enzymatic hydrolysis of benzylpenicillin (71) and in fermentations carried out in the absence of side chain precursors

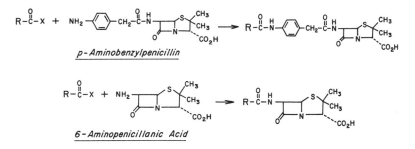

p-Aminobenzylpenicillin

6-Aminopenicillanic Acid

Figure 15.   Preparation of semisynthetic penicillins

(*72, 73*). The significance of these pregnant observations had escaped scientists engaged in antibiotic research at the time.)

Meanwhile, the Beecham group discovered 6-APA independently in the course of studying the biosynthesis of *p*-aminobenzylpenicillin. This discovery also followed from the observation that in precursor-starved fermentations a material was formed which contained the β-lactam function but which was not biologically active (*74*). The Beecham fermentation method provided the first practical means for obtaining large quantities of 6-APA. Although it had previously been argued by some that this structure was too labile to be isolable, once the existence of 6-APA was generally recognized, enzymatic methods for its preparation were quickly perfected in a number of laboratories (*75, 76, 77, 78, 79*).

The discovery of 6-aminopenicillanic acid presented the medicinal chemist with an exceptional opportunity. It was now possible to vary the acyl moiety of penicillins at will to identify and elaborate those structural and physical characteristics which controlled therapeutically relevant properties such as acid stability, oral absorption, serum protein binding, penicillinase resistance, and gram-negative activity. Virtually every new acylpenicillanic acid synthesized retained some biological activity. Acid stable homologs of phenoxymethylpenicillin were the first of the semisynthetic penicillins to be reported and to reach clinical use (Figure 16) (*80*). It was later shown that the acid stability of penicillins can be correlated with the strength of the acid corresponding to the acyl moiety (*81*), a finding consistent with Abraham's postulation that the electronic properties of the phenoxy substituent are responsible for the acid stability of phenoxymethylpenicillin (*82*).

Since, in general, only monosubstituted acetic acid derivatives served as penicillin biosynthetic precursors, one of the prime structural variations made feasible for the first time by partial synthesis was that of di- and trisubstitution at the α-position of the acyl substituent. All of the semisynthetic penicillins which have become important in medical practice are in fact disubstituted at the carbon α to the amide carbonyl. Such compounds provided important insights relating structure to a number of biologically important properties. As the chain length of α-alkyl substituents on phenoxymethylpenicillin was increased, so was the efficiency of oral absorption, the serum half-life, and the degree of serum binding. *In vitro* potency toward penicillin-sensitive bacteria was not altered greatly in the simple homologs; however, it was observed that as the bulk of the α-substituent was increased, this endowed the molecule with a small but significant degree of resistance to destruction by benzylpenicillinase—the enzyme responsible for the resistance of many *Staphylococcus aureus* strains to benzylpenicillin. α-Phenoxyisobutylpenicillin was able to protect mice against an infection caused by a benzylpenicillin-resistant *S. aureus*.

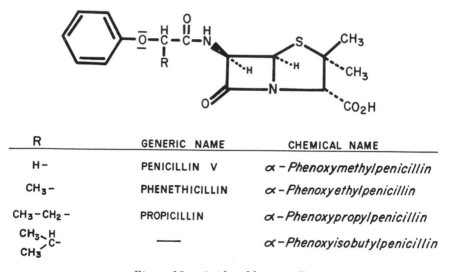

R	GENERIC NAME	CHEMICAL NAME
H–	PENICILLIN V	α - *Phenoxymethylpenicillin*
CH₃–	PHENETHICILLIN	α - *Phenoxyethylpenicillin*
CH₃–CH₂–	PROPICILLIN	α - *Phenoxypropylpenicillin*
CH₃ H CH₃ ⟩C–	——	α - *Phenoxyisobutylpenicillin*

Figure 16.   Acid-stable penicillins

Recognition that the occurrence of increased penicillinase resistance accompanied increased steric bulk about the α-position provided a powerful rationale for directed synthesis: insights gained from studies of steric hindrance of organic reactions were directly applicable to drug design. The end result was a qualitative change in efficacy spectrum compared with benzylpenicillin (83). Analog synthesis progressed through trisubstituted methylpenicillins, such as triphenylmethylpenicillin (84) to the disubstituted aryl and heteroarylpenicillins such as methicillin and oxacillin (Figure 17) (85, 86). Methicillin and the oxacillin family have become the mainstays of the clinical armamentarium used against penicillinase-producing *S. aureus*.

Several factors must have suggested the preparation of α-aminobenzylpenicillin (ampicillin) (87) to the Beecham group. It was α-substi-

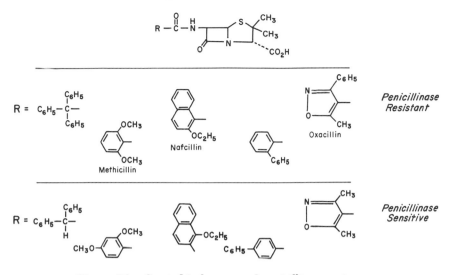

Figure 17.   Steric hindrance and penicillinase resistance

tuted, it could be expected to be acid stable, and evidence was already in hand that amino substituted penicillins (*p*-aminobenzylpenicillin, penicillin N) possessed enhanced activity against gram-negative bacteria (Figure 18). Ampicillin extended the range of chemotherapeutic efficacy of the penicillins to many of the gram-negative bacteria. This qualitative improvement in *in vivo* performance depended upon high quantitative improvement over the weak *in vitro* activity of benzylpenicillin against the same organisms. It now appears that the physical properties of ampicillin facilitate its passage relative to that of benzylpenicillin, through

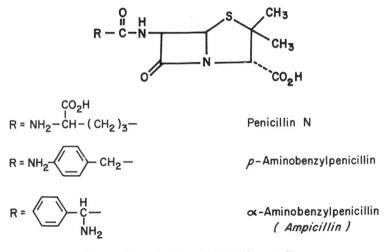

Figure 18.   Amino-substituted penicillins

the cell wall of *Escherichia coli*, for both are potent inhibitors of the isolated transpeptidase enzyme—which is a major site of penicillin action (*88*).

Further studies of α-substituted benzylpenicillins led to the independent discovery by Pfizer and Beecham chemists of carbenicillin (α-carboxybenzylpenicillin) (Figure 19) (*89, 90*), in which the gram-negative spectrum is extended still further (to *Pseudomonas aeruginosa* and the ampicillin-insensitive indole-positive *Proteus* species).

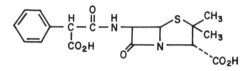

Figure 19. Carbenicillin

Structural Modification by Biosynthetic Methods. The structure of useful antibiotics can be altered by means other than chemical synthesis and transformation. It has already been pointed out that the first structurally modified penicillin to achieve widespread clinical use was the biosynthetic phenoxymethyl penicillin. A majority (67%) of the respondents believe that modification of the structures of presently used antibiotics by manipulation of biosynthetic pathways will be a fruitful approach to discovery of new antibacterial antibiotics in the coming decade. Among the possible variations of this approach are: simple utilization of precursors by antibiotic-producing microorganisms (as in the case of phenoxymethylpenicillin), utilization of precursors by mutants having specific metabolic blocks (as in the preparation of modified neomycins by Shier, Rinehart, and Gottlieb) (*91*), use of inhibitors of specific enzymatic reactions (as in the formation of 6-demethylchlortetracycline by a chlortetracycline producer in the presence of ethionine) (*92*), use of various biological means of combining genetic material of different organisms at least one of which is an antibiotic producer (*e.g.*, syncytic recombination, transformation, transduction and lysogenic conversion) (*93*), and mutation of antibiotic producers (as in the preparation of 6-demethylchlortetracycline (*94*) and rifamycin SV (*95*).

In principle, biosynthetic methods can provide structural variants that are inaccessible or very difficultly accessible by chemical methods; on the other hand, except where incorporation of a wide variety of precursors is possible these methods do not now provide a means for directly making pre-selected changes in structure. Enzymatic or microbiological transformation of antibiotics is a related approach that in principle can bring about selective and specific structural changes. Although this method was used with success in the steroid field, it has not yet provided significant drug discoveries in the antibiotic field. It has received relatively little attention.

Structural Modification of Toxic or Poorly Efficacious Antibiotics. Modification of toxic or poorly efficacious antibiotics does not quite gain majority support of the panel as a fruitful discovery approach for the next decade (Table VII). The author joins the minority (~40%) of respondents on this question.

If a drug fails to meet present day standards because of low *in vitro* potency, metabolic, or chemical instability, poor oral absorption or high degree of serum and tissue binding, experience teaches that the prospects for improvement *via* structural modification are good—if systematic structural modification with retention of biological activity is feasible. The clinically established semisynthetic cephalosporins, rifamycin SV and rifampicin represent precisely this kind of improvement, while laboratory data indicate that it has also been achieved in the coumermycin series as well (*96, 97*).

Table VII.   Ranking of Discovery Potential of Approaches to Antibacterial Drug Discovery

Approach	*Rank*[a]	*Percent Judging Approach Fruitful*
Preparation of structural analogs of useful antibiotics by chemical or other means	1	83
Isolation of new microbial metabolites	1	92
Preparation of structural analogs of toxic or poorly efficacious antibiotics by chemical or other means	2	42
Directed synthesis of organic compounds based upon a biochemical rationale	3	[b]
Empirical screening of organic compounds unrelated to existing antibiotics	4	[b]

[a] The over-all rank was derived from individual rankings by use of a weighted scoring system.
[b] Appropriate question was not asked; however, 65% of the respondents judged that the search for new microbial metabolites will represent a better approach to the discovery of antibacterial drugs having novel structure, mode of action, and range of efficacy.

SEMISYNTHETIC CEPHALOSPORINS. Once the structure of cephalosporin C became known (*98*), attempts were made to find chemically modified analogs having superior biological properties. This was successfully achieved with the synthesis of cephalothin, cephaloridine, cephaloglycine, and cephalexin (Figure 20). In the first two, *in vitro* potency was enhanced as much as 10,000 fold (*99*), in the latter two oral absorption

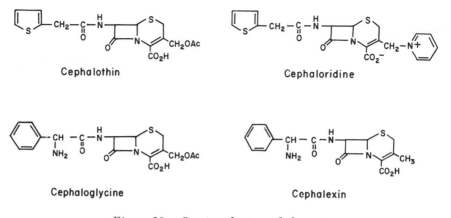

Cephalothin   Cephaloridine

Cephaloglycine   Cephalexin

Figure 20.   Semisynthetic cephalosporins

was achieved (*100*). The starting point for this research was quite different from that for the semisynthetic penicillins. The parent compound was too weakly active to merit clinical application although qualitatively, its biological properties elicited interest; it was active against both gram-positive and gram-negative bacteria and was resistant to benzylpenicillinases.

Here as with the tetracyclines, the solution of difficult chemical problems was a prerequisite to successful new drug discovery. At first the counterpart of 6-aminopenicillanic acid could be made only in very low yields by chemical hydrolysis. A practical enzymatic hydrolysis of cephalosporin C to 7-aminocephalosporanic acid (7-ACA) was not found. R. B. Morin and co-workers provided the elegant solution (Figure 21) (*101*), which made the preparation of 7-ACA and semisynthetic cephalosporins possible on a practical scale. The impetus to persevere in this

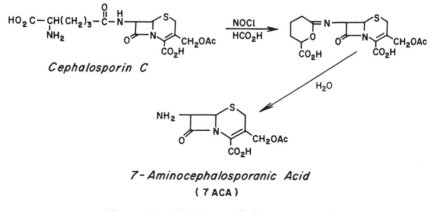

Cephalosporin C

7- *Aminocephalosporanic Acid*
(7 ACA)

Figure 21.   7-Aminocephalosporanic acid

endeavor was indubitably provided by the knowledge that superior semi-synthetic penicillins had been derived from 6-APA. If cephalosporin C had been the only β-lactam antibiotic isolated from microbial sources, it is questionable whether β-lactam antibiotics of either microbial or semisynthetic origin would be in clinical use today. One must now ask whether there exist neglected antibiotics which are as promising as cephalosporin C as starting points for structural modification and whether, by the criteria now used to evaluate newly discovered antibiotics, the potential value of a cephalosporin C (discovered in isolation) would be recognized.

SEMISYNTHETIC RIFAMYCINS. The degree and variety of the improvements that can be made in an antibiotic that has no clinical utility *per se* are well illustrated by the semisynthetic rifamycins (Figure 22) (*102*). The microbial metabolite, rifamycin B, is unstable in aqueous solutions exposed to oxygen and owes most, if not all, of its apparent activity to the corresponding 1,4-quinone, rifamycin S. Reduction of this quinone

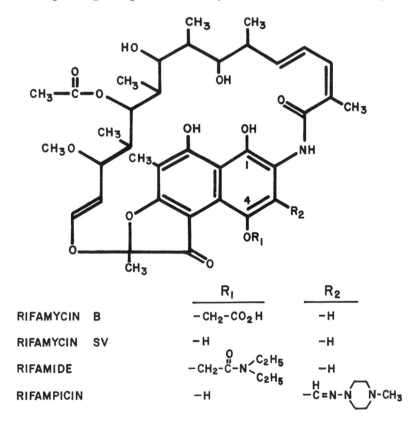

		R$_1$	R$_2$
RIFAMYCIN	B	$-CH_2-CO_2H$	$-H$
RIFAMYCIN	SV	$-H$	$-H$
RIFAMIDE		$-CH_2-\overset{O}{\overset{\|}{C}}-N\overset{C_2H_5}{\underset{C_2H_5}{<}}$	$-H$
RIFAMPICIN		$-H$	$-\overset{H}{\overset{\|}{C}}=N-N\diagup\diagdown N-CH_3$

Figure 22.   The rifamycins

provided rifamycin SV, a parenteral drug which is clinically used primarily against gram-positive and biliary tract infections. The biological consequences of a wide variety of additional structural changes were surveyed, and active structures capable of systematic variation were identified.

Study of the N,N-dialkylrifamycinamides showed that, generally speaking, increased drug lipophilicity is accompanied by a decreased rate of biliary excretion, increased biological half-life and increased chemotherapeutic efficacy after oral administration, relative to parenteral. Rifamide (rifamycin B N,N-diethylamide) which has achieved significant clinical use has a therapeutic index superior to that of rifamycin SV. The 3-formylrifamycin SV hydrazones provided compounds exhibiting good oral absorption, long biological half-life, low biliary excretion rate, and excellent chemotherapeutic action vs. gram-positive and *Mycobacterium tuberculosis* experimental infections. Rifampicin, which is the optimum member of the series, represents an important new addition to the armamentarium of antitubercular drugs.

That structural variation of congeners can spell the difference between drugs of little or no clinical utility and drugs of wide applicability can also be seen by comparing the properties of various members of antibiotic classes isolated solely from microbiological sources. Some of these cases are summarized in Table VIII.

The deoxystreptamine aminoglycoside antibiotics catenulin (paromomycin), neomycin, kanamycin, and gentamicin qualitatively share ototoxicity, nephrotoxicity, and antibacterial activity; the first named however is used only for intestinal infections (amoebic and bacterial), the second is used primarily for local and intestinal infections while kanamycin which combines lower nephro- and ototoxicity with good activity

Table VIII. Congeners of Antibacterial Antibiotics with Improved Biological Properties

Antibiotic Class	Inferior Member	Superior Congener	Improvement
Polymyxins	polymyxins A, C, D	polymyxins B, E	safety
Aminoglycosides	catenulin (paromomycin	neomycin	efficacy
	neomycin	kanamycin	safety
	kanamycin	gentamicin	spectrum, efficacy
Macrolides	picromycin	erythromycin, oleandomycin	safety, efficacy
Steroids	helvolic acid, cephalosporin P_1	fusidic acid	efficacy
Lincomycins	celesticetin	lincomycin	safety

vs. E. coli, Proteus sp. and *S. aureus* is a useful parenteral drug. In turn, gentamicin by virtue of increased potency *vs.* gram-positive and gram-negative bacteria (espccially *Pseudomonas aeruginosa*), has both an improved therapeutic index and spectrum of *in vivo* efficacy compared with kanamycin. In the cyclic polypeptide class, polymyxins B and E are substantially less nephrotoxic than the congeners A, C, and D which are not used clinically. Erythromycin, lincomycin and fusidic acid followed congeners that never reached medical use. The improvements embodied in the later discovered analogs are indicated in Table VIII. In principle, the same sorts of improvements should be achievable by chemical modification of some presently known but unused antibiotics. One obvious reservation should be pointed out; improvement of the therapeutic index of an antibiotic with retention of activity may be impossible where the mechanism of toxicity is related to the mechanism of action. This is true, for example, of the actinomycins.

Guiding Principles for Structural Modification of Existing Antibiotics. Some general principles emerge from the foregoing discussion of drug discovery *via* structural modification of existing antibacterial antibiotics (presently useful or otherwise).

(1) Drug discovery usually requires prior mastery of the chemistry of the parent antibiotic structure: reasonably facile methods for making selective and systematic structural modifications must be perfected. A versatile intermediate from which a variety of congeners may be synthesized is exceedingly useful in this regard.

(2) The testing of new congeners must take imaginative cognizance both of the obvious shortcomings of the prototype drug and its therapeutically marginal but intrinsically desirable properties (*e.g.*, the weak *in vitro* activity of benzylpenicillin *vs.* gram-negatives). Quantitative enhancement of such properties can effect a qualitative change in the range of therapeutic efficacy. Potentially important properties may be overlooked in the absence of such testing.

(3) Changes in therapeutically relevant properties such as resistance to chemical or enzymatic inactivation, *in vitro* potency, degree of serum protein binding, rate of excretion, etc. can usually be correlated with changes in specific structural and/or physical properties. Such correlations provide the best guidance presently available to the medicinal chemist for the design of congeners in which optimization of a particular biological property is sought.

(4) Substantial improvement of therapeutic index is often possible either by enhancement of therapeutic potency, reduction of intrinsic toxicity, or both. If the molecular mechanisms of toxicity and activity are the same the prospect for improvement in therapeutic index is poor. An understanding of these mechanisms is thus important.

Isolation of New Microbial Metabolites. Surprisingly, this discovery approach is placed on a par with chemical modification of useful antibiotics as the most promising for the next decade (Table VII). This is the judgment of the panel despite the disparate records of the two approaches over the past decade (Figure 1). This judgment implies a recognition that improvements in biological properties *via* structural modification of a given type of antibiotic do have practical limits. Microbial metabolism is still viewed as the best potential source of structurally and mechanistically novel antibacterial agents (65% agreement).

The rational bases for the expectation that examination of microbial fermentations can provide important new antibacterial antibiotic discoveries have already been explored. For some of the respondents there is also an element of faith involved. What is expected is not rebirth of the era of prolific discoveries but the isolation and recognition in the next decade of a few significantly improved congeners of antibiotics already in use, a few antibiotics belonging to new structural classes which will have important therapeutic advantages, and a few new prototype structures worthy of chemical modification.

Synthesis of Organic Compounds Structurally Unrelated to Antibiotics. The majority of respondents ranked directed synthesis based upon a biochemical rationale as a relatively unpromising discovery approach. I believe, however, that the increasingly detailed insights (which have come in large part through the study of antibiotic mechanisms of action) concerning such basic processes as bacterial cell wall, protein, and nucleic acid synthesis will provide guidance for antibiotic analog design that is distinct from and complements that derived strictly from structure–activity correlations. Empirical screening of organic compounds was rated the least promising of the five approaches considered. No approaches distinctly different from those listed in Table VII were proposed by respondents.

Projection of Antibacterial Drug Discoveries, 1970–1980

As a logical sequel to the ranking of the discovery potential of the five approaches to antibiotic drug discovery listed in Table VII, the panel was asked to predict in what drug categories discoveries of major, substantial, or marginal importance would be made in the next decade. Generally, the expectations summarized in Table IX are consistent with the previously discussed judgments of approach. Thus 93% of those (approximately 60 persons) willing to assume the role of oracle, expect that new drugs structurally related to antibacterial antibiotics now in use will constitute discoveries of major or substantial importance. The ranking of specific classes is as follows: (1) cephalosporins, (2) penicillins, (3) *ansa*macrolides, and (4) aminoglycosides. A majority of the respondents expect important discoveries to be made in each of these classes.

Table IX. Predicted Importance of Antibacterial Drug Discoveries 1970–1980[a]

	Substantial or Major Discovery	Marginal Discovery	No Significant Discovery
Presently used antibacterial antibiotics	93	5	2
cephalosporins	68	20	12
penicillins	61	18	21
ansamacrolides (rifamycins)	54	32	14
aminoglycosides	52	29	19
macrolides	44	40	16
lincomycins	35	43	22
tetracyclines	29	34	37
polymyxins	10	20	70
Presently unknown class of microbial metabolites	80	7	13
A synthetic drug unrelated in structure to existing antibiotics	49	16	35
Presently known toxic or marginally effective class	39	34	27

[a] Numbers represent percentage of respondents making designation.

Eighty percent of respondents predict that presently unknown classes of microbial metabolites will provide discoveries of major or substantial importance, while only 39% expect that a presently known toxic or marginally effective class will do so. Forty-nine percent expect that a synthetic drug unrelated in structure to existing antibiotics will constitute an important discovery. This prediction is somewhat at variance with the judgment (already discussed) that modification of toxic or marginally effective antibiotics is superior as a research approach to empirical screening of organic compounds and biochemically based directed synthesis.

Microbial Metabolite Drugs of Diverse Application, 1939–1970

To this point, the discussion has been concerned exclusively with antibacterial antibiotics. Historically, these were the first to gain widespread use, they have been the most studied, and they are the most numerous. General principles of drug discovery derived from a consideration of this class should be applicable to other classes as well.

The selective toxicity of antibiotics is, of course, not confined to bacterial pathogens. Some of the earliest discovered antibiotics possessed other types of activity. Thus griseofulvin (1939) and nystatin (1951) are antifungal agents, and the actinomycins (1940) are antineoplastic as well as antibacterial. The action of the broad-spectrum antibiotics (chloramphenicol and the tetracyclines) extends to some protozoa, mycoplasma, rickettsia, spirochetes, and the so-called large viruses of the lymphogranuloma type. Antibiotics are presently the dominant agents used for therapy of diseases caused by fungi and all of the organisms just mentioned save protozoa; they are becoming an increasingly important factor in cancer chemotherapy. In the animal health field, hygromycin (103) and destomycin (104) are anthelmintic agents for swine and chickens, and monensic acid (105) is under development as an antiprotozoal (coccidiostatic) agent for use in chickens. Moenomycin (106), virginiamycin (107), the mikamycins (108) and zeranol (109) are being used as animal growth promotants.

As the discovery rate of clinically accepted antibacterial microbial metabolites has fallen, that for microbial metabolites having other types of useful biological activity has remained at a fairly constant level (Table X). Examination of the structures of the microbial metabolites whose primary use is not as chemotherapeutic antibacterial agents shows that most do not belong to any of the major structural classes of antibacterial antibiotics. Furthermore, representatives of useful new classes have been discovered within the past decade. New structures will be found when microbial fermentations are tested for new types of biological activity.

Table X. Microbial Metabolites with Useful Antifungal, Antiparasitic, or Antineoplastic Activity

Metabolite	Biological Activity	Year of First Literature Report
Griseofulvin	antifungal	1939
Fumagillin	antiprotozoal	1949
Nystatin	antifungal	1950
Paromomycin	antiprotozoal	1952
Trichomycin	antifungal/antiprotozoal	1952
Candicidin	antifungal	1953
Sarkomycin	antineoplastic	1953
Dactinomycin	antineoplastic	1954
Amphotericin B	antifungal	1956
Mitomycin C	antineoplastic	1957
Hygromycin B	anthelmintic	1958
Pimaricin	antifungal	1958
Chromomycin A_3	antineoplastic	1960
Hamycin	antifungal	1960
Mithramycin	antineoplastic	1962
Daunomycin	antineoplastic	1964
Pyrrolnitrin	antifungal	1964
Destomycin	anthelmintic	1965
Bleomycin	antineoplastic	1966
Monensic acid	antiprotozoal	1968
Adriamycin	antineoplastic	1969

Clearly, microbial metabolism should be considered a potential source of drugs for a variety of uses. One question that arises in this connection concerns the relative frequency with which different types of activity occur. A few authors have approached this question by analyzing the types of biological activity reported for known antibiotics. Data abstracted from Kurylowicz (*110*) and Berdy and Magyar (*30*) are shown in Table XI.

Table XI.   Reported Incidence of Inhibitory Action of Known Antibiotics

I[a]		*II*[b]	
Gram-positive bacteria	37%	*Staphylococcus aureus*	60.5%
Gram-negative bacteria	15%	*Escherichia coli*	29.2%
Acid fast bacteria	16%	*Mycobacterium sp.*	25%
Fungi and yeasts	20%	*Candida albicans*	25%
		dermatophyta	16%
Protozoa	4%	protozoa	11%
Viruses	3%	viruses	7%
Tumors[c]	21%	tumors	4%
		helminths	0.2%

[a] W. Kurylowicz (*109*).
[b] J. Berdy and K. Magyar (*30*).
[c] Reported as cytostatic activity.

The majority of the panel believes, however, that the frequency with which a particular type of biological activity has been discovered has been determined to an important extent by the frequency with which effective tests have been made for such activity; (90% agreement). In turn, this frequency has been determined largely by the availability of (1) a high capacity reproducible test system suitable for use with fermentation broths and (2) rapid, sensitive methods for detecting and assaying biologically active materials and thus for guiding purification and isolation (96% agreement). In general, microbial metabolites have been tested narrowly for biological activity (84% agreement), presumably because specific laboratories have concentrated on specific types of activity which were considered important and which could be detected by available *in vitro* methods. Because of this, useful drugs have undoubtedly been missed. I do no think the position of the panel is that all types of biological activity occur with equal frequency. Indeed, the published studies (*e.g.,* those of Avraamova *et al.* and of Burkholder) in which large numbers of isolates have been tested for different types of activity indicate otherwise (*111, 112*). Until, however, large numbers of isolates are tested in various media by equally sensitive detection methods for a variety of biological activities, no accurate estimate of the intrinsic frequencies can be made.

The Future Role of Microbial Metabolites in Drug Research

The panel agreed (81%) that in the next decade microbial metabolites will continue to provide significant discoveries not only in areas of human medicine and animal health in which drugs of microbiological origin have been prominent in the past 30 years but also in new fields. Table XII tabulates the judgments of the panel concerning the importance that secondary microbial metabolites will have among new drug discoveries in major fields of chemotherapy and in the realm of physiologically active drugs. The panel's overview of the role which microbial metabolites will play in the new drug discoveries of the next decade is: among antibacterial and antifungal drugs, a continuing major role; among antiprotozoal and animal growth stimulating drugs, an increasingly important role; among antineoplastic, antiviral and anthelmintic drugs, a significant but not major role. Most interesting is the view of 46% of the respondents that microbial metabolites will be among the substantial or most important discoveries of drugs having physiological actions. When the time period considered is 20 years, this percentage rises to 74% and exceeds that for antineoplastic and antiviral drugs. (Although this subject is beyond the scope of this paper, it is expected that microbial metabolites will also provide new herbicides, insecticides, fungicides, and plant growth regulators in the future.)

What is the basis for the view that microbial metabolite drugs will leap the bounds of infectious disease and cancer chemotherapy to which they seemingly have been confined since 1940? Just as it was clear prior to 1940 that microorganisms produce a variety of antibacterial and anti-

Table XII.   Predicted Importance of Microbial Metabolite Discoveries 1970–1980 by Drug Category

Drug Category	Among Most Important Discoveries	Among Substantial Discoveries	Among Minor Discoveries	Not Among Significant Discoveries
Antibacterial	39	61	0	0
Antiprotozoal	14	54	12	20
Antifungal	20	54	16	10
Antiviral	31	18	13	38
Antineoplastic	27	18	16	39
Animal growth stimulant	22	55	7	16
Anthelmintic	10	35	20	35
Drugs having physiological actions[a]	22	24	3	51

[a] For example, drugs acting on the central nervous system, cardiovascular system, respiratory system, diabetes, rheumatoid arthritis, etc.

fungal substances, today it is clear that microorganisms produce a variety of metabolites (in addition to vitamins and ergot alkaloids) which affect or have the potential to affect physiological processes in man and animals. (This subject has recently been reviewed by Perlman and Peruzzotti (*113*).) The examples cited in Table XIII demonstrate this point. The situation is, of course, not strictly parallel to that of 1940 because physiologically active substances discovered today will not enter a therapeutic vacuum as did new antibacterial drugs 30 years ago. Chemical modification of new lead structures may be required before new drugs actually emerge.

Table XIII. Microbial Metabolites having Demonstrated or Potential Physiological Activity

Compound	*Type of Biological Activity*	*Reference*
Fusaric acid	hypotensive, dopamine-β-hydroxylase inhibition	(*120*)
Colisan	antispasmodic	(*121*)
Monorden	sedative	(*122–4*)
Muscarine	parasympathomimetic	(*125*)
Slaframine	parasympathomimetic	(*126, 127*)
Serotonin	biogenic amine	(*128, 129*)
Psilocybin and Psilocin	hallucinogenic	(*128, 130*)
HO-2135	serotonin antagonism	(*131*)
Nigrifactin	antihistaminic, hypotensive	(*132*)
Zeranol	estrogenic, anabolic	(*109*)
Mycophenolic acid	immunosuppressive	(*133*)
Ergosterol	pro-vitamin D	(*134*)
Leupeptins	plasmin and trypsin proteolysis inhibition, thrombokinase inhibition	(*135*)
Pepstatin	pepsin inhibition	(*136, 137*)
Chymostatin	chymotrypsin inhibition	(*138*)
Desferrioxamine-B	therapeutic for bronze diabetes, hemochromatosis, and acute iron poisoning (*via* iron chelation)	(*139*)

Japanese workers are at the forefront in the search for physiologically active microbial metabolies. Their detection methods are worthy of note for lack of satisfactory testing methods has long hampered this search. Umezawa and his co-workers used *in vitro* enzyme inhibition tests to detect fusaric acid, pepstatin, chymostatin, and the leupeptins. Nigrifactin was discovered by Terashima and co-workers by seeking in experimental fermentations, materials having the chemical properties of alkaloids.

Further examples of the occurrence of useful or potentially useful physiological activity among microbial metabolites are emerging from observations of secondary biological properties of antibiotics. Thus, some of the antifungal polyene macrolides (candicidin, amphotericin B, filipin) have been reported to reduce serum cholesterol levels and prostate gland volume in dogs (*114, 115*). Griseofulvin has been reported to have anti-inflammatory activity (*116, 117, 118*) and mithramycin, in addition to its beneficial effect upon testicular tumors, is antihypercalcemic. It is interesting that the polyene macrolides deplete cholesterol, mithramycin depletes calcium, and desferrioxamine B (Table XIII) depletes iron, in view of the fact that these microbial metabolites form complexes with the same materials *in vitro*.

Conclusion

For the foreseeable future, important new drug discoveries will be derived from products of microbial metabolism. If the full potentialities of this discovery source are to be realized, discovery processes will have to be refined and broadened in scope. These are some of the challenges and opportunities that I see for the decade ahead:

(1) The standards for acceptance of new antibacterial drugs are now exceedingly high and will become even more demanding. The remaining unsatisfied therapeutic needs constitute difficult targets for drug therapy. In view of this, relatively few newly discovered microbial metabolites will qualify *per se* for commercialization and general clinical application in this field. Preliminary testing of new microbial metabolites should then identify both potential drugs and prototype structures whose biological and chemical properties justify structural modification designed to upgrade biological performance. The roster of previously discovered, structurally novel but unused antibiotics should be reexamined for substances of the latter type. Application of biochemical tests for mechanism and selectivity of action should help determine which prototypes hold the most promise.

(2) Antibiotics provide some of the best opportunities for understanding drug action in intimate detail. Research directed toward improvement of a therapeutically important property of an antimicrobial agent should seek an understanding of the critical determinant(s) of that property. Thus to increase *in vitro* potency one may need to increase resistance to enzymatic destruction, increase rate of penetration of the cell wall or membrane, or increase intrinsic potency at the molecular site of action. Where antimicrobial drug action can be studied at the molecular level, the opportunity should be grasped to learn as much as possible about the effect of changes in electrical, geometrical, and chemical properties on this action. Without a full understanding of the nature of and requirements for fruitful drug–receptor interactions, neither basic biochemical studies nor x-ray visualization of receptors will provide the key to rational design of drugs.

(3) The systematic structural variation needed for drug discovery studies will often be impossible without mastery of complex chemistry

and without the perfection of simple and versatile synthetic methods applicable to important drug types. Were such syntheses now available for β-lactams, macrolides, and aminoglycosides, they could provide presently inaccessible structural variants for biological study. This is a challenge to which academic organic chemists might well respond.

(4) Microorganisms that are more difficult to collect, isolate, and grow should be examined, including those that have resisted artificial cultivation in the past. Examination of experimental microbial fermentations must become more thorough and imaginative to detect minor active components, substances formed only under unusual conditions, and substances having diverse biological activities. Media and conditions that are optimal for formation of an antibacterial metabolite may well not be optimal for formation of substances having other types of activity. Sensitive and specific *in vitro* tests indicative of potential physiological activity should be perfected and applied as screening tools. New technology such as high pressure liquid chromatography should be adapted to the rapid isolation of relatively pure components from microbial fermentations thus facilitating the isolation and *in vivo* testing of potential physiologically active components. Coupling of the most rapid and efficient separation and identification techniques with computer analysis of data will be required.

In conclusion, a simple truth bears repetition which has been amply demonstrated in the discovery endeavors reviewed in this paper. Those who make landmark discoveries have minds receptive to the precedent-breaking significance occasionally contained in unconventional, obscure, anomalous, or neglected observations, interpretations, and hypotheses. They break the intellectual bonds imposed on most of us by immersion in immediate technical problems and by acceptance of current scientific rationalizations, fashions, and dogmas.

In considering the developments cited here that have appeared so obvious after the fact (*e.g.*, the recognition of useful antibiotics and the isolation and use of 6-aminopenicillanic acid), what important advances now lie before all of us, unrecognized but easily attainable if only we could remove the scales from our eyes? For the present, I join Louis Pasteur in his lament "Messieurs, c'est les microbes qui auront le dernier mot."

Acknowledgment

The author expresses his appreciation to all who so enthusiastically and painstakingly replied to the questionnaire, to his colleagues, Walter Celmer, Frank Sciavolino, John Routien, Kenneth Butler, and Max Miller for the ideas, information, and advice which they generously contributed during the preparation of this manuscript, and finally to Blanche Bralich, Raymond Sumner, and Daniel Gillen for their invaluable aid in the compilation of questionnaire replies, validation of references, and preparation of tables and figures.

Literature Cited

(1) Dubos, R. J., *Proc. Soc. Exp. Biol. Med.* (1939) **40**, 311.
(2) Schatz, A., Bugie, E., Waksman, S. A., *Proc. Soc. Exp. Biol. Med.* (1944) **55**, 66.
(3) Waksman, S. A., Woodruff, H. B., *Proc. Soc. Exp. Biol. Med.* (1940) **45**, 609.
(4) Waksman, S. A., Woodruff, H. B., *Proc. Soc. Exp. Biol. Med.* (1942) **49**, 207.
(5) Chain, E., Florey, H. W., Gardner, A. D., Heatley, N. G., Jennings, M. A., Orr-Ewing, J., Sanders, A. G., *Lancet* (1940) **2**, 226.
(6) Fleming, A., *Brit. J. Exp. Pathol.* (1929) **10**, 226.
(7) Waksman, S. A., "Microbial Antagonisms and Antibiotic Substances," The Commonwealth Fund, New York, 1945.
(8) Florey, H. W., Chain, E., Heatley, N. G., Jennings, M. A., Abraham, E. P., Florey, M. E., "Antibiotics," Vol. I, Oxford University Press, London, New York, Toronto, 1949.
(9) Consden, R. A., Gordon, A. H., Martin, A. J. P., *Biochem. J.* (1944) **38**, 224.
(10) Boer, C. de, Dietz, A., Wilkins, J. R., Lewis, C. N., Savage, G. M., *Antibiot. Annu.* (1955) **1954-55**, 831.
(11) Hoeksema, H., *J. Amer. Chem. Soc.* (1964) **86**, 4224.
(12) Hoeksema, H., Bannister, B., Birkenmeyer, R. D., Kagan, F., Magerlein, B. J., MacKellar, F. A., Schroeder, W., Slomp, G., Herr, R. R., *J. Amer. Chem. Soc.* (1964) **86**, 4223.
(13) Mason, D. J., Dietz, A., Boer, C. de, *Antimicrob. Ag. Chemother.—1962* (1963) **554**.
(14) Burton, H. S., Abraham, E. P., *Biochem. J.* (1951) **50**, 168.
(15) Chain, E., Florey, H. W., Jennings, M. A., Williams, T. I., *Brit. J. Exp. Pathol.* (1943) **24**, 108.
(16) Godtfredsen, W. O., Daehne, W. Von, Vangedal, S., Marquet, A., Arigoni, D., Malera, A., *Tetrahedron* (1965) **21**, 3505.
(17) Godtfredsen, W. O., Jahnsen, S., Lorck, H., Roholt, K., Tybring, L., *Nature (London)* (1962) **193**, 987.
(18) Hallsall, T. J., Jones, E. H., Lowe, G., Newall, C. E., *Chem. Commun.* (1966) 68.
(19) Iwasaki, S., Sair, M. I., Igarashi, H., Okuda, S., *Chem. Commun.* (1970) 1119.
(20) Oxley, P., *Chem. Commun.* (1966) 729.
(21) Waksman, S. A., Horning, E. S., Spencer, E L., *J. Bacteriol.* (1943) **45**, 233.
(22) Cooper, D. J., Marigliano, H. M., Yudis, M. D., Traubel, T., *J. Infec. Dis.* (1969) **119**, 342.
(23) Ogawa, H., Ito, T., Kondo, S., Inoue, S., *Ibid.*, Ser. A (1958) **11**, 169.
(24) Umezawa, H., Ueda, M., Maeda, K., Yagishita, K., Kondo, S., Okami, Y., Utahara, R., Osato, Y., Nitta, K., Takeuchi, T., *J. Antibiot.*, Ser. A (1957) **10**, 181.
(25) Weinstein, M. J., Luedemann, G. M., Oden, E. M., Wagman, G. H., *Antimicrob. Ag. Chemother—1963* (1964) 1.
(26) Bycroft, B. W., Cameron, D., Croft, L. R., Johnson, A. W., *Chem. Commun.* (1968) 1301.
(27) Finlay, A., Hobby, G. L., Hochstein, F. A., Lees, T. M., Lenert, T. F., Means, J. A., P'An, S. Y., Regna, P. P., Routien, J. B., Sobin, B. A., Tate, K. B., Kane, J. H., *Amer. Rev. Tuberc.* (1957) **63**, 1.
(28) Herr, E. B., Jr., *Antimicrob. Ag. Chemother.—1962* (1963) 201.
(29) Lechowske, L., *Tetrahedron Letters* (1969) 479.
(30) Berdy, J., Magyar, K., *Process Biochem.* (1968) **3** (10), 45.

(31) Perlman, D., "Antibiotics," p. 11, Rand McNally, Chicago, 1970.

(32) Miller, I. M., Stapley, E. O., Chaiet, L., *Bacteriol. Proc.* (1962) 32.

(33) Stapley, E. O., Miller, T. W., Jackson, M., *Antimicrob. Ag. Chemother.* —*1968* (1969) 268.

(34) Mallams, A. K., Jaret, R. S., Reimann, H., *J. Amer. Chem. Soc.* (1969) **91**, 7506.

(35) Waksman, S. A., *Advan. Appl. Microbiol.* (1969) **11**, 1.

(36) Bartz, Q. R., Controulis, J., Crooks, H. M. Jr., Rebstock, M. C., *J. Amer. Chem. Soc.* (1946) **68**, 2163.

(37) Peck, R. L., Hoffhine, C. E. Jr., Folkers, K., *J. Amer. Chem. Soc.* (1946) **68**, 1390.

(38) Tatsuoka, S., Kasuka, T., Miyake, A., Inoue, M., Hitomi, H., Shiraishi, Y., Iwasaki, H., Imanishi, M., *Pharm. Bull.* (1957) **5**, 343.

(39) Coghill, R. D., Stodola, F. H., Wachtel, J. L., "The Chemistry of Penicillin," H. T. Clark, J. R. Johnson, R. Robinson, Eds., p. 680, Princeton University Press, Princeton, 1949.

(40) Controulis, J., Rebstock, M. C., Crooks, H. M. Jr., *J. Amer. Chem. Soc.* (1949) **71**, 2463.

(41) Long, L. M., Troutman, H. D., *J. Amer. Chem. Soc.* (1949) **71**, 2469, 2473.

(42) Rebstock, M. C., Crooks, H. M. Jr., Controulis, J., Bartz, Q. R., *J. Amer. Chem. Soc.* (1949) **71**, 2458.

(43) Smadel, J. E., "Chloromycetin (chloramphenicol)," T. E. Woodward, C. L. Wisseman, Eds., p. xi, Medical Encyclopedia, Inc., New York, 1958.

(44) Cutler, R. A., Stenger, R. J., Suter, C. M., *J. Amer. Chem. Soc.* (1952) **74**, 5475.

(45) Robinson, F. A., "Antibiotics," Pitman, New York, 1953.

(46) Boothe, J. H., Morton, J. II, Petisi, J. P., Wilkinson, R. G., Williams, J. H., *J. Amer. Chem. Soc.* (1953) **75**, 4621.

(47) Conover, L. H., U.S. Patent **2,699,054** (Jan. 11, 1955).

(48) Conover, L. H., Moreland, W. T., English, A. R., Stephens, C. R., Pilgrim, F. J., *J. Amer. Chem. Soc.* (1953) **75**, 4622.

(49) Hochstein, F. A., Stephens, C. R., Conover, L. H., Regna, P. P., Pasternack, R., Brunings, K. J., Woodward, R. B., *J. Amer. Chem. Soc.* (1952) **74**, 3708.

(50) Hochstein, F. A., Stephens, C. R., Conover, L. H., Regna, P. P., Pasternack, R., Gordon, P. N., Pilgrim, F. J., Brunings, K. J., Woodward, R. B., *J. Amer. Chem. Soc.* (1953) **75**, 5455.

(51) Stephens, C. R., Conover, L. H., Hochstein, F. A., Regna, P. P., Pilgrim, F. J., Brunings, K. J., Woodward, R. B., *J. Amer. Chem. Soc.* (1952) **74**, 4976.

(52) Stephens, C. R., Conover, L. H., Pasternack, R., Hochstein, F. A., Moreland, W. T., Regna, P. P., Pilgrim, F. J., Brunings, K. J., Woodward, R. B., *J. Amer. Chem. Soc.* (1954) **76**, 3568.

(53) Minieri, P. P., Firman, M. C., Mistretta, A. G., Abbey, A., Bricker, C. E., Rigler, N. E., Sokol, H., *Antibiot. Annu.* (1955) **1953-54**, 81.

(54) Blackwood, R. K., Beereboom, J. J., Rennhard, H. H., Schach von Wittenau, M., Stephens, C. R., *J. Amer. Chem. Soc.* (1963) **85**, 3943.

(55) Stephens, C. R., Beereboom, J. J., Rennhard, H. H., Gordon, P. N., Murai, K., Blackwood, R. K., Schach von Wittenau, M., *J. Amer. Chem. Soc.* (1963) **85**, 2643.

(56) Woodward, R. B., "Perspectives in Organic Chemistry," A. Todd, Ed., p. 160, Interscience, New York, 1956.

(57) Stephens, C. R., Murai, K., Rennhard, H. H., Conover, L. H., Brunings, K. J., *J. Amer. Chem. Soc.* (1958) **80**, 5324.

(58) McCormick, J. R. D., Jensen, E. R., Miller, P. A., Doerschuk, A. P., *J. Amer. Chem. Soc.* (1960) **82**, 3381.
(59) Martell, M. J. Jr., Boothe, J. H., *J. Med. Chem.* (1967) **10**, 44.
(60) Schach von Wittenau, M., Supplement to *Chemotherapy* (1968) **13**, 41.
(61) Schach von Wittenau, M., Delahunt, C. S., *J. Pharmacol. Exp. Ther.* (1966) **152**, 164.
(62) Schach von Wittenau, M., Yeary, R., *J. Pharmacol. Exp. Ther.* (1963) **140**, 258.
(63) Scriabine, A., Schach von Wittenau, M., Yu, M., Furman, J., *Chemotherapia* (1964) **8**, 85.
(64) Behrens, O. K., Corse, J., Edwards, J. P., Garrison, L., Jones, R. G., Soper, R. F., Van Abeele, F. R., Whitehead, C. W., *J. Biol. Chem.* (1948) **175**, 793.
(65) Brandl, E., Margreiter, H., *Oesterr. Chem. Ztg.* (1954) **55**, 11.
(66) Stewart, G. T., "The Penicillin Group of Drugs," p. 21, Elsevier, New York, 1965.
(67) Sheehan, J. C., "Amino Acids and Peptides with Antimetabolic Activity," G. E. W. Wolstenhome, C. M. O'Connor, J. A. Churchill, Eds., p. 258, London, 1958.
(68) Sheehan, J. C., Henery-Logan, K. R., *J. Amer. Chem. Soc.* (1959) **81**, 5838.
(69) Burger, A., "Medicinal Chemistry," Vol. II, p. 880, Interscience, New York, 1951.
(70) Hockenhull, D. J. D., Ramachandran, K., Walker, T. K., *Arch. Biochem.* (1969) **23**, 160.
(71) Sakaguchi, K., Murao, S., *J. Agr. Chem. Soc. Jap.* (1950) **23**, 411.
(72) Kato, K., *J. Antibiot. Ser. A* (1953) **6**, 130, 184.
(73) Kato, T., *Kagaku (Tokyo)* (1953) **23**, 217.
(74) Batchelor, F. R., Doyle, F. P., Nayler, J. H. C., Rolinson, G. N., *Nature (London)* (1959) **183**, 257.
(75) Batchelor, F. R., Chain, E. B., Richards, M., Rolinson, G. N., *Proc. Roy. Soc., Ser. B* (1961) **154**, 522.
(76) Claridge, C. A., Gourevitch, A., Lein, J., *Nature (London)* (1960) **187**, 237.
(77) Huang, H. T., English, A. R., Seto, T. R., Shull, G. M., Sobin, B. A., *J. Amer. Chem. Soc.* (1960) **82**, 3790.
(78) Kaufmann, W., Bauer, K., *Naturwiss.* (1960) **47**, 474.
(79) Rolinson, G. N., Batchelor, F. R., Butterworth, D., Cameron-Wood, J., Cole, M., Eustace, G. C., Hart, M. V., Richards, M., Chain, E. B., *Nature (London)* (1960) **187**, 236.
(80) Perron, Y. G., Minor, W. F., Holdrege, C. I., Gottstein, W. J., Godfrey, J. C., Crast, L. B., Babel, R. B., Cheney, L. C., *J. Amer. Chem. Soc.* (1960) **82**, 3934.
(81) Doyle, F. P., Nayler, J.) H. C., Smith, H., Stove, E. R., *J. Chem. Soc. (London)* (1961) **191**, 1091.
(82) Abraham, E. P., *G. Microbiol.* (1956) **2**, 102.
(83) Gourevitch, A., Hunt, G. A., Luttinger, J. R., Carmack, C. C., Lein, J., *Proc. Soc. Exp. Biol. Med.* (1961) **107**, 455.
(84) Brain, E. G., Doyle, F. P., Hardy, K., Long, A. A. W., Mehta, M. D., Miller, D., Nayler, J. H. C., Soulal, M. J., Stove, E. R., Thomas, G. R., *J. Chem. Soc. (London)* (1962) 1445.
(85) Doyle, F. P., Long, A. A. W., Nayler, J. H. C., Stove, E. R., *Nature (London)* (1961) **192**, 1183.
(86) Doyle, F. P., Nayler, J. H. C., Waddington, H. R. J., Hanson, J. C., Thomas, G. R., *J. Chem. Soc. (London)* (1963) 497.
(87) Doyle, F. P., Fosker, G. R., Nayler, J. H. C., Smith, H., *J. Chem. Soc. (London)* (1962) 1440.

(88) Izaki, K., Matsuhashi, M., Strominger, J. L., *Proc. Nat. Acad. Sci. (U.S.)* (1966) **55**, 656.
(89) Acred, P., Brown, D. M., Knudsen, E. T., Rolinson, G. N., Sutherland, R., *Nature (London)* (1967) **215**, 25.
(90) Hobbs, D. C., U.S. Patent 3,142,673 (July 28, 1964).
(91) Shier, W. T., Rinehart, K. L. Jr., Gottlieb, D., *Proc. Nat. Acad. Sci. (U.S.)* (1969) **63**, 198.
(92) Hendlin, D., Dulaney, E. L., Drescher, D., Cook, T., Chaiet, L., *Biochim. Biophys. Acta* (1962) **58**, 635.
(93) Elander, R. P., "Fermentation Advances," D. Perlman, Ed., p. 89, Academic, New York, 1969.
(94) McCormick, J. R. D., Sjolander, N. O., Hirsch, U., Jensen, E. R., Doerschuk, A. P., *J. Amer. Chem. Soc.* (1957) **79**, 4561.
(95) Lancini, G., Hengeller, C., *J. Antibiot.* (1969) **22**, 637.
(96) Keil, J. G., Hooper, I. R., Schreiber, R. H., Swanson, C. L., Godfrey, J. C., *Antimicrob. Ag. Chemother.—1969* (1970) 200.
(97) Price, K. E., Chisholm, D. R., Leitner, F., Misiek, M., *Antimicrob. Ag. Chemother.—1969* (1970) 209.
(98) Abraham, E. P., Newton, G. G. F., *Biochem. J.* (1961) **79**, 377.
(99) Chauvette, R. R., Flynn, E. H., Jackson, B. G., Lavagnino, E. R., Morin, R. B., Mueller, R. A., Pioch, R. P., Roeske, R. W., Ryan, C. W., Spencer, J. L., Van Heyningen, E., *Antimicrob. Ag. Chemother.— 1962* (1963) 687.
(100) Wick, W. E., *Appl. Microbiol.* (1967) **15**, 765.
(101) Morin, R. B., Jackson, B. G., Flynn, E. H., Roeske, R. W., *J. Amer. Chem. Soc.* (1962) **84**, 3400.
(102) Sensi, P., Maggi, N., Furesz, S., Maffia, G., *Antimicrob. Ag. Chemother. —1966* (1967) 699.
(103) Mann, R. L., Bromer, W. W., *J. Amer. Chem. Soc.* (1958) **80**, 2714.
(104) Kondo, S., Sezaki, M., Koike, M., Shimura, M., Akita, E., Satoh, K., Hara, T., *J. Antibiot. Ser. A* (1965) **18**, 38.
(105) Shumard, R. F., Callender, M. E., *Antimicrob. Ag. Chemother.—1967* (1968) 369.
(106) Bauer, F., Dost, G., *Antimicrob. Ag. Chemother—1965* (1966) 749.
(107) Somer, P. de, Dijck, P. van, *Antibiot. Chemother. (Washington, D. C.)* (1955) **5**, 632.
(108) Arai, M., Nakamura, S., Sakagami, Y., Fukuhara, K., Yonehara, H., *Jap. J. Med. Prog., Ser. A* (1956) **9**, 193.
(109) Urry, W. H., Wehrmeister, H. L., Hodge, E. B., Hidy, P. H., *Tetrahedron Letters* (1966) 3109.
(110) Kurylowicz, W., *Rev. Immunol.* (1960) **30**, 253.
(111) Avraamova, O., Gavrilina, G. X., Sveshnikova, M., *Bull. Moscow Naturalists, Ser. Biol.* (1953) **58**, 83.
(112) Burkholder, P., *J. Bacteriol.* (1946) **52**, 503.
(113) Perlman, D., Peruzzotti, G. P., *Advan. Appl. Microbiol.* (1970) **12**, 277.
(114) Gordon, H. W., Schaffner, C. P., *Proc. Nat. Acad. Sci. (U.S.)* (1968) **60**, 1201.
(115) Schaffner, C. P., Gordon, H. W., *Proc. Nat. Acad. Sci. (U.S.)* (1968) **61**, 36.
(116) Cochrane, T., Tullet, A., *Brit. Med. J.* (1959) **2**, 286.
(117) D'Arcy, P. F., Howard, E. M., Muggleton, P. W., Townsend, S. B., *J. Pharm. Pharmacol.* (1960) **12**, 659.
(118) Gentles, J. C., *Nature (London)* (1958) **182**, 476.
(119) Celmer, W. D., Sobin, B. A., *Antibiot. Annu. 1955-1956* (1956) 437.
(120) Hidaka, H., Nagatsu, T., Takeya, K., Takeuchi, T., Suda, H., Kojiri, K., Matsuzaki, M., Umezawa, H., *J. Antibiot.* (1969) **22**, 228.
(121) Leon, S. A., Bergmann, F., *Isr. J. Chem.* (1965) **2**, 325.

(122) Delmotte, P., Delmotte-Plaquée, J., *Nature (London)* (1953) **171**, 344.
(123) Mirrington, R. N., Ritchie, E., Shoppee, C. W., Taylor, W. C., Sternhell, S., *Tetrahedron Letters* (1964) 365.
(124) McCapra, F., Scott, A. I., Delmotte, P., Delmotte-Plaquée, J., Bhacca, N. S., *Tetrahedron Letters* (1964) 869.
(125) Bowden, K., Mogey, G. A., *J. Pharm. Pharmacol.* (1958) **10**, 145.
(126) Aust, S. D., Broquist, H. P., *Nature (London)* (1965) **205**, 204.
(127) Rainey, D. P., Smalley, E. B., Crump, M. H., Strong, F. M., *Nature (London)* (1965) **205**, 203.
(128) Benedict, R. G., Brady, L. R., "Fermentation Advances," D. Perlman, Ed., p. 63, Academic, New York, 1969.
(129) Tyler, V. E. Jr., *Science* (1958) **128**, 718.
(130) Hofmann, A., Heim, R., Brack, A., Kobel, H., *Experimentia* (1958) **14**, 107.
(131) Arai, T., Hayama, T., *Jap. J. Med. Progr.* (1962) **49**, 813.
(132) Kaneko, Y., Terashima, T., Kuroda, Y., *Agr. Biol. Chem.* (1968) **32**, 783.
(133) Mitsui, A., Suzuki, S., *J. Antibiot.* (1969) **22**, 358.
(134) Oxford, A. E., Raistrick, H., *Biochem. J.* (1933) **27**, 1176.
(135) Aoyagi, T., Takeuchi, T., Matsuzaki, A., Kawamura, K., Kondo, S., Hamada, M., Maeda, K., Umezawa, H., *J. Antibiot.* (1969) **22**, 283.
(136) Morishima, H., Takita, T., Aoyagi, T., Takeuchi, T., Umezawa, H., *J. Antibiot.* (1970) **23**, 263.
(137) Umezawa, H., Aoyagi, T., Morishima, H., Matsuzaki, M., Hamada, M., Takeuchi, T., *J. Antibiot.* (1970) **23**, 259.
(138) Umezawa, H., Aoyagi, T., Morishima, H., Kunimoto, S., Matsuzaki, M., Hamada, M., Takeuchi, T., *J. Antibiot.* (1970) **23**, 425.
(139) Moeschlin, S., Schnider, U., *N. Engl. J. Med.* (1963) **269**, 57.
(140) Rinehart, K. L. Jr., *J. Infec. Dis.* (1969) **119**, 345.

RECEIVED November 24, 1970.

4

Organic Synthesis as a Source of New Drugs

JOHN H. BIEL and YVONNE C. MARTIN

Experimental Pharmacology Division, Abbott Laboratories,
North Chicago, Ill. 60064

The identification of the infectious disease process by Pasteur, the subsequent formulation by Paul Ehrlich of the concepts of selective toxicity and rational drug design, and the coming of age of organic chemistry provided the imaginative impetus to the spectacular series of drug discoveries which ushered in the era of modern medicine. This paper reviews the evolutionary process of synthetic drug discovery, probes the circumstances that contributed to its success, and finally attempts to predict on the basis of current trends the future course synthetic drug research must take to remain a viable factor in the therapy of human disease.

The purpose of this chapter is not to give an exhaustive review of synthetic drugs as they were developed over the past century, but rather to delve into the "anatomy of synthetic drug discovery," probing into the events that triggered such discoveries and the creative reverberations emanating from them which gave birth to the main stream of modern drug therapy.

Particular stress is placed on the sequential interdependence of certain drug fields as well as the importance of the state of the biological art in recognizing a drug discovery or at least facilitating it. Thus, the major tranquilizers and antidepressants were a synthetic consequence of research on antihistamines which, in turn, had its origin in the biological hypothesis that histamine might be the causative agent in allergic responses. However, the utility of the psychotropic drugs would have gone largely unnoticed had it not been for the willingness of at least part of the psychiatric profession to concede that a "chemical" treatment of mental illness was indeed worthy of in-depth investigation.

The "leitmotif" of this chapter that biological concepts beget synthetic drug discoveries which, in turn, give rise to new biological discoveries and concepts and that these exert a positive feed-back on the creation of new structural drug prototypes, is shown schematically in Figure 1.

81

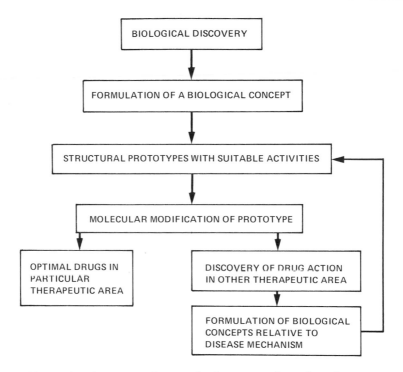

Figure 1.   Sequence of events leading to synthetic drug discovery

For illustrative examples we resorted to those classes of drug structures which spawned the largest variety of chemical therapeutic areas—namely the sulfonamides, antihistaminics, and adrenergic neurotransmitters.

Biochemical and molecular pharmacology as those disciplines which have assumed increasing importance in modern drug design comprise the last part of this chapter.

Paul Ehrlich's Contribution

In 1899 when Paul Ehrlich came face to face with the German chemical industry and saw the profusion of synthetic antipyretics, anesthetics, and analgetics, he decided that if it were possible to synthesize substances that differentiated between various cells in man, it should be possible to synthesize simple substances which would differentiate between man and his parasites.

From his pursuit of this goal was born the concept of selective toxicity, receptor theory, side chain theory, intrinsic activity, and affinity. Ehrlich was a prophet of almost biblical proportions, and much of what he predicted intuitively continues to be confirmed experimentally through the availability of highly sophisticated tools. The fundamental concepts which evolved from his speculative thinking are shown in Figures 2 and 3.

The "biological concept" (Figure 2) of selective toxicity served as a powerful stimulus not only in the development of the antimicrobial and insecticidal drugs but even more spectacularly in the therapeutic approach to endogenously induced diseases—*i.e.*, the selective interaction with certain target tissues without affecting other organ or cellular systems. It gave rise to a number of theoretical subconcepts which attempted to deal with drug design on a physical chemical rather than a purely intuitive or empirical basis.

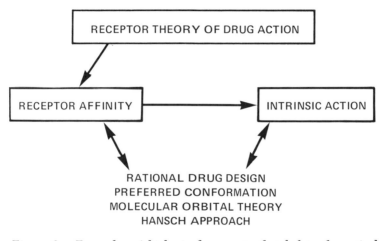

Figure 2. Examples of biological concepts that led to theoretical considerations in drug design

Ehrlich realized at the outset that a drug effect consisted of two phases. First, interaction of certain functional groups of the drug molecule with specific sites on the cell surface rather than with the whole cell; these sites (receptors) were so constituted as to have a high affinity for the prosthetic groups of the drug thereby forming a tightly bonded complex. From this and Langley's earlier hypothesis evolved the receptor theory which formed the basis for rational drug design since successful drug–receptor interaction was thought to be caused mainly by the shape (conformation) of the presenting drug molecule and the physical chemical forces of attraction generated between the invading substance and the appropriate cell receptor.

Secondly, Ehrlich realized that the mere interlocking of the drug with the cell receptor was not sufficient for producing a drug effect since bacteria could be stained without being killed. Hence, he postulated not only a haptophoric (anchoring) but also a toxophilic (poisoning) moiety

in the molecular structure of the drug. The combination of the therapeutic agent with the cell receptor was in itself considered harmless but
served to bring the toxophilic portion of the drug close enough to the
cell to either poison it or produce a pharmacologic effect. From similar
considerations Ariens and van Rossum developed, 50 years later, the
useful concept of affinity and intrinsic activity as determinants of the
nature of a drug effect.

A second major impetus to modern drug development came from the
demonstration of the chemical nature of neurotransmission and from the
identification of histamine as the chemical mediator in the production of
certain allergic responses.

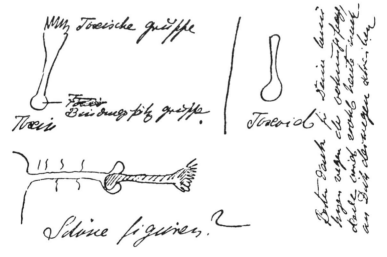

A. Albert, "Selective Toxicity"

*Figure 3.   Ehrlich's explanation of immunochemistry in his own
symbols, 1898* (35)

The results of these two approaches to drug design—namely the
discoveries that easily synthesized organic substances could cure the
diseases caused by virulent pathogens and that major physiological processes and responses were under the control of chemicals of simple structure—came during the period when synthetic organic chemistry was
unfolding to its full bloom. It was only natural that these three areas of
research should converge to usher in the exciting and unbelievably productive era of modern synthetic drug therapy.

One of the results of these early studies was the observation that
drug structures active in one disease area would, through molecular
modification, yield potent therapeutic agents in totally unrelated fields
of pathologic disorders.

The Sulfonamides

This group of drugs affords a familiar but illuminating illustration to the multifacted nature of drug discovery. The search by Domagk (*1*) for azo dyes (based on Ehrlich's affinity theory) that might be effective antibacterial agents ultimately resulted in 1935 in the discovery of Prontosil which protected mice against lethal streptococcal infections. Since this drug is inactive *in vitro*, Fourneau, Tréfouel, Nitti, and Bovet tested it in a reducing medium (*2*). This experiment was based on Ehrlich's earlier findings that pentavalent arsenic had to be reduced to trivalent arsenic *in vivo* before its bactericidal action was evident. The isolation, identification, and synthesis of the active metabolite, sulfanilamide, produced a structural prototype which ultimately led to major breakthroughs in the therapy of infectious, cardiovascular, and diabetic disease (Figure 4). In addition, other structural off-shoots provided anticonvulsant and uricosuric drugs.

These successes would have been impossible without the concurrent and requisite biological discoveries. For example, the development of the carbonic anhydrase inhibitors, which are used to treat congestive heart failure, resulted from the following sequence of biological observations:

(1) The demonstration of clinical acidosis and alkaline urine following sulfanilamide administration in 1937 (*3*).

(2) The discovery of carbonic anhydrase (CA) in the kidney in 1941 (*4*).

(3) The inhibition of CA by sulfanilamide and other sulfonamides in 1940, 1948 (*5, 6*).

(4) The establishment of the role of CA in the reabsorption of Na^+ as $NaHCO_3$ and depression of this function by sulfanilamide in 1945 (*7*).

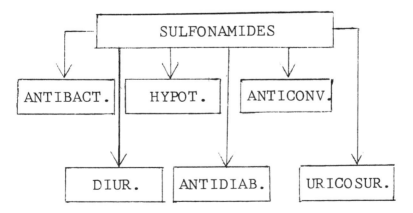

Figure 4. Schematic representation of the therapeutic areas which evolved from sulfonamide research

(5) The demonstration that sulfanilamide produced increased diuresis and natriuresis in 1949 (8).

Thus the "requisite biological discovery" triggers synthetic drug development. The rationalized scheme of this process is summarized in Figure 5. Both a motivating stimulus and an adequate biological test are necessary to encourage the medicinal chemist to persist in the sort of synthetic investigations which finally led to the discovery of the thiazides by Novello, Sprague, Beyer, and Baer (9, 10, 11). Similarly, the clinical observation by Janbon of the hypoglycemic properties of an isopropyl-thiadiazole derivative of sulfanilamide caused Loubatières to initiate the series of studies which culminated in the development of the sulfonyl ureas, an important class of hypoglycemic agents.

Thus Ehrlich's original concept that dyes having a high inffinity for bacteria could be modified structurally to make them bactericidal set off a series of chemical and biological events which resulted in heavy inroads into some major disease categories. A testable theory thus resulted in new biological information which led to a second testable theory.

The Antihistamines

The brilliant series of researches by Barger and Dale, Dale and Laidlaw, and Lewis and his colleagues established histamine as the endogenous "noxious" agent released during certain types of cell injuries and hypersensitivity antigen-antibody reactions. These observations set the stage for the birth of the antihistamines and helped to usher in the era of the psychotherapeutic drugs which have revolutionized the treatment of the mentally ill.

The ease with which the effects of histamine could be demonstrated in animals and isolated organs provided a golden opportunity for a massive and rapid screening effort for substances which would antagonize these actions. Bovet felt intuitively that the aminoethyl side chain in histamine was essential for cell receptor interaction and proceeded to select drugs with this side chain. He chose those molecules substituted with bulky phenyl groups in the hope that these groups would shield the receptors from the approaching histamine.

The size of the allergy market and the ease of synthesis and testing made this an extremely attractive area for research in molecular modification. As in the case of the sulfonamides, histamine antagonists provided inroads into disease areas never heretofore thought of as being amenable to chemical attack (Figure 5). The sequence of events leading to the discovery of these drugs is again revealing.

(1) The isolation of an active endogenous principle.

(2) Chemical and pharmacologic characterization.

(3) Identification of the noxious agent (substance "H") with histamine—*i.e.*, identification of the pathogen.

(4) The use of the concept of competitive inhibition of the histamine receptors as an approach to the therapy of allergy.

(5) Molecular design and modification to obtain an optimum therapeutic response. (The structure of the pathogen serves as a model for drug selection and design.)

(6) Progressive molecular modification leads to modification of pharmacologic response.

(7) The state of the medical art and philosophy of therapy had advanced sufficiently to allow recognition and exploitation (*i.e.*, discovery) of the therapeutic potential of the new drugs by the "primed" clinical investigator.

The necessary ingredients for successful drug discovery are thus close intermeshing of chemistry, pharmacology, and clinical medicine. However, the state of the art in each discipline must be sufficiently advanced to allow the simultaneous convergence of the three disciplines toward the creation of novel therapy.

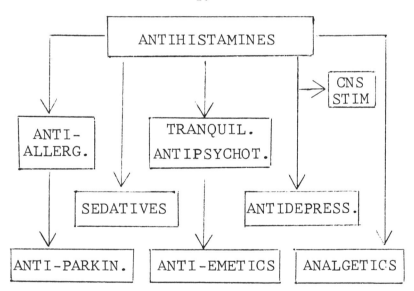

Figure 5.   Schematic representation of the therapeutic areas that evolved from research on antihistaminic drugs

The Neurotransmitters as a Source of New Synthetic Drugs

Up to this point rationally guided empiricism dominated synthetic drug development. The isolation and characterization of endogenous substances of a simple chemical nature, their identification as neurotransmitters of autonomic and possibly central nervous system function, the elucidation of the biosynthetic pathways, and isolation of the enzymes responsible for their biogenesis not only shed a good deal of light on the mechanism of action of existing drugs but opened up greater opportunities for rational drug design. Such substances are summarized in Figure 6.

Drug development in this area took the path of either potentiating, mimicking, or inhibiting neurotransmitter action or blocking the biosynthetic pathways at various steps in the sequence, thereby elucidating the role of a specific neurotransmitter in regulating nervous function and establishing the dependence of certain drugs on these transmitters for their action. In addition, the manipulation of these transmitters gave some hint as to the etiology of certain disease processes, particularly in cardiovascular, mental, and neurological diseases.

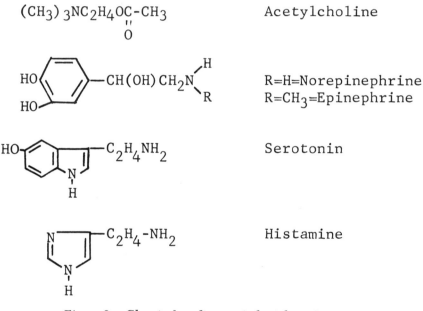

$$(CH_3)_3NC_2H_4OC\text{-}CH_3 \qquad\qquad \text{Acetylcholine}$$
$$\overset{\shortparallel}{O}$$

R=H=Norepinephrine
R=CH$_3$=Epinephrine

Serotonin

Histamine

Figure 6.   Chemical mediators of physiologic functions

Of key importance was the pioneering work of Barger and Dale which established the β-phenethylamine skeleton as the structural prototype for drugs affecting the adrenergic nervous system (Figure 7). From this evolved, through molecular modification, the central stimulant and anorexic agent, amphetamine, and the antiasthmatic drug, isoproterenol.

The second impetus in this field came from the elucidation of the metabolic pathways leading to the endogenous synthesis of norepinephrine (NE) and its ultimate oxidative degradation. The availability of specific enzyme inhibitors capable of blocking (a) the m-hydroxylation of tyrosine to 3,4-dihydroxyphenylalanine (DOPA), (b) the decarboxylation of

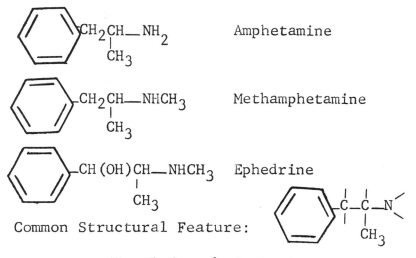

Figure 7.   Sympathomimetic amines

DOPA to 3,4-dihydroxyphenethylamine (dopamine), (c) the β-oxidation of dopamine to norepinephrine (NE), and (d) the inactivation of NE to [3]O-methylnorepinephrine (normetanephrine) or vanillyl mandelic acid (VMA), shed considerable light on the functional role of these neurotransmitters and their precursors (Figure 8).

Inhibition of the rate-limiting step in dopamine and NE synthesis, the *m*-hydroxylation of tyrosine to DOPA, may still offer an approach to the treatment of hypertension and certain types of mental illness (Fig-

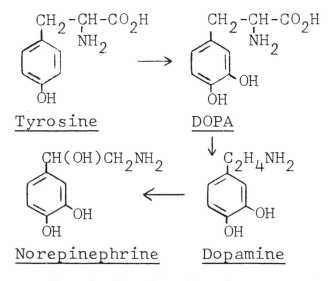

Figure 8.   Biosynthesis of neurohormones

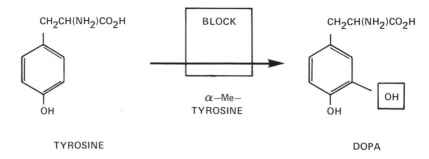

Figure 9.   The rate-limiting step in NE biosynthesis

ure 9). Search for DOPA decarboxylase inhibitors led to the widely used antihypertensive drug, α-methyl DOPA (Aldomet) (Figure 10). While its mechanism of action is probably not caused by enzyme inhibition, it does apparently compete with NE centrally in the form of its de-carboxylated and β-hydroxylated metabolites, α-methyldopamine and α-methyl NE. This competition could be for binding sites, neuronal release from binding sites, transmission of a nerve stimulus, interaction with common receptor sites, or the production of negative feedback resulting in the shutting off of NE biosynthesis. Such compounds which are structurally closely related to the neurotransmitters and have similar affinities for various neuronal sites but lack the intrinsic activity of the neurotransmitters have been called "false" or "surrogate" neurotrans-mitters by Carlsson and Kopin. This concept has given rise to the evalu-

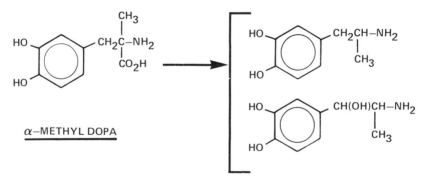

Figure 10.   Metabolites of α-methyl DOPA which could act as false neuro-transmitters.   α-Methyl DOPA acts in the form of its decarboxylated metabolites.

Possible mechanisms of actions are: (a) competitive displacement of NE from binding sites; (b) false neurotransmitter with respect to release on sympathetic stimulation and adrenergic receptor interaction; (c) false neurotransmitters with respect to causing negative feedback on CA biosynthesis. In its clinical action it is widely used as an antihypertensive.

ation of such old compounds as metaraminol and *p*-hydroxynorephedrine in hypertension. While they do lower blood pressure, the initial sympathomimetic pressor effect at least in the case of metaraminol precludes the use of the drug as an antihypertensive agent. However, other compounds with less intrinsic sympathomimetic activity should enjoy antihypertensive activity equal to or greater than that of α-methyl DOPA.

(1) DESTRUCTION OF ADRENERGIC RECEPTORS

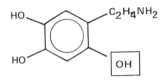

SELECTIVE DESTRUCTION OF SYMPATHETIC NERVE ENDINGS.

(2) POTENT COMT INIIIBITOR

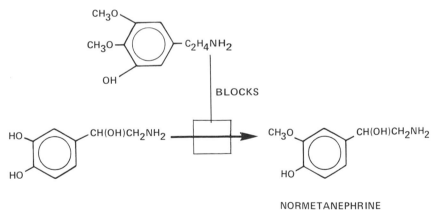

NORMETANEPHRINE

Figure 11.   Effects of some derivatives of dopamine

The intriguing concept of the false transmitters generated a renewed effort of synthesizing and evaluating hundreds of β-phenethylamine derivatives. One of the more interesting research tools that emerged from such molecular modifications is 6-hydroxydopamine (Figure 11) which, in low doses, preferentially depletes neuronal NE storage sites and in higher doses also empties the dopaminergic storage vesicles. Ultimately, with repeated dosing the terminal adrenergic and dopaminergic nerve endings are destroyed and need six weeks to be regenerated. This agent is, therefore, a powerful tool for the study of adrenergic and dopaminergic nervous function.

In 1948 Ahlquist proposed his basic hypothesis of α- and β-drenergic receptors to explain the dualistic properties of epinephrine. Some 15 years later this concept bore fruit in the development of the β-adrenergic blocking drugs as represented by propranolol, MJ 1999, alprenolol and Practolol (ICI 50172) (Figure 12).

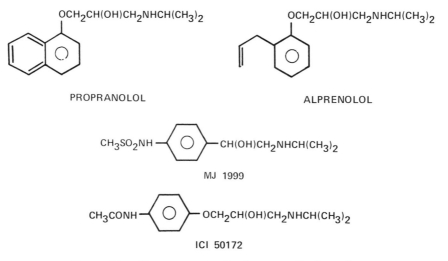

Figure 12.   Representative β-adrenergic blocking drugs

These drugs are potent anti-arrhythmic agents, and some of them enjoy wide use in the treatment of angina pectoris, at least outside the United States. They appear to act as a "governor" on the heart, preventing adrenergically mediated "overshoots" in cardiac activity in response to emotional or physical stress. They have brought Ahlquist's original concept to a significant fruition. Again a biological premise triggered molecular modification of existing structures and "primed" the pharmacologic investigator to recognize and confirm experimentally the original postulate.

DOPA and dopamine (Figure 13) lay dormant for many years. While they were thought to be metabolic precursors of norepinephrine, no particular function was ascribed to them. Dopamine had been shown to be simply a lesser amine of lesser potency and stability than NE. However, in the hands of a few inquisitive investigators, these two compounds were to create a major breakthrough in medical history. Hornykiewicz was the first to demonstrate cardiovascular effects of dopamine different from NE in guinea pigs, where it lowered instead of raised blood pressure. Subsequently, he discovered significantly decreased brain levels of dopamine in the neostriatum and substantia nigra of recently deceased Parkinson patients. With the theory of the biochemical nature of neuro-

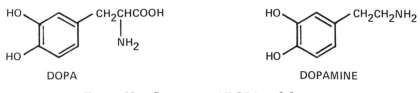

Figure 13.   Structures of DOPA and dopamine

transmission as a background, Hornykiewicz felt justified in correlating a biochemical deficiency with a neurological disease syndrome, similar to insulin in diabetes. As replacement therapy Hornykiewicz and Birkmeyer gave the precursor of dopamine, DOPA, which was resistant to monoamine oxidase attack and capable of penetrating the blood-brain barrier. His results were inconclusive in proving the hypothesis, mainly because (as it turned out later) the large doses used just were not high enough. It remained for Cotzias to develop a safe dosage regimen that enabled one to titrate gradually the Parkinsonism patient to effective dosage levels as high as 8 grams/day, producing a significant improvement in two-thirds of the cases treated.

Goldberg postulated the presence of dopaminergic receptors in the renal arteries on the basis of the ability of dopamine to dilate the renal arteries and the inability of α- or β-adrenergic blocking drugs to antagonize this action. However, drugs that produce iatrogenic Parkinsonism such as haloperidol or spiroperidol are capable of blocking the renal vasodilatory effect of dopamine.

Hence, the demonstration of discrete dopaminergic receptors (Figure 14) opens up a whole new field of investigation to explore the role of dopamine in the central and peripheral nervous system with respect to mental, cardiovascular, and neurological disturbances.

The Role of Biochemical Pharmacology in Drug Discovery

By 1950 biochemical pharmacology had become a discipline in its own right. It had its beginning in drug metabolism and disposition, a science that developed rapidly during World War II and was responsible for resurrecting the antimalarial agent, Atabrine, on the basis of Brodie's findings that this drug was originally given on an incorrect dosage schedule. From the chemical determination of drug in serum it was found that 0.8 gram of drug should be given the first day, 0.3 gram/day thereafter.

Biogenic Amines. With the tools for biochemical pharmacology thus forged, Brodie's attention now turned to endogenous levels of serotonin and NE. The discovery of reserpine's profound depleting activity on brain serotonin and NE and its potent tranquilizing action suggested a correlation between the two phenomena—*i.e.*, that a biochemical change could

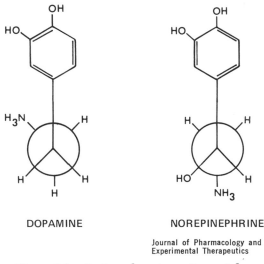

DOPAMINE   NOREPINEPHRINE

Journal of Pharmacology and
Experimental Therapeutics

Figure 14.   Preferred conformations of dopa-
mine and norepinephrine (view down the line
of the carbon-carbon single bond) (36)

give rise to a behavioral depression. Almost concurrently, the work by
Biel *et al.* (*16*) with sympathomimetic amines had led them to investigate
an analogous series of hydrazines to enhance the potency and duration
of this important class of drugs (Figure 15). These authors felt that the
hydrazines would be less prone to metabolic attack by MAO on the basis
of Zeller's work with hydrazides which actually inhibited this enzyme
irreversibly. The fortuitous discovery of mood elevation of the antitu-

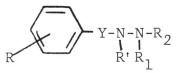

a.   Replacement of 'NH$_2$' by 'NH-NH$_2$'

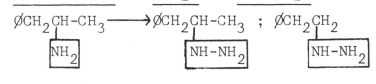

b.   Isosteric replacement of 'CH$_2$' by 'NH'

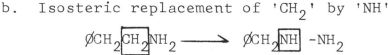

Figure 15.   Potent antidepressants (neurotic and psychotic depressions)

bercular drug, iproniazid, in tubercular patients coupled with Zeller's demonstration of its moderately potent MAO inhibitory properties prompted Brodie to measure NE and serotonin brain levels following the administration of iproniazid and the potent MAO inhibitor, α-methylphenethylhydrazine (Figure 16). He found that both drugs increase brain amine levels by 200–300% (Table I) and predicted that in contrast to reserpine they should have behavioral stimulant properties. This was confirmed quickly by Kline who demonstrated the potent antidepressant activities of these agents in severely depressed patients.

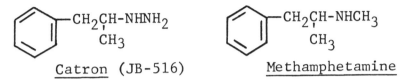

Figure 16.   *Structures of Catron (JB-516) and methamphetamine*

Table I.   Brain Levels of Serotonin and Norepinephrine After Five Days of Daily Administration of Three MAO Inhibitors

Drug	Dose, mg/kg s.c. rabbits	NE Levels, γ/gram tissue	Serotonin Levels, γ/gram tissue
Controls	—	0.40	0.58
Isoniazid	50.0	0.40	0.58
Iproniazid	5.0	0.43	0.60
Iproniazid	10.0	1.1	0.92
JB-516	1.0	0.95	1.6

At this point Brodie formulated his unifying hypothesis that serotonin and NE were responsible for controlling brain function and that mental illness might be a consequence of a chemical imbalance in central neurotransmitter amines. The stage was thus set for the medicinal chemist to design molecules which would affect brain amine levels in such a way as to alter the emotional state.

Reserpine and the MAO inhibitors thus afforded the medical breakthrough to the chemical treatment of mental illness and established a rational basis for synthetic drug design of antipsychotic and antidepressant drugs. New types of biochemical and pharmacological screening procedures were developed as a result of Brodie's work, and the 1960's were to become the era of the biogenic amines.

The biochemical pharmacologist who had generated a powerful new methodology to detect minute quantities of endogenous hormones in brain and the medicinal chemist with his almost uncanny ability to come up with the proper chemical tools at the appropriate moment worked in concert to establish the important concept of biochemical correlates of human behavior and emotional disturbances. Together they teamed up to create a new field of therapy.

A direct consequence of work on the aralkylhydrazines was the development of aralkylhydrazino acids. Biel and Drukker (17) synthesized them because they wanted to produce higher brain levels of the aralkylhydrazines and thus overcome the peripheral side effects of these drugs such as liver involvement and orthostasis. Unlike the corresponding amino acids, however, these acids neither penetrated the brain nor were they decarboxylated to generate MAO inhibitors. They were, however, potent DOPA decarboxylase inhibitors, particularly the Merck drug, α-methyl-N-aminodopa (MK-485) (Figure 17).

This drug or the Roche compound, Ro 4-4602, when administered concomitantly with DOPA, lowered the required anti-Parkinsonism dose of DOPA 6–10-fold. Thus, many of the severe peripheral side effects engendered by the usual massive does of DOPA, including emesis and orthostasis, are mitigated.

The model scheme (Figure 18) developed by Iversen illustrates some of the theories which have been advanced to explain the action of the tricyclic antidepressant and antipsychotic drugs, as well as that of reserpine, amphetamine, and the false neurotransmitters.

Brodie demonstrated that the tricyclic antidepressants do not reverse reserpine depression if the animal has been depleted of both dopamine and NE; hence, he concluded that their action depends on the presence

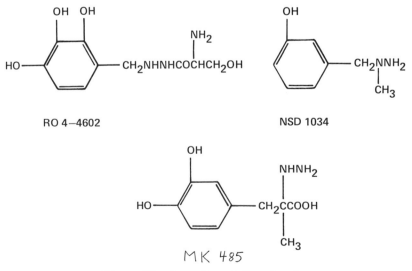

Figure 17.   Inhibitors of decarboxylase

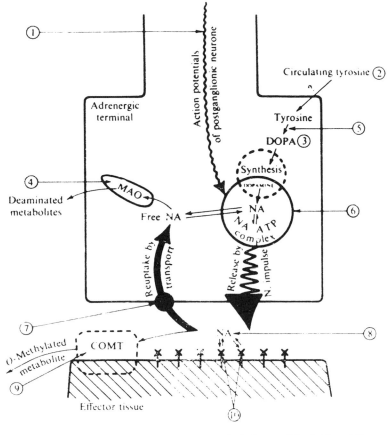

L. L. Iversen, "The Uptake and Storage
of Noradrenaline in Sympathetic Nerves"

*Figure 18.   Schematic of neuronal pathways in drug-biogenic amine
interaction* (15)

of threshold amounts of these two biogenic amines. Axelrod showed that the tricyclic antidepressants inhibit the re-uptake of adrenergically released NE into neuronal storage sites at the level of the neuronal membrane; thus, the adrenergic receptors are presented with increased quantities of the neurotransmitter. Amphetamine both released NE from its storage sites and prevented its re-uptake. As a result there is an initial volley of stimulation arising from large amounts of NE at the receptors. However, the stimulation of neuronal release added to the inhibition of neuronal uptake ultimately results in NE depletion and a loss of efficacy of the amphetamines. Furthermore, certain metabolites formed from amphetamine, presumably *p*-hydroxynorephedrine, act as a "surrogate" neurotransmitter to block adrenergic transmission. Both factors limit the action of amphetamine and render it useless for the chronic treatment of mental depression. The MAO inhibitors inhibit the metabolic destruction of dopamine, NE, and serotonin (5-HT), and their antidepressant effects may be explained on the basis of an overflow of adrenergic amines which activate the CNS.

Since the two major side effects of the tranquilizers are orthostatic hypotension and Parkinsonism (caused by dopaminergic blockade), they are thought to be centrally potent adrenergic and/or dopaminergic blocking agents. Thus, the adrenergic receptors are shielded from excess stimulation by the neurotransmitters.

Reserpine is a potent biogenic amine depletor by two mechanisms: (1) by impairing dopaminergic, noradrenergic, and serotoninergic binding sites and (2) by inhibiting the uptake of dopamine into the storage compartments where it would normally be converted to NE and stored as a tight complex of ATP:3NE:0.08 Mg^{2+}.

Lithium ion, the anti-manic agent, is said to facilitate the intraneuronal release of NE making it an easy prey to MAO attack, thus causing neuronal depletion. Biochemically, this can be demonstrated by the appearance of increased amounts of oxidative metabolites such as VMA.

False neurotransmitters could act at various neuronal levels: by inhibiting the uptake of NE, by interfering with sufficient release of the true transmitter, or by operating as stimulators of negative feedback of dopamine and NE biosynthesis.

These hypothetical models of the mechanism of action of the psychotropic drugs have been extremely useful not only in suggesting new methods of screening for drugs which would have been termed inactive by classical pharmacologic testing methods but also in stimulating the medicinal chemist to design drugs which might fulfill the requisite biochemical criteria.

Drug Metabolism Approach

Thus biochemical pharmacology did much to further the concept of rational drug design. It helped to explain why certain moieties in a drug molecule were critical to its action. Drug metabolism has also contributed greatly to our understanding of species differences in drug efficacy and potency as well as toxicological responses.

We have already discussed the use of DOPA and α-methyl DOPA as the protected precursors of the active amine metabolites and resorting to the use of DOPA decarboxylase inhibitors in making possible the administration of greatly lowered doses of the "none-too-innocuous" DOPA.

Allopurinol, a close structural analog of hypoxanthine, prevents the oxidative conversion of the latter to uric acid and has become one of the most effective agents in the treatment of gout (Figure 19).

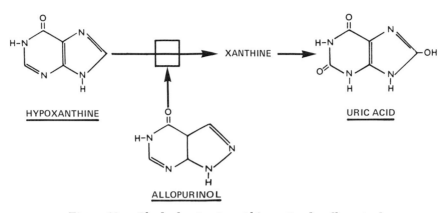

HYPOXANTHINE   URIC ACID

XANTHINE

ALLOPURINOL

Figure 19.   Blockade of uric acid formation by allopurinol

Advantage of species differences in metabolism was taken with the synthesis of malathion which is attacked by esterases in mammals and excreted rapidly as the diacid before conversion of the innocuous thiophosphate to the toxic phosphate. Insects have very low levels of esterases, and metabolism to the lethal "oxo" metabolite can occur unimpeded (Figure 20).

Drug metabolism studies demonstrated ether cleavage in the 4-position of 3,4,5-trimethoxyamphetamine, a potent hallucinogenic drug, to the inactive 4-hydroxy-3,5-dimethoxyamphetamine. The synthesis of the much less readily metabolized 4-methyl derivative resulted in a drug which had 10 times the potency of the parent structure (Figure 21).

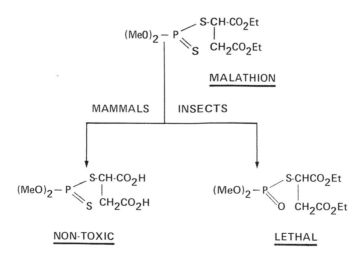

MALATHION

MAMMALS   INSECTS

NON-TOXIC   LETHAL

Figure 20.   Metabolism of malathion in mammals and insects

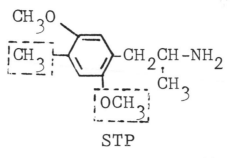

STP

Science

*Figure   21.   An   amphetamine-derived
hallucinogen (37)*

Effect of dose:
   3 mg/man: euphoria
   *3–10 mg/man: pronounced hallucinogenic
   effects for more than 8 hours, 100 times
   as strong as mescaline, 1/30 as strong
   as LSD*

Another drug designed on biochemical principles was ethacrynic acid (Figure 22). Organic mercurials produce their diuretic effect by combining with the sulfhydryl groups of renal tubular enzymes and by this means prevent reabsorption of water and sodium. This drug was designed with a dichlorophenoxyacetic acid moiety which has a high affinity for renal tissue and an activated double bond which reacts with the critical sulfhydryl groups of the renal enzyme systems, resulting in the most potent diuretic agent ever synthesized.

The science of enzymology has contributed many ideas to drug design. There is an obvious analogy between the receptor and the enzyme and between the drug and the inhibitor or substrate. In addition, many drugs owe their pharmacologic effect to enzyme inhibition. A particularly good example of these interrelationships is the design of 2-pyridine aldox-

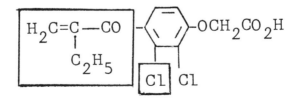

Ethacrynic
Acid

Figure 22.   Drug-designed diuretic

ime methiodide (PAM) for the reactivation of alkylphosphate-inhibited acetylcholinesterase by Wilson and Ginsberg (*18*). At the time it was known that the enzyme contained two sites (Figure 23). The first is an anionic site which binds quaternary ammonium structures. The second is the esteratic site which interacts with the esteratic function of acetyl-choline. During hydrolysis the basic group of the enzyme is acylated to form an acyl-enzyme intermediate. The acyl-enzymes formed from normal substrates hydrolyze rapidly to regenerate the original enzyme. However, the acyl-enzymes formed from the phosphate inhibitors are not hydrolyzed readily. This forms the basis for the mechanism of action of these inhibi-tors. Wilson and Ginsberg reasoned that the first prerequisite of a reac-tivator of the inhibited enzyme would be a quaternary ammonium group

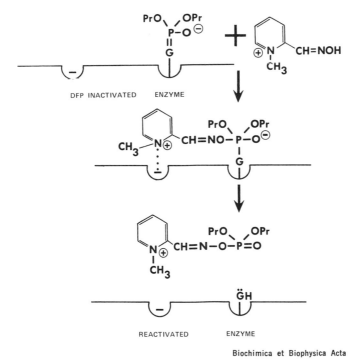

Biochimica et Biophysica Acta

Figure 23.   The reactivation of alkylphosphate-inhibited cholinesterase by 2-pyridine aldoxime methiodide (18)

which would thus fit into the anionic site and act as an anchoring group. They also knew that nicotine and picolinohydroxamic acids were mod-erately potent reactivators. Thus, they reasoned the second prerequisite of a reactivator was a nucleophilic group which could react with the inhibitor bound to the esteratic site. They designed and synthesized 2-pyridine aldoxime methiodide. On testing it, they discovered that the enzyme activity was regenerated in less than one minute. By careful reasoning they had synthesized only one compound and discovered a reactivator 50,000 times more potent than the best previously known.

This conforms to Ehrlich's earlier picture of an antibacterial drug model requiring both a haptophoric (anchoring) and toxophilic (bactericidal) moiety to interact with and destroy the pathogen. Ariens and van Rossum's concept of two stages in drug action—receptor affinity (anchoring of drug molecule) and intrinsic activity (drug potency)— represents a more sophisticated version of this same postulate. It explains strikingly how a weak drug with high receptor affinity can block out or displace a highly potent agent with weak receptor affinity. Thus harmaline, a reversible and moderately potent MAO inhibitor, can block the action of an extremely potent, irreversible MAO inhibitor, such as pheniprazine or tranylcypromine.

The Physical Chemical Approach to Drug Design

The search for physical chemical correlates of drug action began as early as 1899 with the Meyer-Overton theory which stated that the potency of an anesthetic was directly proportional to its oil:water partition coefficient. The more lipid soluble the compound was, the more readily it was thought to penetrate the central nervous system.

A useful technique for analyzing structure–activity relationships which has come into use within the past five or so years is that pioneered by Corwin Hansch (19). Its underlying concept is that the relative biological activity of a derivative depends on the difference in hydrophobic, electronic, or steric factors between the derivative and the parent compound. The contribution of each effect to activity is assumed to be independently additive so that one has a linear free energy relationship. Equations of the form below are expected:

$$\log \frac{1}{BR} = k + a \log P + b (\log P)^2 + c\sigma + d E_s$$

BR is the relative biologic activity under investigation, for example the molar ED_{50} or the percent response at a given dose. Log P is the logarithm of the octanol–water partition coefficient, σ is the approprite Hammett signa constant (electronic in nature), and E_s is the Taft steric parameter. With the important demonstration by Hansch that the partition coefficient is often an additive constitutive property, all of the physical parameers may be obtained from the literature. A second important contribution by Hansch is the recognition that the use of statistical techniques is essential to the analysis of quantitative structure–activity relationships. To develop an equation such as that above, one feeds the appropriate data into a multiple regression program on the computer. Standard statistical tests are then used to isolate the parameters which are important for each series. Thus, one would obtain the correlation coefficient, r for the whole equation as well as values of the F and t parameters to test the statistical significance of each term and the whole equation if n, the number of compounds, is known. There are many examples of such correlations in the literature; we discuss here those which have proved to be of predictive value.

In 1964 Hansch and Fujita (20) studied the structure–activity relationships of the thyroxine-like activity of nine halogen-substituted thyroxine analogs. From their results they suggested that the *tert*-butyl analog should also show thyroxine activity. This compound was synthesized (21) and found to be as potent as the most active halogen compound.

Fuller, Marsh, and Mills (22) applied the Hansch approach to a series of 16 N-(phenoxyethyl)cyclopropylamines which are monoamine oxidase (MAO) inhibitors. The activity is expressed as pI_{50}, the negative logarithm of the concentration of the derivative which inhibits MAO 50%. They used a dummy variable, γ, to designate the steric effects of meta substitution. Their results are summarized in Figure 24.

On the basis of the equations developed two additional compounds were synthesized and tested. The p-amino analog was expected to have moderate activity whereas the p-phenyldiazo derivative had a predicted pI_{50} value higher than any in the initial series. These predictions were nicely confirmed.

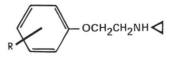

EQUATIONS FOUND

$$pI_{50} = 0.865\gamma + 0.209\pi + 1.547\sigma + 5.928 \quad r = .91 \quad n = 16$$

PREDICTIONS

	calc.	obsd.
4 N = NC_6H_5	7.28	7.56
4 NH_2	4.57	4.40

Journal of Medicinal Chemistry

Figure 24.   Inhibition on monoamine oxidase by N-
(phenoxyethyl)cyclopropylamines (22)

A number of studies have compared the use of the multiple regression technique using semiempirical parameters such as π and σ, and parameters calculated for the particular molecules from molecular orbital theory. Hermann, Culp, McMahon, and Marsh (23) studied the relationship between the maximum velocity of acetophenone substrates for a rabbit kidney reductase. These workers were interested in the reaction mechanism, and two types of quantum chemical calculations were made: (1) extended Huckel treatment, and (2) complete neglect of differential overlap (CNDO/2). Hydride interaction energy and approaching transition-state energies were calculated from the CNDO/2 treatment. All these parameters plus π and σ values were then subjected to regression analysis. The best results are presented in Table II.

Table II.   Structure-Activity Relationships among 10 Acetophenone Substrates for a Rabbit Kidney Reductase (Purified) (23)

Sigma and Pi	r^2
$\log k_0 = 2.09\ \sigma + 0.414\ \pi + 1.10$	.79
Sigma	
$\log k_0 = 2.04\ \sigma + 1.17$	.75
Eigenvalue Difference LEMO	
$\log k_0 = 0.346\ \Delta E + 1.04$	.74
Electron Density Near Carbonyl	
$\log k_0 = 1.13\ E_c + 1.32$	.72
Incipient Transition State Energy Differences	
$\log k_0 = 0.588\ \delta_E + 1.07$	.66

Although it is an unfair summary of this elegant work, it is obvious that a chemist interested in designing a better substrate for this enzyme would prefer to use the first equation listed since this equation fits the data the best and the parameters are easy to obtain.

P. R. Andrews (24) also used both quantum chemical methods (Extended Huckel Theory and CNDO/2) to calculate dipole moments and atomic charges on various atoms and groups of atoms for a series of anticonvulsants. There was no correlation between any of these parameters and the anticonvulsant activity of the compounds. In more recent work, Lien (25) has shown that the activity is explained by the partition coefficient (Table III).

Again the advantage of the simple parameters is evident, both in that they are more predictive and in that they are much less expensive to obtain.

Table III.   Anticonvulsant Activity of 11 Compounds (25)

Dipole Moment   r

$\qquad \log 1/c = -0.51 \, \mu + 4.09$ .221

Charge on "Biological Active Center"

$\qquad \log 1/c = -1.04 \, (EHT) + 3.51$ .371

Partition Coefficient

$\qquad \log 1/c = -0.242 \, (\log P)^2 + 1.30 \log P + 2.33$

$\qquad (optimum = 2.67)$ .948

In 1969, Clayton and Purcell (*26*) studied the structure–activity relationships of some 1-decyl-3-carbamoylpiperidines against butyryl-cholinesterase. The equations in Figure 25 were found. In this case the activity is presented as the pI_{50}, the negative logarithm of the concentration of derivative which inhibits butyrylcholinesterase 50%. The parameter σ^* is the Taft substituent constant which depends only on the net polar effect of the substituent. One compound of moderate activity was omitted from the calculations. The calculated equation was then used to predict the activity of this compound. The predicted pI_{50} was 5.00, that observed was $5.01 \pm .03$. In fact, the activity of these compounds depends so strongly on the partition coefficient that the use of the much simpler equation (Equation 2) predicts the activity nearly as well.

These calculations are of special interest because Purcell and co-workers have been interested in the structure–activity relationships of this series of compounds for several years and have compared several approaches to structure–activity relationships with the same compounds. Earlier they (*27, 28*) reported on detailed studies of the effect of partition coefficients (benzene–water), electric moments, and electronic structures on the relative activity of the congeners. Purcell (*28*) used Huckel molecular orbital theory to calculate the net charges on all the atoms of each compound. The only apparent success was the apparent correlation of the net charge at the amide nitrogen atom with activity. This was later shown to be caused by the statistically significant correlation between the π value and the net charge on the nitrogen atom (*29*).

Recently Wohl (*30*) reported on extensive studies on the competitive antagonism of Ca^{2+}-induced rat aortic vasoconstriction *in vitro* by a series of 36 benzothiadiazines. The Extended Hückel Theory (EHT) was used to calculate the preferred tautomer in solution, and charges, etc., on all atoms. The final equation was fairly successful in predicting the activity of several moderately potent compounds not included in the original regression.

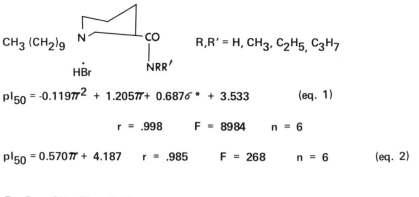

$$pI_{50} = -0.119\pi^2 + 1.205\pi + 0.687\sigma^* + 3.533 \qquad \text{(eq. 1)}$$

$$r = .998 \qquad F = 8984 \qquad n = 6$$

$$pI_{50} = 0.570\pi + 4.187 \qquad r = .985 \qquad F = 268 \qquad n = 6 \qquad \text{(eq. 2)}$$

For R = CH_3, R' = C_2H_5

(NOT INCLUDED IN ABOVE EQUATION)

observed pI_{50} = 5.01 ± .03

calculated pI_{50} = 5.00   equation 1

5.04   equation 2

Journal of Medicinal Chemistry

Figure 25.   Butyryl cholinesterase inhibitory potency of carbamoylpiperi-dines (26)

A different use of molecular orbital calculations, one that does not use multiple regression analysis, is that pioneered recently by Kier (*31*). In this approach the Extended Hückel Theory is used to calculate the preferred conformation of each of several potent drugs of different structure but with a common pharmacologic activity. The drug receptor is then mapped by considering those portions of the various drugs molecules which present nearly identical patterns of like-charged atoms. Kier has mapped the receptors for acetylcholine, nicotine, serotonin, histamine, steroids, and α-adrenergic agents. Although no new drugs have been reported to result from such considerations, the method is a fascinating one and may prove successful in this sense in the future. An obvious limitation on any quantum chemical calculation is cost. The EHT calculation for a single conformation is relatively inexpensive, of the order of $10–$20; however, if a molecule has several groups which can rotate independently, computer time can become long and costly. Molecules in which the distance between the important atoms is fixed would be the most expeditious choice for a test of a predicted arrangement of atoms.

The Hansch and Kier approaches are obviously different. First, the Hansch approach can consider activity of a drug in a whole animal—*i.e.,* the equation can include terms which reflect relative penetration of the drug to the receptor. Quantum mechanical approaches in general are concerned only with the reaction of the drug with the receptor. In the multiple regression technique one treats data on the same biological test on at least six compounds whereas for the preferred conformation method one needs to know the general type of pharmacologic activity of two or three molecules of different structure. Built into the Hansch approach is a statistical test of the theory whereas none is appropriate for the Kier method. The cost of computer time is small for multiple regression analyses whereas to do EHT calculations to arrive at a preferred conformation can quickly become very costly. The Kier approach will obviously fail when the drugs in question produce an effect by a nonspecific interaction (such as for the anesthetics) rather than by engaging a specific receptor. There is no guarantee that it is the preferred conformation of a drug which interacts with the receptor. However, if the Kier approach is proved successful, it should become a powerful tool for designing compounds of more radically different structure for "leads." The Hansch technique would then be used to optimize the desirable features, decrease toxicity, etc. The most obvious limitation of any structural approach is that its success depends on a proper and reliable pharmacologic test. The appropriateness of the biological model for particular disease state will determine the ultimate clinical usefulness of any drug.

When the chemist is designing a series of drugs to be synthesized, he should plan the compounds so that the most useful series for Hansch-type structure activity analyses is prepared. Four criteria should be considered: (1) in general, only compounds for which physical parameters such as π and σ are known should be included; (2) no two compounds should be made which have essentially duplicate physical properties; (3) the series should be planned so that the various physical parameters are not highly correlated with each other; and (4) the widest possible variation in each parameter should be included. For example, in the list of aromatic substituents in Table IV, 13 groups are included (*32, 33, 34*). For variety in the π term one would want to include amino and *tert*-butyl as well as the unsubstituted compound and probably also hydroxyl and iodo. To gain enough variety in the σ term, one should also include trifluoromethyl. For a large group (minimum E_s) acetamido would be desirable. Thus from a set of 13 compounds seven have been chosen as being the most desirable to synthesize. Notice that certain compounds duplicate information from others—*e.g.*, methoxy has the same σ value as hydroxy, the same π value as H, and the same E_s as amino. Similarly, ethyl has the same σ value as *tert*-butyl, the same π value as trifluoromethyl, and an E_s value close to that of iodo. Thus, methoxy and ethyl need not be included in the sample. By careful planning the chemist

**Table IV. Representative Parameters for Typical Aromatic
(p-Substituted) Functional Groups**

	π	σ	E_s
—H	0	0	1.24
—OH	−.61	−.37	Variable
—OMe	−.04	−.27	.69
—NH$_2$	−1.63	−.66	.63
$\begin{matrix} & \text{O} \\ & \| \\ \text{—NH—CMe} \end{matrix}$	−.79	0	−2.13
—Cl	.70	.23	.27
—Br	1.02	.23	.08
—I	1.26	.18	−.16
—F	.15	.062	.78
—Me	.51	−.17	0
—Et	1.00	−.15	−.07
—tert-Bu	1.6	−.15	−1.54
—CF$_3$	1.0	.54	−1.16

can thus design a series with a large variety in each parameter and yet
not an endless list of possibilities to synthesize. Once the first set of compounds has been tested and the structure–activity relationships analyzed,
additional compounds might be necessary to test other parameters.

Summary and Conclusions

The sequence in synthetic drug development has not changed greatly
over the past 60 years since Ehrlich's monumental contribution to modern
medicine. The first step is usually the discovery of a biological phenomenon or the promulgation of a novel and often unifying biological concept
which can be translated and exploited chemically. With the stimulus thus
given and the seed newly planted, the medicinal chemist then proceeds
to shape the kinds of substances suggested by the original concept of
disease. The tools that he is likely to use will depend on the state of the
art of the allied disciplines as well as the nature of the biological discovery and the subsequent hypothesis. Being the adaptive animal that
he is, he will quickly become conversant with the biological climate into
which he has been thrust or in which he wants to become purposely
involved. In either case, he really has no choice but to become involved
if he wants to make a meaningful contribution. Medicinal chemistry has
no place in itself. It is a discipline which depends totally on biological
input because if there is no biological problem, there is no need for
medicinal chemistry. Thus, the tools that the medicinal chemist will select
for challenging and unravelling natural processes will reflect the depth
of his understanding of the biological phenomenon to which he chooses

to address himself. For instance, what is the nature of the inflammatory process? If it is an autoimmune response, it may require an immuno-suppressive agent. If it is caused by an invading pathogen, the approach may be entirely different. If it is the result of a stress-induced deficiency, replacement therapy is indicated. Often the shrewd and astute chemist will be able to outguess his biological colleague and create the tools that will lead to a better understanding of biological phenomena, such as mental illness or congestive heart failure.

The Future of the Synthetic Approach in Drug Research. One may wonder whether there are enough combinations left in organic chemistry to come up with novel drug molecules. That is like asking how much more new music can be composed because there are only a handful of basic notes, and ultimately there must be a limit to the number of musical variations that can be gleaned from them. No one, however, appears to be concerned about this eventuality and it is hard to conceive that it could ever happen. Styles in music as well as in science change drastically and quickly. The medicinal chemist must remain highly adaptable and responsive to the changing scientific and even cultural environment without following every fad blindly.

Twenty years ago the likelihood of an antianxiety, a mood-elevating, or an antifertility pill being accepted by the medical profession or the general public would have seemed remote. Today these drugs constitute almost a half billion dollar business.

To be sure, many good drugs are now available to treat diseases in a palliative fashion, and it becomes increasingly difficult to come up with superior medications. However, our technology has advanced so rapidly that new drug entities can be synthesized and screened faster and in a more sophisticated manner to produce novel therapeutic types. The bio-medical sciences are supplying clues to the possible etiology of a disease process with greater dispatch than ever thought possible.

However, there are areas of concern for the future of synthetic drug research. One comes from the discipline that represented the foundation of medicinal chemistry—namely organic chemistry. This discipline is moving steadily away from the area of synthesis toward mechanistically oriented horizons. Medicinal chemistry will have to take over and continue to refine the art of organic synthesis.

Our young graduates have become increasingly reluctant toward the "instinctive" empirical approach of molecular modification. They are much more inclined toward the rational, mathematical, and computer oriented type of research. This is fine as long as it is based on sound biochemical and pharmacologic principles and is not oblivious to the fact that there still is a living organism to be treated that is sufficiently complex to defy mathematical typing. Over-reliance on pure rationale is as dangerous as blind adherence to indiscriminate and unsophisticated molecular modification. Properly balanced, the two styles of research are eminently compatible.

Pharmacology, too, is changing from the classical to the biochemically and molecular biologically oriented approach. The medicinal chemist should familiarize himself with these new concepts and philosophies lest he become obsolete by a rapidly developing dynamic discipline.

Synthetic medicinal chemistry can remain one of the major cornerstones to drug discovery since it is the very structure of a new drug which will ultimately determine its success in human therapy. Yet the optimum structure of a novel therapeutic agent must reflect the input from many allied disciplines besides organic chemistry.

The proper orchestration of all these contributing instruments of modern science, as well as his own creativity and imagination, will in the end decide whether the medicinal chemist will continue to be a significant composer and arranger in the turbulent field of drug discovery.

Literature Cited

(1) Domagk, G., *Deut. Med. Wochschr.* (1935) **61**, 250.
(2) Fourneau, E., Trefouel, J., Nitti, F., Bovet, D., *C. R. Soc. Biol.* (1936) **122**, 652.
(3) Southworth, H., *Proc. Soc. Exptl. Biol. Med.* (1937) **36**, 58.
(4) Davenport, H. W., Wilhelmi, A. E., *Proc. Soc. Exptl. Biol. Med.* (1941) **48**, 59.
(5) Krebs, H. A., *Biochem. J.* (1948) **43**, 525.
(6) Mann, T., Keilin, D., *Nature* (1940) **146**, 164.
(7) Pitts, R. F., Alexander, R. S., *Am. J. Physiol.* (1945) **144**, 239.
(8) Schwartz, W. B., *New Engl. J. Med.* (1949) **240**, 173.
(9) Sprague, J. M., *Ann. N.Y. Acad. Sci.* (1958) **71**, 328.
(10) Novello, F. C., Bell, S. C., Abrams, E. L. A., Ziegler, C., Sprague, J. M., *J. Org. Chem.* (1960) **25**, 970.
(11) Beyer, K. H., Baer, J. E., *Progr. Drug Res.* (1960) **2**, 9.
(12) Loubatières, A., *Ann. N.Y. Acad. Sci.* (1957) **71**, 4.
(13) Goodman, L. S., Gilman, A., "The Pharmacologic Basis of Therapeutics," 3rd ed., p. 615, Macmillan, New York, 1965.
(14) Bovet, D., Staub, A., *C. R. Soc. Biol.* (1937) **124**, 547.
(15) Iversen, L. L., "The Uptake and Storage of Noradrenaline in Sympathetic Nerves," p. 217, Cambridge University Press, 1967.
(16) Biel, J. H., Nuhfer, P. A., Conway, A. C., *Ann. N.Y. Acad. Sci.* (1959) **80**, 568.
(17) Biel, J. H., Drukker, A. E., unpublished work.
(18) Wilson, I. B., Ginsberg, S., *Biochem. Biophys. Acta* (1955) **18**, 168.
(19) Hansch, C., "Annual Reports in Medicinal Chemistry, 1966," N. Cain, Ed., p. 347, Academic, New York, 1967.
(20) Hansch, C., Fujita, T., *J. Am. Chem. Soc.* (1964) **86**, 1616.
(21) Jorgenson, E. C., Reid, J. A. W., *J. Med. Chem.* (1965) **8**, 533.
(22) Fuller, R. W., Marsh, M. M., Mills, J., *J. Med. Chem.* (1968) **11**, 397.
(23) Hermann, R. B., Culp, H. W., McMahon, R. E., Marsh, M. M., *J. Med. Chem.* (1969) **12**, 749.
(24) Andrews, P. R., *J. Med. Chem.* (1969) **12**, 761.

(25) Lien, E., *J. Med. Chem.* (1970) **13,** 1189.
(26) Clayton, J. M., Purcell, W. P., *J. Med. Chem.* (1969) **12,** 1087.
(27) Purcell, W. P., Beasley, J. G., Quintana, R. P., Singer, J. A., *J. Med. Chem.* (1966) **9,** 297.
(28) Purcell, W. P., *J. Med. Chem.* (1966) **9,** 294.
(29) Martin, Y. C., *J. Med. Chem.* (1970) **13,** 145.
(30) Wohl, A., *Mol. Pharmacol.* (1970) **6,** 189.
(31) Kier, L. B., "Fundamental Concepts in Drug-Receptor Interactions," J. F. Danielli, J. F. Morgan, and D. J. Triggle, Eds., Academic, New York, 1970.
(32) Fujita, T., Iwasa, J., Hansch, C., *J. Am. Chem. Soc.* (1964) **86,** 5175.
(33) Cohen, S. G., Streitwieser, A., Taft, R., "Progress in Physical Organic Chemistry," Vol. 2, p. 334, Interscience, New York, 1964.
(34) Kutter, E., Hansch, C., *J. Med. Chem.* (1969) **12,** 647.
(35) Albert, A., "Selective Toxicity," 4th ed., p. 105, Methuen, London, 1968.
(36) Kier, L. B., Truitt, E. B., *J. Pharmacol. Exp. Therap.* (1970) **174,** 94.
(37) Snyder, S. *et al., Science* (1967) **158,** 669.

RECEIVED November 5, 1970.

Discussion

C. J. CAVALLITO

Ayerst Laboratories, 685 Third Avenue, New York, N. Y.

Changes are evolving in health products research, resulting not just from changes in science but from changes in society with which this research is inextricably bound. What kinds of changes influence the science of drug research and discovery? Major factors include the need for new drugs, the standards for acceptance of new drugs, methodology in research and development, and sources of support for research. The rational exploitation of new drug leads has become a somewhat sophisticated operation. Training of scientific personnel has undergone changes, but time does not permit discussion of this influence. Probably the least changed factor is the most important in the discovery of that which is truly novel—namely, our dependence on the individual in research. All these factors contribute to changes in the balance between opportunities and risks in discovering new drugs.

Needs for New Drugs

A review of the drug contributions of the past 35 years shows that the priorities of needs for new drugs during this period have undergone continuing changes as a result of many contributions in various fields of therapy. This is not to say that we have provided perfect drugs in such fields. Differences among individuals or in the same individual at different times alone may make it impossible to create the "perfect" drug. The availability of reasonably satisfactory products and the diminishing returns in exploiting earlier leads has reduced interest in a number of drug classes, such as antihistamines, antispasmodics, barbiturates, etc. Some drug categories—e.g., hypotensive ganglionic blocking agents and mercurial diuretics—have been superseded by more desirable classes of drugs. Since one does not create new vitamins or mineral requirements, the tremendous contributions in nutritional research of 1935–1950 are not repeatable. A similar situation exists with many hormones. More recently developed major therapeutic classes, such as psychotherapeutic agents, continue to attract considerable research effort. Important unmet needs remain in such areas as drugs for cancer, certain virus diseases, and diseases associated with aging or degenerative changes. Not surprisingly, most of the major diseases for which new drug needs now are greatest are those for which useful drugs are much more difficult to discover and develop. With our motivation to survive, there will always be the challenge to extend life expectancy. More important, I believe, will be the need for new drugs to make our present life tenures more physically and mentally acceptable.

Although we can identify drug classes in which major advances were made in the past, we do recognize that sometimes solutions are not permanently achieved. The need for new drugs may be revived in areas in which we thought satisfactory ones had been provided. For example, the development or identification of resistant or new infectious organisms can create needs for new antibiotics and chemotherapeutic agents. Antimalarial research was re-intensified for such reasons after about 20 years of dormancy.

Need as a motivation for drug research in an area also may become better recognized with the discovery of therapeutic opportunities. Meprobamate and chlorpromazine not only fulfilled certain needs but helped identify other potentials in the broad field of psychotherapeutics.

In considering the needs for new drugs from a therapeutic perspective, we have little basis for preferring nature or synthesis as a primary source. A disease resulting from an imbalance in amount or function of a physiological substance will attract initial emphasis on natural products research. The skills of the chemist now are such that programs originating as natural products investigations often quickly shift in emphasis to programs of synthesis. This results from the ability of the chemist more quickly to isolate and to elucidate the structure of a complex molecule as well as to adapt synthetic skills to its reproduction or modification. Natural products research effort has been cyclical, both qualitatively and quantitatively, particularly in the pharmaceutical industry. Antibiotic's search and research were most extensively conducted in the 1940's through mid-1950's although continued at an appreciable level in some laboratories in subsequent years. Dr. Conover's survey represents an interesting cross section of current opinions in this field. The application of *Rauwolfia* and its alkaloids in modern medical practice gave natural products research a world-wide boost in the early to mid-1950's, just on the heels of intensified interest in steroids. Dr. Conover's paper details an interesting analysis of similarities and differences in the evolution of steroid and prostaglandin research. A major difference which motivated the early widespread research in the steroid field was a clearer identification of therapeutic potentials for steroids than for prostaglandins. The discovery of anti-inflammatory properties of corticosteroids intensified research in the early 1950's; however, therapeutic endocrinological applications of steroids had served as inducements in the late 1930's and 1940's. The early prostaglandin research was conducted intensively in relatively few laboratories and with assumption of higher risks with less probability of development of a useful drug. In cancer chemotherapy, the limited successes of any product to date, natural or synthetic, dampens the ardor of natural products search. Still, there is a feeling we should persevere, not with the hope of finding *the* drug, but yet another drug, even if it be only a modest contribution in this frustrating field of research.

Regulatory Standards

The standards for acceptance of new drugs became more demanding during the early 1960's. The Food and Drug Administration (FDA), by its requirements for proof of efficacy before a new drug is marketed, has been a principal factor in pressing for new performance guidelines. The pharmaceutical industry in the 1950's was carried away with new product introductions, particularly combination products, some of questionable advantage. In the 1960's we witnessed a regulatory over-reaction to this, which is continuing into the 1970's. Those of us in research certainly find more personally rewarding the opportunity to generate truly useful new drugs, but we are concerned lest well-intentioned statutes or regulations are interpreted and implemented in a manner incompatible with that which is possible in the laboratory or in clinical practice. This will be of growing concern in the future.

Methodology in Research and Development

The advances in research methodology and instrumentation of the past 25 years not only have made some aspects of drug research much more efficient but have permitted the resolution of problems virtually unsolvable a few years ago. Separation, isolation, and analysis have become possible for quantities and kinds of compounds previously unapproachable. The chemist engaged in synthesis has had available an increasingly greater variety of intermediates, chemical methodology, equipment, and techniques to expand his horizons. From a biological perspective, monitoring instrumentation in pharmacology has improved, and increasingly sophisticated biochemical equipment and techniques are utilized in both micro- and macrobiology. Among natural products, advances in the vitamin and hormone fields during the 1930's and 1940's were assisted materially by the availability of bioassays for these substances. Today we could isolate and determine the structure of the vitamins far more quickly than was possible in the 1930's and 1940's; however, their functional identification still depends on appropriate biological or biochemical test models.

An important factor which can influence relative interest in natural sources *vs.* synthetics as test objects for biological screening is the effort required to prepare a natural product for testing. *In vitro* antibacterial tests can be carried out inexpensively with crude extracts containing a virtual microcosm of chemical components. Screening for properties which demand animal test systems, however, generally requires more elaborate pretreatment of a natural product with separation or concentration of components to be tested.

A continuing problem in methodology is that of devising more reliable laboratory models to detect chemical substances potentially useful in treating some condition in man. In pre-technological societies, by plan or accident, man usually was the direct test species which led to discovery of useful or poisonous natural products. Laboratory model systems have served us well in some instances, inadequately in others. *In vitro* screening in the 1940's developed into a major activity with the search for new antibiotics. Since the mid-1950's interest in screening large numbers of compounds for potential psychotherapeutic properties led to some interesting exercises. We have slugged the mouse with large doses of compounds and watched him run, jump, stagger, convulse, collapse, sleep, or die while his fur, tail, ears, eyes, and bowels are read for signs in a fashion reminiscent of the seers of old who read the future from the entrails of animals. Yet, for the truly unusual discovery or lead, so often we have continued to depend on man himself to display the unexpected during the course of assessing the expected. We then go back to trying to relate the new observation in man to some response in the animal. The net result is that with our laboratory screening methodology, we increase our skills in detecting new drugs with properties similar to those we already have. Considerations of methodology also bring us to differences of opinion as to the relative value of general screening of many compounds, screening of selected compounds for a limited number of activities, mission-oriented synthesis, and biochemical mechanistic rational design in drug research. As a compromise, most industry laboratories engage to some extent in each activity.

In evaluating drugs in man, there also have been improvements in methodology, particularly in the design of better controlled experiments and the use of statistical techniques to interpret the data. This has been more significant in disease conditions in which subjective factors may obscure the interpretation of results. However, in some major diseases, as for example atherosclerosis, osteoporosis, and connective tissue degenerations, the absence of reliable qualitative measures for early identification of the disease state and quantitative measures for comparing improvements or deteriorations have become a much more serious limitation than they were 10 years ago. The requirement for proof of efficacy of a new drug in man in certain disease conditions becomes almost hopeless if one attempts, for example, to demand a similar degree of confidence in measuring improvement in treating osteoporosis vs. treating pneumonia. For almost a decade, the FDA has been demanding evidence of drug efficacy, without exercising a concomitant diligence in helping to develop realistic guidelines for acceptable evidence.

The importance of man as a test medium for discovering the unexpected is well documented. Since 1962 the transition from laboratory to man has become increasingly complicated, and with proportionately fewer new investigational drugs being evaluated in man, chance alone will permit fewer opportunities to discover the unexpected.

Sources of Support for Research

The amount and distribution of support for health research have changed tremendously in the last 20 years, and such shifts cannot help but influence the processes of new drug discovery. The pharmaceutical industry in the United States increased its research dollar expenditures approximately 12-fold between 1950 and 1970. Between 1947 and 1967, the federal government increased its medical research expenditure some 50-fold through both intramural and extramural programs. Increasing costs of doing research during this period, of course, resulted in less than a proportionate increase in research effort. In the pharmaceutical industry, the growth of the 1950's encouraged and sustained rapidly increased research effort; in the 1960's the distribution of effort by discipline changed appreciably with the medicinal chemist finding himself a less dominant factor in the over-all research and development process. In academia, the infusion of federal funds in the 1950's to mid-1960's led to some ways of life that have been undergoing agonizing reappraisals during the past three years. The end results of this are not yet clear. We can be fairly certain, however, that whether it be in industry or academia, health-related research will need to be responsive to changing criteria for support.

It has become fashionable, not only among some scientists, but even security analysts and many regulatory people, to attribute the decline of new drug introductions in the 1960's to an alleged depletion of our store of basic knowledge from which new drugs are discovered. How strange that knowledge was "used up" faster by industry in increasing research expenditures 12-fold in the period that the federal health research budget rose some 50-fold. Arguments presented before Congress during budget hearings led one to expect that these federal expenditures would support the generation of new basic knowledge which could lead to new agents for treating disease. Certainly important new knowledge was generated in this period. I do not believe that the major drug discoveries of the 1940's and 1950's were any more derived from a surplus of basic knowledge than any depletion of such knowledge by the 1960's was responsible for the reduction in new drug output in that decade. Depletion of basic knowledge appears to be a simplistic explanation for a far more complex phenomenon. This brings us to some comments on the rational approach to drug research and discovery.

The Rational Approach

We have heard, and will continue to hear, considerable discussion about how increasingly rational drug research and discovery will be in the future. In fact, Dr. Biel makes us appear to have been quite rational for some time. Expressions such as "rational approaches" and "store of basic knowledge" probably have little definitive meaning out of context. Basic research and rational approaches are not precisely definable expressions and mean different things to different people. The distinction between "basic" and "applied" research may sometimes be as much a reflection of the limitations in imagination and experience of the individual scientist as in his research mission. The truly novel concept usually occurs to the individual, not to a committee or a team, and a great deal of individuality of style remains in the conception and conduct of research. Obviously, there is no one way in which to make new drug discoveries. An expression which of itself is neither good nor bad is "molecular modification." This has been referred to more snidely as "molecular manipulation" and has been looked upon as some sort of second-rate research indulged in by the pharmaceutical industry. Molecular modification as an approach to drug development or new drug discovery has been staunchly defended by most medicinal chemists, with the recognition that individuals vary considerably in level of creativity expressed in its exercise. In judging creativity by hindsight, novelty must be assessed in the context of the situation at the time of a discovery. The most unobvious can become generally self-evident soon after its discovery.

In treating specifically with medicinal chemists, one might identify individual creative or productive types in some such manner:

The Intuitive Discoverer. This is the individual who designs or discovers molecules with unusual or interesting biomedical properties through some conceptual hypothesis, projected from minimal available data (which hypothesis may or may not be valid in retrospect).

The Deductive Discoverer. This individual designs or discovers molecules with unusual or interesting biomedical properties by developing a sequentially logical rationale, founded on a solid base of data. In some aspects, he is similar to the intuitive discoverer, except that the latter requires less information from which to project his concepts.

The Analytical Rationalizer. This individual usually does not create new molecules or discover drugs but explains why or how those discovered by others work.

The Imitator. The imitator looks to others for the discovery of new leads, then quickly enters the field with some structural modifications, hoping to carve out a piece of patentable novelty before the field is saturated.

The Plodder. This is the chemist who turns. out large numbers of modifications of a prototype molecule and hopes the biologist will make a discovery for him. He may feel secure with a particular preparative reaction, or intermediates may be readily available.

Before judging too hastily the relative merits of the contributions of individuals in the classification, it should be recognized that degree of novelty of a discovery and its utility or usefulness do not necessarily go hand in hand. The imitator or plodder may make useful, practical, competitive contributions. The intuitive or deductive discoverer may add to so-called "basic knowledge" without necessarily creating a useful product and thus lay the foundation for the work of others. The analytical individual may not make a drug discovery directly, but he may provide a better interpretative framework for organizing and understanding existing information. Most individuals are a mixture in different proportions of these stylized types. My point is, to each his own style, depending on his training, experience, interests, imagination, and motivations—yet each can add to the drug discovery processes. Among biologists, we especially cherish those individuals who appreciate the significance of an observation, particularly the unexpected, in terms of potential application in an area of need.

The discovery process for a new drug may be considered broadly in terms of two kinds of research; that in which one is exploring for a new lead, and research directed to the exploitation of leads. In exploring for leads by selecting or designing new compounds for evaluation, the intuitive and deductive approaches are still largely relied on. In contrast, exploration for leads by routine indiscriminate screening of many preparations is more mechanical. If the availability of many compounds assured success, the large chemical companies would have had a different record of performance in entry into the pharmaceutical industry. The medicinal chemist must be competent in organic chemistry to execute his ideas, but he can benefit from some biological background if he is to increase his efficiency in designing potential drugs. In drug discovery, we are much more adept at rationally exploiting a lead than in exploring for one. This is semantically logical since a rational approach to a discovery implies a more extended systematic sequence of operations. However, by the time we have systematically achieved a goal, it no longer appears to have the novelty implied in the observation which is derived from more exploratory, less predictable approaches. When we refer to rational approaches in drug design, however, these are not always predominantly biochemical in nature. For the discovery of new leads, we have depended strongly on the biologist and medical scientist; the exploitation of leads has been the principal theater of operation of the organic medicinal chemist. The value of the clinical investigator in discovering a lead should not be underestimated. Leads to new potential applications of a drug prototype frequently have been derived from man when a drug designed for one purpose demonstrated unexpected properties. Having observed these in man, we then go back to the laboratory and attempt to design animal model systems that will correlate with the properties observed in man. In time we tend to forget that some compound was not discovered through a laboratory animal test, but rather the animal tests evolved following discovery of the properties of the compound in man. The value placed on some animal test systems in retrospect is reminiscent of the confidence with which biochemical principles and sophisticated physical parameters now appear to be considered as guides to new drug discoveries. In evaluating the usefulness of approaches to drug research, it is important to distinguish between that which is of value in retrospectively rationalizing and that which truly aids prediction. Systems are most valuable which permit us to reach farthest into the unknown, with reasonable accuracy, from the most limited base of existing knowledge. This is extremely difficult to quantify in exploring for a research lead since virtually by definition, degree of novelty is gauged by level of unpredictability.

Dr. Kupchan alluded to major contributions of drugs from plants since 1800. Many of these useful drugs served as prototypes for synthetic congeners; however, these leads were exploited during a period in which their actions could be described partly by gross pharmacological effects but not in terms of events at the molecular level. In reference to his newer research, there is evidenced the interest of the medicinal chemist in seeking mechanistic common denominators at the molecular level as a guide for exploiting a lead. Dr. Kupchan states, "Several observations have focused attention on the importance of the conjugated α-methylene lactone function for the biological activity of . . . lactones. Furthermore, the results support the view that the α-methylene lactones may exert their effects on cells by interacting with sulfhydryl enzymes that regulate growth." With some nostalgia, I recall relating a similar impression in a review in Volume I of "Medicinal Chemistry" about 20 years ago in which some α-methylene lactones from plants discovered in the 1940's were held out to be an attractive area of research as sulfhydryl inhibiting antibiotics. Although we have known something about the reactions of these lactone types at the molecular level for over 25 years, the field has, for other reasons (such as toxicity) progressed more slowly in leading to useful new drugs than have some natural product prototypes for which we know almost nothing of interactions at the molecular level. Thus, although information of a molecular reaction mechanism may be useful in exploiting a drug lead, it is not a guarantee of success.

With reference to the value of enzymological mechanistic concepts in leading to new drug discoveries, a number of examples are cited by the authors. I recall the tremendous interest in the latter 1950's in monoamine oxidase (MAO) inhibition as a route to drug design. Inhibition of MAO was observed among tuberculostatic, antidepressant, and antihypertensive drugs. After a time, we began to suspect that there might be little relationship between the useful properties we were seeking and potency as MAO inhibitors. Today we are more apt to test interesting drug leads against MAO with the hope that the agent is *not* an inhibitor. There appears to be considerable doubt that α-methyl DOPA acts as an antihypertensive agent by inhibition of DOPA decarboxylase. There are a number of illustrations of drugs with biochemical properties which are not necessarily biochemical causes of the desired effect. Care must be used in relating enzymological mechanisms to a phenomenon before enough appropriate molecular modifications of the drugs are available for correlation. This also is an area in which one must guard against supporting rather than testing a hypothesis.

As we compare the papers which discuss the sources of new drugs— past, present, and future with those on the significance of rational drug design we are presented with some accomplishments of the past in contrast to challenging approaches of the future. We could smugly point to the former group with pride of proved accomplishment or equally smugly to the latter as guiding the way to a more sophisticated, less bumbling approach to future discovery. For those who subscribe strongly to approaches of the past, we should caution that those procedures most widely followed usually provide us with the greater number of discoveries but not necessarily in proportion to effort expended either in the past or future. For those who embrace allegedly more sophisticated physical chemical and mechanistic approaches to drug design, let us distinguish between those exercises that are intellectually stimulating in helping clarify relationships retrospectively and those which are more helpful in leading to useful new drugs. Here too, in our comparison of past, present, and future, distinction should be made between procedures that permit a more efficient exploitation of a lead *vs.* discovery of a lead. We are becoming increasingly effective in exploiting leads and in using teams to do this. In the discovery of a lead, we depend more on the individual. The truly innovative person, by his very nature, is more difficult to describe in terms of a neat, predictable mode of operation. He is apt to be a keen observer who can envision the possible relationship between some phenomenon and an unsolved problem or need, and he uses his knowledge without being too inhibited by it in exploratory research.

Whether by past, present, or future approaches, molecular design or selection in drug discovery usually involves the use of hypotheses in planning the research. A hypothesis can be a useful tool or a straight jacket, depending on how we use it. Working hypotheses can help us to design a research plan. Hypotheses obviously vary in initial basis of data support, but the major danger is that individuals become emotionally attached to them. More effort may be expended in supporting hypotheses than in testing them. Support may take the form of selective use of data from the literature, and the preparation of more compounds, or conduct of additional experiments, likely to support the hypothesis. It may be more productive and less illusory to try to disprove the hypothesis, and if it survives such efforts, it gains more in value as a basis for future experimental design.

The planning of a productive program in new drug research involves the consideration of opportunity and risk factors. This involves a continually changing set of parameters. The fulfillment of a therapeutic need results in some reduction of opportunity for new drugs in that field with competitive standards becoming more difficult to achieve. The resolution of some disease conditions can increase the need for attention, and thus the opportunities, in other directions. For example, cardiovascular diseases gain in relative importance as infectious diseases are better controlled. We hear on occasion that the easier problems have been solved; however, advances in methodology permit us to solve complex problems more readily. It costs a great deal more in time and money to develop a new drug, but it is also subject to less rapid competitive displacement or obsolescence. On the whole, however, resource risk factors appear to have been growing faster than new drug development opportunities during the past decade and probably will continue to do so. The medicinal chemist today must be far more astute in assessing risks and opportunities than ever before. He usually is at the origin of a protracted chain of events which may consume from 5 to 10 years and as many millions of dollars from the time he prepares a compound of possible interest to its introduction in a competitive marketplace. Many disciplines, potentials for failure, and frustrations beyond his control lie between his efforts and the consummation of his aspirations.

As we read the contributions in this volume, let us search for suggestions as to how we can improve the balance between opportunity and risk in drug research in an ever changing scene. New drug discovery requires a considerable element of luck. What we are seeking are ways of improving our odds of being lucky in a game in which the stakes are high. We must be alert constantly to better ways of playing the drug discovery game, but we should not fall victims to illusions of how we wish drugs could be discovered rather than how they are more apt to come about. A valuable sobering guide would be a collection of accurate, unglamorized accounts of the actual sequence of events unrationalized by hindsight that led to novel drug discoveries. From such expositions selected from the past 35 years, we might better assess the impact of changing influences in drug discovery and the extent to which we might expect changes in the next 10 to 15 years.

RECEIVED November 5, 1970.

Physicochemical Approaches to Drug Design

WILLIAM P. PURCELL and JOHN M. CLAYTON

Department of Molecular and Quantum Biology, College of Pharmacy,
University of Tennessee Medical Units, Memphis, Tenn. 38103

*One of the most potentially successful approaches to drug
design is the attempt to place correlations between changes
in molecular structure with changes in biological activity on
a quantitative and predictive level. While qualitative efforts
have been made in this area by chemists and pharmacologists for over 100 years, more recent progress illustrates the
potential of regression analyses, molecular orbital calculations, and parameterization using various physicochemical
measurements. The mathematical and linear free-energy related models along with their modifications and applications
are reviewed. It is concluded that quantitative structure-
activity studies hold some promise for the future in designing
therapeutic agents without exhaustive synthetic work and
pharmacological screening.*

For over 100 years chemists and pharmacologists have been intrigued
by observed changes in biological effects of chemical congeners paralleling somewhat minor alterations in molecular structure. Following
many successes and failures since the initial work, this interest continues
to increase among medicinal chemists as the level of sophistication of the
methods for studying and "isolating" these substituent effects in drug
design improves. Of ultimate interest is the utilization of these techniques
to achieve a rational, custom design of therapeutic agents along with the
elucidation of activity mechanisms at the submolecular level (1).

It is necessary to point out initially that in a report of this type it
would be virtually impossible to include every work that has been significant to the development of the methods presented here. While the
authors have attempted to give a representative sample of these contributions, they have not attempted an exhaustive review. In view of the
numerous literature examples of the application of physicochemical meth-

ods to drug design, the interested reader is referred to more thorough treatments of the methodology (*1–3*) and reviews of the recent literature (*4–8*).

In the late 1860's Crum-Brown and Fraser demonstrated that gradual alterations in molecular structure of certain drugs coincided with changes in their elicited biological responses (*9*). These observations led to the postulate that the activity of a drug (ϕ) was a function of its structural features (C) (Equation 1).

$$\phi = f(C) \tag{1}$$

Further, experimental work on narcotic agents in 1893 led Richet to postulate that the degree of activity of the compounds was inversely related to their water solubilities (*10*). Meyer and Overton expanded this work just at the turn of the twentieth century to show that the narcotic activities of certain congeners paralleled their oil/water partitioning properties (*11–15*). Of course, this parameter was designed to simulate the *in vivo* condition of the drug's partitioning between an aqueous biophase and a lipophilic site of action. In 1907, Fühner quantitatively approximated the biological responses of a homologous series of narcotics (*16, 17*). He demonstrated that the decrease in equiresponse concentrations of these compounds followed a geometric progression [1, 1/3, $(1/3)^2$, $(1/3)^3$, etc.] as the number of carbon atoms increased in the series.

In further investigations of the relationship between other physicochemical properties of molecules and their biological responses, Traube in 1904 observed a correlation between surface tension and narcotic action (*18*). These data led Warburg to postulate a mechanism of narcotic action for these agents in 1921 (*19*). Similarly, in 1917 Moore noted that the boiling points of a series of insecticide fumigants paralleled their toxicities (*20, 21*).

An important observation in structure–activity studies was made by Ferguson in 1939 when he demonstrated an interrelationship among much of the earlier work (*22*). Equation 2 was postulated to describe the biological responses of several congeneric series, where C_i is the concen-

$$C_i = kA^m_i \tag{2}$$

tration of congener i necessary to elicit a defined response, A_i is a physicochemical or descriptive parameter for the compound (*e.g.*, partition coefficient or number of carbon atoms in a side chain), and k and m are constants for the series. Since C_i is usually less than 1, the negative logarithm of Equation 2 leads to Equation 3, which is more useful in quantitative structure–activity studies and is a basis for similar work today (*23, 24, 25*).

$$\log \frac{1}{C_i} = - \log k - m \log A_i \tag{3}$$

Further applications of physicochemical parameters to biological activities were made by McGowan (*26, 27, 28*). He has successfully correlated the biological activities of selected series of molecules with their molecular volumes or parachors.

Further major contributions to, development of, and applications of quantitative structure–activity correlations began in 1956 with the work of Bruice and co-workers (*29*). Their empirical, mathematical method was applied to the correlation of thyroxine-like activities of a series of congeners with the sum of constants assigned to different substituents of the molecules. Using Equation 4 they obtained excellent correlations

$$\log \% \text{ thyroxine-like activity} = k\Sigma f + c \tag{4}$$

between calculated and observed activities. In Equation 4, $\Sigma f = (f_X + f_{X'} + f_{OR'})$ where f_X, $f_{X'}$, and $f_{OR'}$ are entirely empirical and were selected similar to the method of Hammett for the evaluation of sigma constants. Subscripts X, X', and OR' represent substituent positions of the molecular structures of interest (*29*).

Free and Wilson gave a more general description of this mathematical (empirical) model in 1964 (*30*). According to their method, the defined biological response (BR) of a congener in a homologous series is equal to the sum of the substituent group contributions to the activity plus that of the parent structure (μ), Equation 5. For example, Purcell has used

$$BR = \Sigma(\text{group contributions}) + \mu \tag{5}$$

this method in studying the anticholinesterase potencies of a homologous series of 3-carbamoylpiperidines (I) (*31*). If a methyl group were sub-

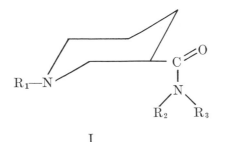

I

stituted at position R_1 and ethyl groups were substituted at positions R_2 and R_3, Equation 5 would become Equation 6, where $[CH_3]_{R_1}$ is the

$$BR = [CH_3]_{R_1} + [C_2H_5]_{R_2} + [C_2H_5]_{R_3} + \mu \tag{6}$$

activity contribution of a methyl group substituted at position R_1, $[C_2H_5]_{R_2}$ represents the activity contributed by an ethyl group substituted at position R_2, and $[C_2H_5]_{R_3}$ stands for the ethyl group at R_3 (*31*).

In view of the assumed equivalency of R_2 and R_3, the linear equation can be simplified by reducing the number of unknowns, and Equation 6 becomes Equation 7. Accordingly, an equation is generated for each compound.

$$BR = [CH_3]_{R_1} + 2[C_2H_5]_{R_2} + \mu \qquad (7)$$

with a measured biological response. In addition, restrictions (symmetry equations) are placed on each nonequivalent substituent position. That is, the summation of the group contributions at each nonequivalent position must equal zero over the entire set of equations (*30*). Thus, for this example, there would be two symmetry equations in addition to the other equations. The simultaneous equations are then solved independently by the method of least squares. Solution of the equations yields the calculated activity contribution of each substituent group as well as that of the parent structure. For comparison with the observed biological activities, the calculated total activity of each molecule can be obtained by summation of these group contributions and μ (*30*). The main purpose of such a treatment is to rank the biological activities of the substituent groups while noting possible structure–activity relationships and to predict the compounds of the series not tested, and possibly not synthesized, which would have the greatest potential for further investigation (*32*).

For a meaningful application of this method, the biological data should meet three basic prerequisites: (1) molecules in the series should be closely similar to increase the probability of their having the same mechanism of action, (2) biological activity data selected should be accurate, quantitative, and measured under uniform conditions for the series, and (3) the group contributions must be intrinsically additive for the chosen activity parameters (*32*). It is also desirable to have a high number of degrees of freedom since the greater the ratio of the number of observations to the number of unknowns, the more reliable are the results (*32*). Recently, the problem of ill-conditioning has been noted when this method is applied to certain series of data (*33*). Explicit conditions for applying the method as well as the statistical interpretation of the results were also defined.

The major limitation of the method lies in the fact that the activity contributions of the substituents must be additive. To date, most literature examples of applications of this method unfortunately have been made by laboratories different from the one which generated the data.

A much more desirable situation exists when data generation and analysis are made by the same laboratory for only then are the nature, limitations, and quantitative reliability of the data fully realized and appreciated.

At about the time of Free and Wilson's work, Kopecky and co-workers introduced a similar mathematical structure–activity model (*34, 35*). They tested four equations (Equations 8–11) for the expression of the quantitative difference between the log LD_{50} values of *p*- (*34*) and *m*- (*35*) disubstituted benzenes and benzene.

$$BA = a_x + a_y \tag{8}$$

$$BA = b_x b_y \tag{9}$$

$$BA = c_x + c_y - d_x d_y \tag{10}$$

$$BA = c_x + c_y + d_x d_y \tag{11}$$

In Equations 8–11 *a*, *b*, *c*, and *d* represent the substituent contribution to the total activity of the compounds while the subscripts *x* and *y* denote the substituent positions on the parent molecule. Neither the additive model (noticeably similar to the Free-Wilson model) (Equation 8), the multiplicative model (Equation 9), nor the combined model (Equation 10) described the biological activity significantly. The combined expression (Equation 11), however, gave a statistically significant correlation between substituent activity and biological response for both the *m*- (*35*) and *p*- (*34*) disubstituted series.

At the time that the basic formulation and testing of the mathematical models of quantitative structure–activity correlations were being made, another type of approach, the linear free-energy related model, was introduced (*2*). Using the basic Hammett equation (*22, 36*) for the chemical reactions of benzoic acid derivatives (Equation 12), several investigators attempted quantitative correlations between physicochemical properties

$$\log (k_X/k_H) = \rho \sigma \tag{12}$$

and biological response (*1, 37*). In Equation 12, k_X and k_H are the equilibrium constants for reactions of substituted and unsubstituted compounds, respectively, σ is a constant which depends entirely on the nature and position of the substituent, and ρ is a constant which depends on the type and conditions of reaction as well as the nature of the compound (*22*). Rewritten as Equation 13, the Hammett equation clearly illustrates

$$\log k_X = \rho \sigma + \log k_H \tag{13}$$

the linear relationship between the substituent constant σ and the logarithm of the reactivity of the compound (k_X) (*1, 38*). Since the logarithm of an equilibrium constant is proportional to the change in Gibbs free energy (Equation 14) (39), Equation 13 and others like it are "free-energy related" (38). In Equation 14, R is the ideal gas constant, $\Delta F°$ is

$$\Delta F° = - RT \ln k \qquad (14)$$

the Gibbs free energy change, T is absolute temperature, and k is the equilibrium constant for the reaction. Applications of this Hammett linear free-energy related equation to several biological systems by various investigators, however, yielded only limited success from about 1952 to 1966 (37, 40–47). Such applications led Hansen to propose a "biological" Hammett equation with a restrictive set of conditions for application (48). Even with these restrictions, however, it has met with only limited success.

The use of the Hammett equation was extended by Zahradník and co-workers to relate other physicochemical parameters of homologous series of compounds to their biological activities (Equation 15) (49). In Equation 15, τ_i is the molar concentration of the ith congener of an

$$\log (\tau_i/\tau_{et}) = \alpha\beta \qquad (15)$$

aliphatic homologous series necessary to elicit a defined biological response, τ_{et} is the molar concentration of the ethyl derivative of the series required to produce a similar response, α is a constant which depends upon the nature of the series of compounds and the biological system, and β is a physicochemical parameter which depends upon the substituent. Various types of β have been used, including the Hammett and Taft constants, on several homologous series in various biological systems (49–52). Again the use of a single parameter, however, to define a biological response has given correlations of limited significance.

Recognizing the physicochemical nature of biological reactions and realizing the importance of partitioning in a drug's reaching its site of action (53, 54), Hansch and co-workers expanded the linear free-energy related expression in 1964 to include additional physicochemical parameters (55, 56, 57). Following the approach of Taft (58) in the linear combination of two constants, they derived a new expression (Equation 16) for the correlation of biological activity with molecular structure in

$$\log (1/C) = k_1\pi + \rho\sigma + k_2 \qquad (16)$$

what is called the "ρ-σ-π equation" (55). C represents the molar concentration of a congener necessary to elicit a defined biological response, π is the substituent partitioning parameter defined as the difference between the logarithms of the octanol/water partition coefficients of the substituted and unsubstituted parent compound in the series (59), σ is the Hammett substituent constant, and k_1, ρ, and k_2 are constants generated by regression analysis of the series. Although all the terms are free-energy related and approximate true thermodynamic constants, the equation is termed "extrathermodynamic" since these parameters are used in systems other than those similar to the systems in which they were determined (55, 60).

After meeting with much success in correlating the structure–response data in a wide variety of systems (7, 61), this basic equation was modified by adding or substituting a variety of parameters in attempts to describe better the activities of numerous compounds. One of the foremost modifications of this basic equation has been the postulate that the biological response to a drug is parabolically and not linearly related to its partitioning properties resulting in the inclusion of a π^2 term (56, 57, 62). Although it may seem that the parameters in Equation 16 are somewhat arbitrary and highly empirical, it can be shown that these variables can be derived from first principles. Justification for them may be apparent when one considers the random walk process by which a drug reaches its site of action. Since the molecule must cross a series of lipoidal membranes or barriers, the elicited response depends more on its concentration at the receptor site than on the quantity of drug administered (56). Therefore, the rate of biological response may be given by:

$$d(\text{response})/dt = ACk_X \qquad (17)$$

where A is the probability of a molecule's reaching its receptor site, C is the concentration of drug administered, and k_X is the equilibrium or rate constant involved at the active site. AC would then represent the effective intracellular concentration of drug. To apply this equation practically, it is necessary to determine experimentally the values of A and k_X (56). It was for this approximate evaluation of A that the π term was derived while k_X was approximated by the Hammett σ parameter (22). If one assumes an optimum π value of π_o for a maximum elicited response and assumes the biological response follows a normal Gaussian distribution with respect to π while other factors are held constant, Equation 18 in which a and b are constants is obtained (56).

$$A = f(\pi) = a \exp\left[-(\pi - \pi_o)^2/b\right] \qquad (18)$$

Expansion of Equation 18 yields Equation 19. Assuming that π_o is con-

$$A = a \exp\left[(-\pi^2 + 2\pi\pi_o - \pi_o^2)/b\right] \qquad (19)$$

stant for a particular series of congeners in the given biological system, one obtains Equation 20, where c and d are constants replacing the terms

$$A = a \exp \left[(- \pi^2 + c\pi + d)/b \right] \tag{20}$$

in π_0. Substituting Equation 20 into Equation 17 yields Equation 21, where the rate of biological response is replaced by a constant, k', since

$$k' = a \exp \left[(- \pi^2 + c\pi + d)/b \right] C k_X \tag{21}$$

one is interested in the response level during a specific time interval rather than its rate. Taking the logarithm of Equation 21 and rearranging the terms gives Equation 22, in which the constants from Equation 21 have

$$\log (1/C) = - k\pi^2 + k_1\pi + k_2 + \log k_X \tag{22}$$

been combined to yield simplified constants, k, k_1, and k_2. Substitution of Equation 12 for $\log k_X$ and incorporating $-\log k_H$, constant for a homologous series, into constant k_2 results in the widely used Hansch equation (Equation 23) (56).

$$\log (1/C) = - k\pi^2 + k_1\pi + \varrho\sigma + k_2 \tag{23}$$

Application of this equation to series of biological data involves the summation of the physicochemical parameters for all of the substituents along with the generation of an equation of the form of Equation 24 for each observation. For example, Hansch and Deutsch have applied

$$\log (1/C) = k\Sigma\pi^2 + k_1\Sigma\pi + \varrho\Sigma\sigma + k_2 \tag{24}$$

this method to study the structure–activity correlations of 2,6-dialkoxy-phenylpenicillins (II) in the presence of serum (63).

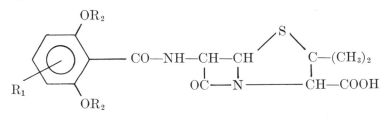

II

When a methyl group is substituted at R_1 with hydrogens at equivalent positions R_2, the resulting ϱ-σ-π equation is Equation 25. Simultaneous

$$\log (1/C) = - k(\pi^2_{CH_3} + 2\pi^2_{H}) + k_1(\pi_{CH_3} + 2\pi_{H}) +$$
$$\varrho(\sigma_{CH_3} + 2\sigma_{H}) + k_2 \tag{25}$$

solution of the equations generated for each of the eight members of this series gives Equation 26. Since the correlation coefficient, r, is a measure

$$\log (1/C) = 0.01\pi^2 - 0.316\pi + 1.76\sigma + 1.853 \quad r = 0.930 \quad (26)$$

of the goodness of fit between the calculated and observed data, the equation appears to describe adequately the biological response parameters (63).

The real value of this extrathermodynamic approach to drug design lies in its flexibility to modification by incorporating or deleting a variety of physicochemical parameters. For example, it may be used to elucidate the mechanism of drug action at the submolecular level by determination of the relative importance of each parameter in describing the biological response. In the above example, Hansch and Deutsch used modifications of Equation 24 in attempts to isolate substituent effects (Equations 27 and 28) (63). Analysis of the data using the π parameter alone (Equation

$$\log (1/C) = k_1\pi + k_2 \tag{27}$$

$$\log (1/C) = k_1\pi + k_2\sigma + k_3 \tag{28}$$

27) yielded $r = 0.823$ while inclusion of σ with π (Equation 28) gave $r = 0.929$. Comparison of the correlation coefficients of Equations 26 and 28 indicates that the π^2 term does not make a significant contribution to the biological response (63). Extension of this idea to another biological system has shown that the electronic parameter σ made a significant contribution to the activity in that particular system (64). This illustrates the problem involved in the proper selection of parameter combinations to describe adequately biological response in different systems.

Another potential use of this linear free-energy related method in custom tailoring a drug is parameter optimization. Once a particular series of data has been analyzed, one may evaluate π_0 for the series and make this the starting point in suggesting molecules for further synthesis and testing. Use of this approach also might indicate that a different series of compounds should be considered if optimum parameters have already been achieved in the compounds tested (1).

As was true in the mathematical approach, one of the foremost limitations of this method is its dependence on accurate, quantitative biological data. In addition, the quantitative nature of the linear free-energy related model is limited by the accuracy of the experimental physicochemical parameters as well as their applicability in systems somewhat distant to those in which they were determined. Although the plot of Hammett σ values gives a distinct break in linear relationship paralleling a sudden change in mechanism of action (38, 65), such a change in biological mechanism of action may not be readily detected in the Hansch analysis. Also, at the present time, there is no apparent means to determine whether an administered drug or some metabolite of this drug is responsible for an elicited response from congener to congener in this approach. Despite these limitations, however, this method does offer a basis or starting point for increasing the level of sophistication and accuracy to describe more adequately the complexity of events surrounding drug response.

In addition to these attempts at quantitative structure–activity model building, a theoretical approach, quantum chemistry, has been used to study chemical compounds of biological interest (1, 3, 66). In this connection, one should mention the major contributions of the Pullmans in applying quantum chemistry to biology since 1950 (67–71). Their work on the possible mechanism of chemical carcinogenesis in terms of quantum mechanical properties as well as calculations on the nucleic acid constituents has provided much of the foundation for the increasing interest in quantum biology. At a somewhat more fundamental level, Löwdin has also been a pioneer in the application of quantum mechanics to problems of biological interest (72). His theoretical calculations of the properties of the nucleic acid base pairs has led to a proposed mechanism of DNA replication.

In 1965 Neely published an example of the utility of molecular orbital theory in correlation studies (73). This study illustrated the use of quantum chemical calculations as an aid in correlating molecular structure of selected organophosphates and carbamates with their cholinesterase inhibitory potencies. Kier has been another pioneer in utilizing quantum mechanics to postulate the nature of biological receptors (74–80). From several types of calculations he has predicted the preferred conformations of isolated molecules of biological interest and related their lowest energy conformations to the nature of their receptors (80).

More recently numerous investigators have made wide use of these basic methods in the physicochemical approach to drug design. Using the mathematical model of Free and Wilson (30), Beasley and Purcell have given the first example of the successful prediction of the activity of a compound before its synthesis (81). In 1965 Purcell reported the predicted butyrylcholinesterase inhibitory potency of 1-decyl-3-(N-ethyl-N-methylcarbamoyl)piperidine hydrobromide, (I, $R_1 = C_{10}H_{21}$, $R_2 = C_2H_5$, $R_3 = CH_3$) (31). Three years later this compound was synthesized and evaluated biochemically. The observed and predicted response values agreed within experimental error (81). Ban and Fujita have also applied this method to the norepinephrine uptake inhibition of selected sympathomimetic amines (82). Again, excellent correlations were obtained between calculated and experimental response values.

More recent efforts have been concerned with attempts to correlate structure with activity, utilizing minor modifications of the linear free-energy related models (4, 5, 6, 8, 83). Although the basic transport and electronic parameters are usually retained, several parameters other than π and σ have been studied. Hansch and co-workers obtained excellent correlations in a wide variety of studies using log P instead of the substituent π parameter where P is defined as the partition coefficient of the compound (*84, 85*). The *in vitro* partitioning system of interest for the *in vivo* simulation continues to be that of octanol and water (*86*). Although other partitioning systems were studied [such as oleyl alcohol/ water (*87*)], very little improvement, if any, has been shown in the correlations using other partitioning systems (*86*). Others have obtained excellent structure–activity correlations by approximating the transport phenomenon with the chromatographic parameter R_m (*88–93*).

More extensive parameter variations have been reported in the approximation of electronic substituent parameters. In addition to the widely used σ value, numerous workers have applied the Taft σ^* parameter (*58, 60*) to aliphatic systems with varying degrees of success (*2, 4, 8, 94, 95*). McFarland has suggested the use of group dipole moments (μ) and electronic polarizability parameters (α) in addition to Hammett σ values to explain better the electronic interactions between drugs and receptors (*96, 97*). He obtained excellent results in correlating inhibitory rate constants of *E. coli* by chloramphenicol analogs (Equation 29) (*96*).

$$\log (1/C) = k_1\pi^2 + k_2\pi + k_3\sigma + k_4\mu + k_5\alpha + k_6 \qquad (29)$$

More recently he has given an extensive derivation of the theoretical basis for including both the μ^2 and α parameters (*97*).

Clayton and Purcell have illustrated the predictive utility of this method when applied to selected butyrylcholinesterase inhibitors (*94*). They obtained quantitative correlations using σ^* values, amide group dipole moments, and μ in addition to hydrophobic parameters. In addition, Hansch and co-workers have used Taft steric parameters (E_s) (*60*) and pK_a values to obtain excellent correlations in various systems (*84*). E_s has recently been shown to be quantitatively related to van der Waal's radii for symmetrical top-like substituents (*98*) while pK_a values have been used as a measure of electron density distributions (*99*). Fukuto and co-workers combined Taft's E_s and σ^* parameters in a physicochemical approach to the mode of action of organophosphorus insecticides (*95*).

Modified Hammett substituent constants (*100*) were used by Garrett *et al.* to describe the bacterostatic activities of a series of sulfanilamides (*101*). Hansch also used the homolytic substituent constants (E_R) of Yamamoto and Otsu (*102*) in analyzing the activity of selected chloramphenicol derivatives (*103*). The resulting correlations led to the hypothesis of a free-radical mechanism of chloramphenicol action. Substituent measures of π electron charge density distributions (σ_i and σ_π)

(*104*) were used by Sasaki and Suzuki to illustrate the dependence of partition coefficients and biological activity on molecular electronic conditions (*105*).

In addition to these, the use of several other thermodynamic substituent constants has been investigated (*1, 4, 106*). For example, Ostrenga used molar attraction constants (*107, 108*), and Turner and Battershell have correlated chemical reactivities, vapor pressures, and partition coefficients of a series of isophthalonitriles with their fungicidal properties (*109*).

Jones and co-workers used regression analyses to study the effects of field constants and resonance parameters (*110*) of some carbamate derivatives on their penetration and detoxication with some success (*111*). Similar studies have also been made by Fukuto and co-workers using selected oximes and their anticholinesterase activities (*112*). Kakeya *et al.* used chemical shifts and valence force constants in addition to other thermodynamic parameters in the structure–activity study of a series of sulfonamide carbonic anhydrase inhibitors (*113*).

The combination of quantum mechanical calculations and the linear free-energy related model has been used recently by several investigators in drug activity studies—*i.e.*, a variety of indices obtained from the quantum chemical calculations has been utilized in these correlations (*4, 8, 114*). For example, Neely and co-workers obtained excellent correlations between the energy of the highest occupied molecular orbital, a relative measure of the ability of a molecule to donate an electron to an acceptor molecule, of a series of imidazolines and their analgetic potencies (*115*).

In an analysis of the linear free-energy relationships in drug–receptor interactions, Cammarata has shown a theoretical interpretation of substituent constants in a biological context (*116, 117*). He has separated the free energy change occurring in a reaction into its electronic, desolvation, and steric components, defined each in terms of its contributions, and approximated these contributions with quantum mechanical indices (*118, 119*). Using atomic orbital coefficients and total electronic charge on certain portions of the molecule, Cammarata obtained excellent correlations between quantum mechanical indices and sulfanilamide activity (*120*). He also suggested the use of π net charge, π-electrophilic and nucleophilic superdelocalizabilities, and energy level differences to interpret drug–receptor interactions. When this approach was applied to selected cholinesterase inhibitors, he obtained very good correlations (*121*).

Hermann *et al.* obtained good correlations between the relative substrate efficiencies of some acetophenones toward rabbit kidney reductase and selected quantum mechanical parameters (*122*). The substituent indices were derived from electron density calculations and energy differences between ground and incipient transition states (*122*). In the study of the DNA intercalation by chloroquine derivatives, Bass *et al.* (*123*) calculated sigma-electron charge distributions and used these in addition to other substituent parameters to investigate a mechanism proposed by O'Brien and Hahn (*124*) for antimalarial activity. The derivation of and rationale behind the inclusion of this term into the Hansch equation were also given (*123*).

It may seem that the various structure–activity models and parameters are not truly so independent as they are presented here. Certainly this suspicion is justified. Recently, Singer and Purcell evaluated the interrelationships among the quantitative structure–activity models and illustrated their similarities (*125*). Also, the parameters used in these models can not be totally independent of one another. One merely attempts to find those parameters which alone or in combination best describe the biological activity. In view of this, Leo *et al.* have reported a comparison of the parameters currently used in studies of this type (*86*).

Apart from their use in linear free-energy related equations, quantum mechanical calculations have been used in other ways in drug design studies. Nagy and Nador found that the central exciting effect of amphetamines increases with a decrease of the negative charge, as determined by quantum mechanical methods, on the second carbon of the benzene ring (*126*). Corcodano calculated the ring carbon reactivity indices of some phenylacetic acid derivatives and showed that this parameter correlates well with their auxinic activities (*127*). Using the Hückel molecular orbital method, Mainster and Memory proposed that superdelocalizability may be used in characterizing chemical carcinogens (*128*).

In other studies, Purcell and Sundaram used the sum of the energy of the highest occupied molecular orbital (HOMO) and that of the lowest empty molecular orbital (LEMO) as a measure of molecular electronegativity when applied to quinolinemethanol antimalarials (*129*). Sharpless and Greenblatt found electron density, LEMO, and pK_a values to correlate well with the acridine toxicities to various microorganisms (*130*). These correlations have led to their postulation of a mechanism of action. In a final example, Andrews used quantum chemical methods to calculate the dipole moments of a series of anticonvulsant drugs and related compounds (*131*). These calculations suggest a mechanism of action for these drugs different from that which had been proposed previously (*132*).

One additional area of increasing interest in the physicochemical approach to drug design is the use of instrumental methods, particularly nuclear magnetic resonance (NMR). Pioneered by Jardetzky and coworkers (*133, 134*), the use of NMR in studies of drug–receptor interactions at the molecular level is showing great promise. This technique is used primarily to follow the change effected in the relaxation rates of the protons of a small molecule upon binding to a macromolecule by observing differential peak broadening of its NMR spectrum. In addition, changes in the chemical shift of the NMR spectrum of the small molecule have been used to investigate substrate–receptor interactions. Thus far, NMR has been applied successfully to the study of enzyme–substrate interactions (135, 136), enzyme–coenzyme interactions (137), and enzyme–inhibitor interactions (136, 138). Although the literature is beginning to show numerous in vitro examples of the utility of NMR in this area, one recent application has used the intact cellular system (139). In this study, Fischer and Jost directly observed the interaction of epinephrine with its receptor site in the mouse liver cell and were able to postulate the nature of the interaction (139). As is the case with the other physicochemical methods, however, the potential of the application of NMR to drug design is great, but much development lies ahead for its realization.

Advances have been and are being made in the physicochemical approaches to drug design. Although progress has been slow in developing quantitative structure–activity relationships because of the complexity of the biological systems underlying an observable response from a drug and there is no promise that these techniques offer a panacea in drug design, there is great potential in "dissecting the role of the important molecular forces at work which yield different biological responses in the series of congeners" (140) and in using physicochemical methods for selecting promising molecules for synthesis and evaluation.

As in virtually all areas of scientific advancement, the various areas of endeavor are at different levels of sophistication. For example, one knows more about the molecular structure of an isolated molecule from instrumental analyses than about the specific interaction of this molecule with a complicated biological system. Illustrating this condition in another way, one could say that the level of sophistication of handling simultaneous equations is greater than the understanding of a parameter from pharmacological testing. It is important, however, to recognize that certain areas will lag behind others as one attempts more rigorous interpretations in interactions between molecules and biological systems. In the authors' opinion, this does not mean that work should stop in one area in order for the level of sophistication to "catch up" in another area. Rather, the entire activity should move along without the investigators' becoming preoccupied with the imbalance of the levels of development of the areas of activity. For example, it is most fortunate that the derivation of the Schrödinger equation (141) did not "wait" for the development of high speed digital computers, which could give practical application to its solution. This analogy holds for drug design. That is, one should continue efforts to put structure–activity relationships on a quantitative level even though there are limitations to the significance of certain biological activity data. As long as the investigators are aware of these limitations, it is appropriate to continue to refine the models.

Few people would have predicted a successful "moon walk," and few would try to predict the time at which new drug molecules can be designed specifically without exhaustive synthetic work and pharmacological screening. The potential of predicting accurately the biological activity of a molecule before its synthesis does appear to exist; only continued work in this area and time will determine whether or not this potential is real.

Acknowledgment

The authors gratefully acknowledge support by the U. S. Army Medical Research and Development Command (DA-49-193-MD-2779), the National Science Foundation (GB-7383), the Cotton Producers Institute, a grant from Eli Lilly Co., and a National Institutes of Health Fellowship (5FO1-GM43,699-02) from the National Institute of General Medical Sciences during the period this manuscript was written.

Literature Cited

(1) Purcell, W. P., Singer, J. A., Sundaram, K., Parks, G. L., in "Medicinal Chemistry, " 3rd ed., A. Burger, Ed., Chap. 10, Wiley, New York, 1970.
(2) Hansch, C., in "Drug Design," Vol. I, E. J. Ariëns, Ed., Academic, New York, in press.
(3) Kier, L. B., Ed., "Molecular Orbital Studies in Chemical Pharmacology," Springer-Verlag, New York, 1970.
(4) Clayton, J. M., Millner, O. E., Jr., Purcell, W. P., *Annu. Rep. Med. Chem.* (1970) **1969**, 285.
(5) Hansch, C., *Annu. Rep. Med. Chem.* (1967) **1966**, 347.
(6) *Ibid.* (1968) **1967**, 348.
(7) Hansch, C., *Proc. Int. Pharmacol. Meet., 3rd* (1968) **7**, 141–167.
(8) Purcell, W. P., Clayton, J. M., *Annu. Rep. Med. Chem.* (1969) **1968**, 314.
(9) Crum-Brown, A., Fraser, T., *Trans. Roy. Soc. Edinburgh* (1868–69) **25**, 151.
(10) Richet, M. C., *C.R. Soc. Biol.* (1893) **45**, 775.
(11) Meyer, H., *Arch. Exp. Pathol. Pharmakol.* (1899) **42**, 109.
(12) Meyer, K. H., Hemmi, H., *Biochem. Z.* (1935) **277**, 39.
(13) Overton, E., *Z. Physiol. Chem.* (1897) **22**, 189.
(14) Overton, E., *Vierteljahresschr. Naturforsch. Ges. Zuerich* (1899) **44**, 88.
(15) Overton, E., "Studien uber die Narkose," p. 45, Fischer, Jena, Germany, 1901.
(16) Fühner, H., *Arch. Exp. Pathol. Pharmakol.* (1904) **51**, 1.
(17) *Ibid.*, p. 69.
(18) Traube, J., *Arch. Ges. Physiol. (Pflügers)* (1904) **105**, 541.
(19) Warburgh, O., *Biochem. Z.* (1921) **119**, 134.
(20) Moore, W., *J. Agr. Res.* (1917) **9**, 371.
(21) *Ibid.* (1917) **10**, 365.

(22) Hammett, L. P., "Physical Organic Chemistry," 1st ed., pp. 184–199, McGraw-Hill, New York, 1940.
(23) Ferguson, J., *Proc. Roy. Soc., London, Ser. B* (1939) **127**, 387.
(24) Ferguson, J., "Mécanisme de la Narcose," p. 25, Centre National de la Recherche Scientifique, Paris, 1951.
(25) Ferguson, J., Pirie, H., *Ann. Appl. Biol.* (1948) **35**, 532.
(26) McGowan, J. C., *J. Appl. Chem., London* (1951) **1**, S120.
(27) *Ibid.* (1954) **4**, 41.
(28) McGowan, J. C., *Nature* (1963) **200**, 1317.
(29) Bruice, T. C., Kharasch, N., Winzler, R. J., *Arch. Biochem. Biophys.* (1956) **62**, 305.
(30) Free, S. M., Jr., Wilson, J. W., *J. Med. Chem.* (1964) **7**, 395.
(31) Purcell, W. P., *Biochim. Biophys. Acta* (1965) **105**, 201.
(32) Purcell, W. P., Clayton, J. M., *J. Med. Chem.* (1968) **11**, 199.
(33) Hudson, D. R., Bass, G. E., Purcell, W. P., *J. Med. Chem.* (1970) **13**, 1184.
(34) Boček, K., Kopecký, J., Krivucová, M., Vlachová, D., *Experientia* (1964) **20**, 667.
(35) Kopecký, J., Boček, K., Vlachová, D., *Nature* (1965) **207**, 981.
(36) Hammett, L. P., *Chem. Rev.* (1935) **17**, 125.
(37) Aldridge, W. N., Davison, A. N., *Biochem. J.* (1952) **51**, 62.
(38) Wells, P. R., "Linear Free Energy Relationships," Academic, London, 1968.
(39) Klotz, I. M., "Chemical Thermodynamics," p. 278, Prentice-Hall, Englewood Cliffs, 1950.
(40) Bender, M. L., Nakamura, K., *J. Amer. Chem. Soc.* (1962) **84**, 2577.
(41) Blomquist, C. H., *Acta Chem. Scand.* (1966) **20**, 1747.
(42) Nath, R. L., Ghosh, N. K., *Enzymologia* (1963) **26**, 297.
(43) Neims, A. H., DeLuca, D. C., Hellerman, L., *Biochemistry* (1966) **5**, 203.
(44) Omerod, W. E., *Biochem. J.* (1953) **54**, 701.
(45) O'Sullivan, D. G., Sadler, P. W., *Arch. Biochem. Biophys.* (1957) **66**, 243.
(46) Sager, W. F., Parks, P. C., *Proc. Nat. Acad. Sci. U.S.* (1964) **52**, 408.
(47) Seydel, J. K., *Mol. Pharmacol.* (1966) **2**, 259.
(48) Hansen, O. R., *Acta Chem. Scand.* (1962) **16**, 1593.
(49) Zahradník, R., Chvapil, M., *Experientia* (1960) **16**, 511.
(50) Chvapil, M., Zahradník, R., Cmuchalová, B., *Arch. Int. Pharmacodyn. Ther.* (1962) **135**, 330.
(51) Zahradník, R., *Arch. Int. Pharmacodyn. Ther.* (1962) **135**, 311.
(52) Zahradník, R., *Experientia* (1962) **18**, 534.
(53) Collander, R., *Trans. Faraday Soc.* (1937) **33**, 985.
(54) Collander, R., *Physiol. Plant.* (1954) **7**, 420.
(55) Hansch, C., *Accounts Chem. Res.* (1969) **2**, 232.
(56) Hansch, C., Fujita, T., *J. Amer. Chem. Soc.* (1964) **86**, 1616.
(57) Hansch, C., Muir, R. M., Fujita, T., Maloney, P. P., Geiger, F., Streich, M., *J. Amer. Chem. Soc.* (1963) **85**, 2817.
(58) Taft, R. W., in "Steric Effects in Organic Chemistry," M. S. Newman, Ed., p. 556, Wiley, New York, 1956.
(59) Fujita, T., Iwasa, J., Hansch, C., *J. Amer. Chem. Soc.* (1964) **86**, 5175.
(60) Leffler, J. E., Grunwald, E., "Rates and Equilibria of Organic Reactions," Wiley, New York, 1963.
(61) Hansch, C., Steward, A. R., *J. Med. Chem.* (1964) **7**, 691.
(62) Hansch, C., Steward, A. R., Anderson, S. M., Bentley, D., *J. Med. Chem.* (1968) **11**, 1.
(63) Hansch, C., Deutsch, E. W., *J. Med. Chem.* (1965) **8**, 705.
(64) Hansch, C., Steward, A. R., Iwasa, J., *Mol. Pharmacol.* (1965) **1**, 87.

(65) Wells, P. R., *Chem. Rev.* (1963) **63**, 171.
(66) Neely, W. B., *Mol. Pharmacol.* (1967) **3**, 108.
(67) Pullman, A., Pullman, B., "Physico-chemical Mechanisms of Carcinogenesis, The Jerusalem Symposia on Quantum Chemistry and Biochemistry, I," p. 9, The Israel Academy of Sciences and Humanities, Jerusalem, 1969.
(68) Pullman, B., "Electronic Aspects of Biochemistry," B. Pullman, Ed., p. 559, Academic, New York, 1964.
(69) Pullman, B., in "Molecular Orbital Studies in Chemical Pharmacology," L. B. Kier, Ed., p. 1, Springer-Verlag, New York, 1970.
(70) Pullman, B., Pullman, A., "Quantum Biochemistry," Interscience, New York, 1963.
(71) Pullman, B., Pullman, A., Umans, R., Maigret, B., "Physico-chemical Mechanisms of Carcinogenesis, The Jerusalem Symposia on Quantum Chemistry and Biochemistry, I," p. 325, The Israel Academy of Sciences and Humanities, Jerusalem, 1969.
(72) Löwdin, P. O., "Electronic Aspects of Biochemistry," Pullman, B., Ed., p. 167, Academic, New York, 1964.
(73) Neely, W. B., *Mol. Pharmacol.* (1965) **1**, 137.
(74) Kier, L. B., *J. Med. Chem.* (1968) **11**, 441.
(75) *Ibid.*, p. 915.
(76) Kier, L. B., *J. Pharm. Sci.* (1968) **57**, 1188.
(77) Kier, L. B., *J. Pharmacol. Exp. Ther.* (1968) **164**, 75.
(78) Kier, L. B., *J. Pharm. Pharmacol.* (1969) **21**, 93.
(79) Kier, L. B., *J. Pharm. Sci.* (1970) **59**, 112.
(80) Kier, L. B., in "Fundamental Concepts in Drug-Receptor Interactions," J. F. Danielli, J. F. Moran, D. J. Triggle, Eds., p. 15, Academic, New York, 1970.
(81) Beasley, J. G., Purcell, W. P., *Biochim. Biophys. Acta* (1969) **178**, 175.
(82) Ban, T., Fujita, T., *J. Med. Chem.* (1969) **12**, 353.
(83) Hansch, C., Deutsch, E. W., Smith, R. N., *J. Amer. Chem. Soc.* (1965) **87**, 2738.
(84) Hansch, C., Lien, E. J., Helmer, F., *Arch. Biochem. Biophys.* (1968) **128**, 319.
(85) Lien, E. J., Hansch, C., *J. Pharm. Sci.* (1968) **57**, 1027.
(86) Leo, A., Hansch, C., Church, C., *J. Med. Chem.* (1969) **12**, 766.
(87) Lien, E. J., *J. Agr. Food Chem.* (1969) **17**, 1265.
(88) Bark, L. S., Graham, R. J. T., *J. Chromatogr.* (1966) **23**, 417.
(89) Biagi, G. L., Barbaro, A. M., Gamba, M. F., Guerra, M. C., *J. Chromatogr.* (1969) **41**, 371.
(90) Biagi, G. L., Guerra, M. C., Barbaro, A. M., Gamba, M. F., *J. Med. Chem.* (1970) **13**, 511.
(91) Boyce, C. B. C., Milborrow, B. V., *Nature* (1965) **208**, 537.
(92) Iwasa, J., Fujita, T., Hansch, C., *J. Med. Chem.* (1965) **8**, 150.
(93) Soczewiński, E., Bieganowska, M., *J. Chromatogr.* (1969) **40**, 431.
(94) Clayton, J. M., Purcell, W. P., *J. Med. Chem.* (1969) **12**, 1087.
(95) Fukuto, T. R., "Residue Reviews," F. A. Gunther, Ed., p. 327, Springer-Verlag, New York, 1969.
(96) McFarland, J. W., *Proc. Nat. Med. Chem. Symp., 11th,* June 1968.
(97) McFarland, J. W., personal communication, March 1970.
(98) Hansch, C., *J. Org. Chem.* (1970) **35**, 620.
(99) Brown, E. V., Kipp, W. H., *Cancer Res.* (1969) **29**, 1341.
(100) Yoshioka, M., Hamamoto, K., Kubota, T., *Bull. Chem. Soc. Jap.* (1962) **35**, 1723.
(101) Garrett, E. R., Mielck, J. B., Seydel, J. K., Kessler, H. J., *J. Med. Chem.* (1969) **12**, 740.
(102) Yamamoto, T., Otsu, T., *Chem. Ind., London* (1967) 787.

(103) Hansch, C., Kutter, E., Leo, A., *J. Med. Chem.* (1969) **12**, 746.
(104) Yukawa, Y., Tsuno, Y., *J. Chem. Soc. Jap., Pure Chem. Sec.* (1965) **86**, 873.
(105) Sasaki, Y., Suzuki, M., *Chem. Pharm. Bull.* (1969) **17**, 1569.
(106) Neely, W. B., Allison, W. E., Crummett, W. B., Kauer, K., Reifschneider, W., *J. Agr. Food Chem.* (1970) **18**, 45.
(107) Ostrenga, J. A., *J. Med. Chem.* (1969) **12**, 349.
(108) Ostrenga, J. A., Steinmetz, C., *J. Pharm. Sci.* (1970) **59**, 414.
(109) Turner, N. J., Battershell, R. D., *Contrib. Boyce Thompson Inst.* (1969) **24**, 139.
(110) Swain, C. G., Lupton, E. C., Jr., *J. Amer. Chem. Soc.* (1968) **90**, 4328.
(111) Jones, R. L., Metcalf, R. L., Fukuto, T. R., *J. Econ. Entomol.* (1969) **62**, 801.
(112) Fukuto, T. R., Metcalf, R. L., Jones, R. L., Myers, R. O., *J. Agr. Food Chem.* (1969) **17**, 923.
(113) Kakeya, N., Aoki, M., Kamada, A., Yata, N., *Chem. Pharm. Bull.* (1969) **17**, 1010.
(114) Martin, Y. C., *J. Med. Chem.* (1970) **13**, 145.
(115) Neely, W. B., White, H. C., Rudzik, A., *J. Pharm. Sci.* (1968) **57**, 1176.
(116) Cammarata, A., *J. Med. Chem.* (1969) **12**, 314.
(117) Cammarata, A., "Molecular Orbital Studies in Chemical Pharmacology," L. B. Kier, Ed., p. 156, Springer-Verlag, New York, 1970.
(118) Rogers, K. S., Cammarata, A., *Biochim. Biophys. Acta* (1969) **193**, 22.
(119) Rogers, K. S., Cammarata, A., *J. Med. Chem.* (1969) **12**, 692.
(120) Cammarata, A., *J. Med. Chem.* (1968) **11**, 1111.
(121) Cammarata, A., Stein, R. L., *J. Med. Chem.* (1968) **11**, 829.
(122) Hermann, R. B., Culp, H. W., McMahon, R. E., Marsh, M. M., *J. Med. Chem.* (1969) **12**, 749.
(123) Bass, G. E., Hudson, D. R., Parker, J. E., Purcell, W. P., *J. Med. Chem.* (1971) **14**, 275.
(124) O'Brien, R. L., Hahn, F. E., *Antimicrob. Ag. Chemother.* (1966) **1965**, 315.
(125) Singer, J. A., Purcell, W. P., *J. Med. Chem.* (1967) **10**, 1000.
(126) Nagy, V., Nador, K., *Arnzeim.-Forsch.* (1967) **17**, 1228.
(127) Cocordano, M., *C.R. Acad. Sci., Paris, Ser. C* (1968) **266**, 897.
(128) Mainster, M. A., Memory, J. D., *Biochim. Biophys. Acta* (1967) **148**, 605.
(129) Purcell, W. P., Sundaram, K., *J. Med. Chem.* (1969) **12**, 18.
(130) Sharpless, N. E., Greenblatt, C. L., *Exp. Parasitol.* (1969) **24**, 216.
(131) Andrews, P. R., *J. Med. Chem.* (1969) **12**, 761.
(132) Perkow, W., *Arzneim.-Forsch.* (1960) **10**, 284.
(133) Jardetzky, O., *Advan. Chem. Phys.* (1964) **7**, 499.
(134) Jardetzky, O., *Naturwissenschaften* (1967) **54**, 149.
(135) Kato, G., *Mol. Pharmacol.* (1969) **5**, 148.
(136) Schmidt, P. G., Stark, G. R., Baldeschwieler, J. D., *J. Biol. Chem.* (1969) **244**, 1860.
(137) Hollis, D. P., *Biochemistry* (1967) **6**, 2080.
(138) Raftery, M. A., Dahlquist, F. W., Parsons, S. M., Wolcott, R. G., *Proc. Nat. Acad. Sci., U.S.* (1969) **62**, 44.
(139) Fischer, J. J., Jost, M. C., *Mol. Pharmacol.* (1969) **5**, 420.
(140) Burger, A., "Fundamental Concepts in Drug-Receptor Interactions," J. F. Danielli, J. F. Moran, D. J. Triggle, Eds., p. 1, Academic, New York, 1970.
(141) Schrödinger, E., *Ann. Phys. (Leipzig)* (1926) **79**, 361.

RECEIVED November 5, 1970.

6

Receptor Mechanisms and Biochemical Rationales

B. BELLEAU[1]

Departments of Biochemistry and Chemistry, Faculties of Medicine and Science, University of Ottawa, Ottawa, Ontario, Canada

The following biochemical aspects of receptor structure and function are analyzed: (a) extra-thermodynamic approaches, (b) kinetic approaches, (c) molecular approaches from the biophysical and biochemical standpoints as applied to cholinergic and adrenergic systems, (d) receptor allosteric or control sites in relation to structure–action relationships and molecular quasi-symmetry in drugs. The following conclusions are drawn: additivity functions based on linear free energy relationships are shown to be uninformative with regard to binding specificities. Agonists and antagonists do not modulate the same physical parameters in receptors. The cholinergic receptor and the anionic regulatory unit of acetylcholinesterase would be structurally analogous or homologous. Neurotransmitter receptors include accessory control sites which reduce the diffusion times of agonists, and which provide additional binding sites for drugs. Because of their topography, these sites would interact preferentially with symmetrical or quasi-symmetrical molecules.

Until about 10 years ago (*1, 2*), neurotransmitter– and drug–receptor interactions had been treated phenomenologically rather than in terms of modern structural chemistry. Since then, progress in receptor chemistry has been too modest to allow clear-cut predictions of immediate tangible value in the field of drug design. Nonetheless, hopes are high presently that the rational design of new therapeutic agents may no longer be a dream—an impression which can markedly affect future experimental approaches to drug discovery. These hopes or expectations are based largely on extrapolations from a variety of extra-thermodynamic

[1] Present address: Department of Chemistry, McGill University, Montreal, Canada.

141

relationships between substituent effects in small molecules (or ligands) and binding on model systems. However, the structural chemistry of the receptors of excitable membranes is as yet poorly understood, and even less is known about the mechanisms underlying their response to ligands. At first, then, the question naturally arises as to what qualitative relevance have studies with model systems to the structure and regulation of membrane receptors? All explanations of the effects of structural or substituent changes on binding or on chemical reactions are always based on some kind of comparison with models, which may be simple or complex. In the latter case, many of the complexities are, so to speak, averaged out in the comparisons, thus allowing for the generation of simple mechanistic pictures. This is the situation, for instance, when the hydrophobic bonding theory (3) is used to explain the inherently complex kinetic responses of enzymes to organic ligands (4, 5). On the other hand, the use of simple models, such as those for substituent effects on hydrophobic transfer forces, may often require more complex and more empirical explanations because several additional simple models (for steric or electronic effects, for example) must be considered simultaneously to achieve correlations with effects on a real system (6). In any event, when structural or substituent effects are explained in terms of the same effects in a model system, the parameters which are compared are always of a thermodynamic nature—usually free energies in the case of ligand–protein or drug–receptor interactions—and so cannot tell us anything about reaction paths, as is well known. Only occasionally have enthalpies and entropies been used in such comparisons (7, 8), an unfortunate omission since they can help narrow the choice of possible interpretations. It is clear, then, that the quality of the answers which studies with model systems can supply depends critically on the nature of the questions which are asked of the model. If non-specific questions are asked, the parameter of specificity, which characterizes real receptor systems (and all life processes, for that matter) can hardly appear in the answers, thus forcing the conclusion that specific drugs may not yet be designed rationally through extrapolations from models which incorporate only what is common to all systems.

Extrathermodynamic Approaches

Often, simple additivity relationships between one thermodynamic property or the other and some suitable substituent properties are found (6), but these relationships are not part of thermodynamics per se (*i.e.*, they are extra-thermodynamic). It is interesting that many linear free energy relationships between affinity for model systems and certain substituent properties could be found (6). Hence, the formal interaction mechanisms deduced from such model studies appear to have an exact counterpart in real systems of very common occurrence. Accordingly, the measured additive effects of ligand–substituents in real complex systems must have some fairly common physical dimensions which, at first approximation, are identical to those controlling the behavior of the simple model systems. Part processes of such wide occurrence can only be driven by component forces which are common to many systems. Clearly, only external forces (such as solute–solvent interactions) apply so indiscriminately, with the consequence that the ligand–substituents will happen to perturb some property which is common to all their macromolecular partners [such as parallel changes in the surface free energy or the volumes of the systems (*see below*)]. In other words, non-specific perturbations will be induced, as is the case in general enzyme–receptor inhibition, by homologous series of substrate analogs (*9, 10*). Ligand-induced losses of a specific receptor or enzyme property (such as catalytic activity) can result from many kinds of unproductive perturbations of the active sites, so that potency in preventing an effector molecule from initiating a specific conformational change has only the dimension of a relative free energy change, which may be subject to modulation simply by changing the substituent interaction with the medium. It follows that the observation of additivity functions based only on ΔG changes cannot serve to identify the binding reaction paths, which must distinguish one receptor system from another, and even though extrapolations of the functions may serve to improve over-all strength of binding, non-specific interactions will tend to dominate the picture. In fact, it is deviations from additivity functions which are indicative of specificity effects, a measure of which is sometimes given by the number of semi-empirical parameters which must be considered simultaneously to achieve correlations with real systems (*6*) The basic question as to whether the respective effects of activators (neuroeffectors) and inhibitors (antagonists) measure the same thermodynamic property did not even attract attention until recently (*10, 11; see below*). Other more suitable models allowing an insight into the molecular mechanisms of receptor responses to neuroeffectors are therefore needed badly (*see below*). Before elaborating on this subject it would be advantageous to describe briefly some recent advances in knowledge of the kinetic behavior of the excitable membrane receptors as it bears on the problem of interaction specificities.

Kinetic Approaches

Little attention need be devoted here to the classical kinetic analyses of drug–receptor interactions as based on the general appearance of dose–response curves. This approach to receptor mechanisms has been documented fully, and no significant progress has been made since which can help achieve an improved understanding in structural terms. This approach has served essentially to show that the response curve of certain membranes to graded increases in ligand concentrations often obeys the Langmuir isotherm (12) and that structurally related drugs can induce different maximal responses (a phenomenon at the origin of the concept of "intrinsic activity") (12). However, it has been noted in recent years (13) that depending on the type of excitable membrane, the dose–response curves can be slightly S-shaped, and sometimes extremely sharp (as in "all-or-nothing responses"). These observations suggest a previously unsuspected property of receptors and associated molecules. By extrapolating from the known behavior of regulatory enzymes (14, 15), a model was proposed where receptor protomers would display cooperative responses typical of highly ordered structures (16). Based on the assumption that the receptor can exist in only two conformational states, a theoretical treatment, using the molecular field approximation (17) of the cooperative conformational transition, allowed the construction of dose–response curves closely approximating certain real situations. As in the case of the theoretical treatment of regulatory enzyme behavior (15), the basic assumption was made that the reversible conformational changes of the protomer pre-exist ligand binding. However, recent experimental evidence has accumulated which casts serious doubt on the validity of this free equilibrium model (18, 19). It now seems more evident that phase-transitions in ordered structures require nucleation, a step which was also incorporated in a recent treatment of oscillating phase transitions as related to cooperative effects in steady-state transport across membranes (20). Nevertheless, cooperativity of receptor units is an important factor in propagating membrane depolarizations and nerve impulses and offers a rational basis for all-or-nothing processes in general. The reality of cooperative phenomena at the receptor level of membrane lattices denies the existence of simple additivity functions between ligand affinities and substituent properties and further suggests that those ligands which may antagonize receptors by cooperative mechanisms (assuming that more than two receptor conformations can display cooperativity) should be sought actively. This aspect of drug research is emphasized below.

Molecular Approaches

Biophysical Aspects. The nature of the molecular responses of receptors to activators (or nucleators) and inhibitors (or antagonists) must be understood in molecular terms if structure–activity relationships are to be rationalized. Phenomenologically, receptor responses are revealed when the nature of the medium in contact with excitable membranes is varied by adding salts, acids, or various organic ligands, thus leading to a sudden change in the physicochemical properties of the membranes. This sharp transition can best be ascribed to conformational changes (which may be cooperative; *see above*) in some special biopolymers, from a physical state which normally braces a structured matrix of liproteins to one which spurs a cascade of biophysical events ultimately producing depolarization of the membrane, and in several cases contraction or relaxation of muscle fibers. The receptors for the neurotransmitters acetylcholine (ACh) and the catecholamine hormones are the best known examples of such specific biopolymers. They are generally believed to be proteins, and the phase transition from the "bracing" state B to the "spurring" state S can be nucleated by ACh and related quaternary salts or by norepinephrine (NE) and some of its analogs. By analogy with the crystallites and other highly ordered polymers, the reversible phase transition B $\rightleftharpoons$ S can give rise to simple sigmoids, whose steepness of slope depends on the degree of cooperativity between the receptors (*see above*). The principles at work may be illustrated by the classical model of the helix-coil transition in polypeptides and proteins (*21*). However, for the case at hand, it is best to imagine that the receptor transition involves a change from one ordered state to another structured one, rather than a random coil which would hardly allow for ready reversibility. Obviously, nucleators of the transition may bind on both the B and S states, and reversal of the transition (S $\rightarrow$ B) may require nucleation by other effectors which may be released in the S state of the receptors. We now come to the case where large groups of ligands or drugs combine with the receptor while being unable to nucleate the transition from the B to the S state. Many of these ligands or drugs prevent the action of nucleators by a process which often follows the law of competitive kinetics (*12*), so that the observed thermodynamic property measured by these mutual exclusion effects has the dimension of a relative ΔG change (in the absence of cooperativity), which being substituent sensitive may allow the generation of extra-thermodynamic relationships (*see above*).

However, the truly important question for the future is: what thermodynamic property is measured by the observed effects of nucleators or agonists? In other words, do nucleators and antagonists modulate the same physical variables? A negative answer appears most likely for the following reason. The seasoned medicinal chemist has frequently observed that an increase in the size or hydrophobic bulk of agonist substituents will often transform them into antagonists (*10, 12*), thus suggesting strongly that an excess of apolar bulk allows the participation of physical variables which are not normally disturbed by the nucleators themselves. Accordingly, agonists and antagonists must produce their effects by way of different physical interaction mechanisms. Hence, if the measured thermodynamic property for antagonist effects is a relative ΔG change, this may not be true for nucleators. In other words, agonist potencies cannot be a simple function of affinity for the receptors, as is frequently implied (12). Rather, assuming that B and S states attain equilibrium, relative nucleator potencies should be a direct function of the position of the conformational equilibrium, so that potency would have the dimension of a conformational free energy change. It is clear, then, that agonist affinities for receptors or model systems [such as acetylcholinesterase (22)] have no bearing on the degree of conformational shift induced by nucleators. Much confusion would be eliminated if these considerations were properly weighted. In contrast to the inhibited physical state of the receptor for which many relatively chaotic, unproductive conformations are possible, it seems probable that the spurred physical state should possess exclusive characteristics uniquely allowing for cooperative behavior (16). Ideally, then, nucleators should all modulate qualitatively similar physical variables since otherwise more than one spurred state would have to be postulated. One key factor which may contribute importantly to the magnification of the unitary molecular response to nucelators is cooperativity between receptor promoters (*see above*), and if we assume that besides the B and S states, additional but unproductive states can also display cooperativity, highly specific and potent therapeutic agents would become accessible. The reality of this possibility appears to be confirmed, at least in principle, by the manner in which the colicin class of antibiotics produce their effects (16, 23).

Other models can be constructed which lead to similar conclusions regarding the divergence of interaction mechanisms for agonists and antagonists. It becomes of considerable interest, then, to discover which measurable physical parameter(s) may have direct relevance to nucleator potencies at the receptor level. At membrane surfaces macromolecular structures such as receptors occur at an aqueous interface. Hence, solute–solvent interactions in both the initial and final states of the binding partners will contribute to the relative thermodynamic stability of the addition complex. For a tightly packed globular lipoprotein, such as is postulated for the receptor, the uptake of a ligand will necessarily produce a volume change which may be positive or negative. The volume change will result in a parallel change in the hydrophobic or hydrophilic area of the receptor "micelle" which is exposed to the solvent and adjacent macromolecules. The receptor–water interfacial tension will therefore be changed by the ligand, and it follows that the surface free energy of the receptor protein must always be changed by the ligands. These ligand-induced volume changes may as well be loosely referred to as conformational perturbations. For convenience, we can easily conceive that antagonists or inhibitors penetrate the surface of the receptor micelle, causing a volume increase, whereas nucleators or agonists may cause, by way of desolvation, a volume contraction which must have a minimum value in order that the desired macroscopic effects may be observed. This model also predicts that different physical variables would control the stability of the "contracted" (or spurred) and the "expanded" (unproductive) states respectively. Now, the change from the initial "braced" state to a uniquely spurred state must occur by way of a stereotyped bond-breaking and bond-making process in which the aqueous interface must participate actively. This suggests that the enthalpies and entropies of binding should be markedly sensitive to structural effects in the nucleators but not the free-energies since the postulated uniqueness of the physical mechanism underlying the volume contractions will lead to compensated fluctuations in the enthalpies and entropies of binding.

These predictions have recently been experimentally verified through extensive thermodynamic studies of quaternary salt binding on the enzyme acetylcholinesterase (AChE) as a model (7). Of considerable interest was the additional finding of a correlation between the enthalpies of salt binding (but not the free energies) and the degree of conformational response of the enzyme (11). It was also noted that physical changes at the aqueous interface appeared to dominate the picture, and evidence was adduced that indeed different physical variables may be modulated by receptor nucleators and antagonists respectively, as required by theory (10). As it turns out, agonist potencies appear to be a function of modulation intensity (or degree of conformational stabilization of the S-state), whereas antagonist potencies are simple functions of the thermodynamic stability of the unproductive addition complexes. Parallel studies with intact membrane preparations will undoubtedly prove fruitful.

Looking ahead, it would seem that drugs capable of inducing receptor rearrangements by cooperative mechanisms would have much greater value in therapeutics. To achieve this, increased attention may have to be paid to protein topography if drug structures are to be designed which are compatible with low energy receptor conformations displaying cooperativity. In this connection, it is not inconceivable that one of the reasons why so many highly active drugs are found among the natural products (such as the alkaloids, for instance) may be related to the fact that as the end products of protein actions themselves, they are necessarily endowed with "built-in knowledge" about protein topography. It may be worthwhile, then, to use the accumulated knowledge about the three-dimensional structures of proteins as a starting point for drug design.

Biochemical Aspects. Although serious efforts have been made over the past few years to isolate and characterize the neurotransmitter receptors by the method of affinity labelling (24, 25), the results have thus far been generally disappointing and ambiguous. The isolation of a muscarone binding protein fraction from electroplax tissue and thought to be distinct from acetylcholinesterase (AChE) has been reported (26), but it is too early to assess the possible significance of these observations. Nevertheless, significant advances in the *in situ* structural chemistry of both the cholinergic and adrenergic systems have been made in recent years, and the observations may suggest new avenues to drug research.

CHOLINERGIC SYSTEMS: DIRECT AND MODEL OBSERVATIONS. Since the background of this subject has recently been covered elsewhere (27), only some of the important new highlights are discussed here. These concern the ACh receptor of electroplax tissue, of the mouse diaphragm and the frog toe muscle, especially in relation to AChE as a model receptor.

New approaches to the chemistry of the eel electroplax receptor have been designed by Karlin (24, 28). It was shown that dithiothreitol (DTT) reduces a disulfide bond at or near the ACh-receptor level, and one of the liberated thiols can be irreversibly alkylated by appropriate thiol reagents carrying a quaternary moiety. The possibility is therefore available of achieving selective affinity labelling of the DDT-generated thiol group, and preliminary experiments along this line have already been carried out (29). Of considerable interest was the observation that the DTT-treated electroplax is activated by hexamethonium instead of being blocked. The reduced receptor can be reconstituted functionally by oxidation with Ellman's reagent. Apparently, these thiol reagents were without effect on solubilized AChE (*see below*, however). It thus appears possible that nucleation of phase transitions by agonists may normally be transmitted from the receptor to the other membrane components by way of disulfide bonds acting as pullers. This suggests that new useful drugs may be designed which would be endowed with specific intrinsic power to affect disulfide links or to engage in disulfide interchange reactions at the receptor level of excitable membranes. This area of medicinal chemistry has hardly been explored, except in the field of radioprotective agents whose mechanisms of action are still poorly understood.

In recent years, much attention has been paid to the role of calcium in receptor phenomena, besides its better known involvement in enzyme activation and contraction of muscle fibers. Earlier observations by Csillik and Savay (30) and Nakamura *et al.* (31) led Tazieff-Depierre and co-workers (32) to study calcium release at the motor end plates of mouse diaphragm in relation to receptor activation and inhibition. Of considerable interest was the observation that whereas membrane depolarizers (carbachol, succinyldicholine, etc) liberate calcium on the motor end plates, non-depolarizers such as *d*-tubocurarine fail to do so. It appeared that the greater the depolarizing potency of the effector, the larger was the amount of calcium liberated. This suggests a new approach to the evaluation of relative potencies through direct chemical methods rather than classical pharmacological procedures. It was also shown that calcium liberation leads to activation of vicinal membrane-bound AChE, whereas certain venom toxins and potassium ions induce calcium release at the muscle fiber level and not on the motor end plates. Hence: in accord with earlier concepts (*see below*), calcium appears to be critically involved in the stabilization of receptor conformation, and its liberation by nucleators would serve the dual purpose of stabilizing the spurred physical state and of activating enzymes controlling glycogenolysis and the contraction of the muscle fibers. It would be of interest, therefore, to design drugs (or protein reagents) which can specifically influence calcium interactions with receptors. Up to now, only non-specific chelating agents have been used, and these mostly as analytical tools. Interestingly, the proposal was recently advanced (*33*) that certain receptor inhibitors of the alkylating variety (quaternary aziridinium salts) may block a calcium binding site (*see below*), thus creating a potentially valuable precedent in the field.

In our own laboratories, the working hypothesis that the anionic site-rich chain of AChE may be conformationally homologous to the ACh receptor (*34, 35, 37*) has now been explored sufficiently to allow a partial resolution of the long standing controversies regarding the relation of the enzyme to the receptor. The following highlights may be worth bearing in mind. The enzyme includes two physically different regions, one which carries unspecific esteratic activity, and another which carries at least four (and probably more) anionic sites, two of which can be covalently masked by the alkylating agent *N,N*-dimethyl-2-phenylaziridinium chloride (DPA) (*36, 37*). The DPA-modified enzyme has increased esteratic activity toward neutral substrates (*38, 39*)—such as indophenyl acetate or IPA—but none whatsoever toward ACh. Two moles of ^{14}C-DPA react per active subunit, and one of the covalently-bound DPA molecules is readily removed at pH 9–9.5, thus leading to a mono-DPA enzyme species which has still higher activity toward IPA but none at all toward ACh (*36*). The bis-DPA enzyme is conformationally unresponsive to decamethonium and *d*-tubocurarine (IPA assay), but the mono-DPA species is as responsive as the native enzyme to the latter drug, while being unaffected by the former (*36*). Hence, depolarizing and non-depolarizing drugs interact with different anionic sites on the anionic chain of AChE, a topographical distinction which conceivably underlies their different modes of action on the motor end plate receptors

(Figure 1). The postulate that depolarizers and non-depolarizers induce divergent conformational responses at the receptor level was confirmed using the conformational responsiveness of the anionic chain of AChE as a model. When AChE is exposed to methanesulfonyl fluoride (MSF), the esteratic site undergoes irreversible sulfonylation, the rate of which is markedly sensitive to quaternary ion interactions with the anionic chain (40). These kinetic effects are thus indicative of conformational changes initiated in the anionic chain (41), and of considerable interest was the finding that whereas alkyl monoquaternary (34) and bisquaternary depolarizers strongly stimulate the rate of the MSF reaction (42), non-depolarizers such as d-tubocurarine and gallamine inhibit the reaction by a non-competitive mechanism (42). Moreover, the strongest kinetic effects were obtained with the best depolarizers of the motor end plate membrane. These model studies prove beyond question that relative affinities as such for AChE (as measured by the ACh assay) are irrelevant when the purpose is to establish the existence of similarities or differences between the anionic chain of the enzyme and the ACh receptors. It is true affinity and the degree as well as nature of the response which have a bearing on drug–receptor interactions, as was pointed out above. Recently, conclusive structural evidence for our anionic chain hypothesis was provided by Leuzinger (43), who showed that his crystalline AChE preparation (44) (65,000 daltons per active subunit) is actually made up of two different chains of equal molecular weights and chemically dis-

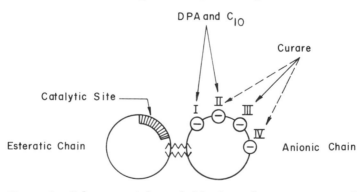

Figure 1. Schematic of the probable physical structure of acetyl-cholinesterase. One physical region carries the esteratic site, which is proximal to one anionic site (Site I); the other region would carry at least four anionic sites, and would be homologous to the acetylcholine receptor of the motor end plate excitable membrane. Sites I and II are masked by DPA, but Site II can be regenerated at alkaline pH. Decamethonium (C_{10}) would interact at least with Sites I and II whereas curare would bind at III and IV, and perhaps at II and III. Most quaternary salt substituents bind on the anionic chain [exo-binding (26, 36, 42, 35)], thus projecting away from the esteratic region.

sociatable by exposure to mercaptoethanol in urea solution. In agreement with hypothesis, only one of the separated chains carries labeled phosphorus after treatment of the native enzyme with radioactive diisopropyl fluorophosphonate (DFP). These new observations thus confirm our hypothesis that AChE is a non-specific esterase on which a conformationally responsive anionic chain acting as an ACh-protoreceptor has been grafted (27), (Figure 1). Indeed, a somewhat analogous conformational responsiveness of the ACh receptor has been chemically demonstrated by Rang and Ritter (45). In addition, both the enzyme and the receptor are modified by thiol reagents (43, 46), contrary to earlier impressions.

From the point of view of drug research, these new advances are of practical significance in a number of ways: the receptor surface for ACh includes several anionic sites, all of which appear to be involved in the cooperative nucleation of the spurred physical state of the receptor. Clearly these sites must be distinguishable by their stereoelectronic requirements so that many structures bearing only a formal resemblance to ACh may be accommodated, which accounts for the wide diversity of drug structures which are capable of inducing curarization or depolarization. The alkaloid *d*-tubocurarine is certainly a distant relative of ACh, and it is doubtful that it could have been designed rationally using the ACh structure as a model. As it turns out, in fact, the model of the ACh interaction with the esteratic chain of the enzyme, on which several interpretations of structure–activity relationships are still based (48) is erroneous since most ACh analogs interact mainly with the anionic chain (exo-binding) (37, 41, 42) (Figure 1), the topography of which has only begun to be explored (36, 45). Until the detailed topographies and specificities of such large binding surfaces are understood, novel effector or inhibitor prototypes endowed with specificity will remain essentially unpredictable. It seems clear that the classical concept, which requires antagonist molecules to occupy the agonist binding sites proper, should be used with extreme caution in view of the multiplicity of binding sites and the wide occurrence of exo-binding at the active site level (11).

We have recently established (B. Belleau, A. Paturet, and M. Saucier, in preparation) that erythrocyte-bound AChE behaves as a genuine allosteric enzyme displaying "explosive" cooperative behavior which suggests that it probably plays a role in the control of membrane configuration. A phase transition must be first nucleated by appropriate effectors before the esteratic center can accept the substrate ACh. We conclude that the regulatory units of membrane-bound AChE possess the biophysical qualifications for a receptor-like role on excitable membranes.

ADRENERGIC SYSTEMS. Over the past few years, significant advances in our understanding of the *in-situ* chemistry of both the α- and β-receptors for catecholamines have been made. We shall examine briefly some of the highlights as they pertain to the structural and conformational properties of these receptors.

The α-Receptor. It appears more and more likely that certain classes of CNS drugs may act partly by influencing the α-receptors (*49*). Hence, the need to achieve better comprehension of drug action at this level. Because membrane-bound ATPases are somehow involved in active transport across membranes (such as the Na^+,K^+-activated ATPase) much speculation on the possible involvement of ATP and ATPases as components of the α-receptor system has been made (*2, 41, 50*). The temptation to visualize ATP as forming part of the binding sites for catecholamines has no doubt been reinforced by the known role of ATP in the binding of catecholamines in the storage granules (*51*), as well as its involvement as substrate for the hormone-sensitive adenylcyclases and the contractile proteins. A tentative connection between catecholamine stereochemistry and receptor-bound ATP was envisaged several years ago (*2*), but the first detailed molecular theory of catecholamine action as based on the "ATP-receptor" picture was advanced by Bloom and Goldman (*50*). As far as the writer is aware, they were the first to present cogent arguments for the central role of calcium as a link between receptor responses and metabolic events, an idea which has since led others to suggest that calcium may indeed act as a second universal messenger (besides cyclic AMP) of membrane events (*52*).

In spite of the elegance of Bloom and Goldman's proposal, various aspects of their models may be questioned. For instance, the assumed central role of ATP as a primary reaction site for catecholamines denies a primary involvement of the receptor protein itself. As far as is known, enzyme inhibitors and activators (with the exception of metal ion chelating agents) act on protein binding sites rather than their cofactors. The drug N-ethoxycarbonyl-2-ethoxy-1,2-dihydroquinoline (EEDQ) (*53*), a selective protein reagent devoid of chemical affinity for nucleotides (*54*), in fact behaves as a selective irreversible inhibitor of the α-receptors (*55*). Partly for these reasons we have conceived an alternative model where both calcium and protein groups would serve as binding sites for catecholamines and inhibitors (*56*). It was proposed that the calcium site would be essential only for catecholamine binding and not for antagonists. Recent experimental evidence was obtained which supports this hypothesis (*57*). However, our model also specified that the receptor might be a calcium-magnesium dependent ATPase on which the terminal phosphate of ATP would come in contact with the ammonium function of catecholamines so that catalysis of ATP cleavage would be somehow involved in the nucleation of a phase transition as well as calcium translocation at the membrane level. [This part of the model may appear unnecessary, and perhaps too speculative, because the nucleation of a phase transition need not be an ATP-requiring process.] In contrast, rapid repolarization may depend on energy supplies in the membrane, but this can hardly concern the catecholamine receptors per se. What may appear worth retaining, however, is the model of the calcium-protein complex in catecholamine nucleation of phase transitions in view of the newly established participation of calcium in the depolarization of the motor end plate receptors. Indeed, it could be shown that calcium is required for norepinephrine (NE) to nucleate the spurred state of the receptor, a physical form which is chemically less reactive than the resting conformation toward phenoxybenzamine (an alkylating agent) (57). Moreover, in the absence of calcium, NE could not protect against inactivation of the receptor by the latter alkylating drug, in accord with the model (57).

The reverse situation, where the spurred state would be chemically more reactive than the braced resting state, thus becomes equally plausible since the reactivity of a binding site may as easily be increased by a change of conformation. In fact, this has been observed for AChE as well as the motor end plate receptor. Therefore, evidence could be obtained which clearly confirms this expectation as regards the adrenergic α-receptor. Kalsner discovered that EEDQ, which induces the formation of an extremely stable amide bond at the active site level of the receptor (55), has its potency markedly enhanced by low concentrations of various phenethylamines including NE, as well as serotonin and even histamine (58). It seems evident that as for the AChE protoreceptor chain and the motor end plate receptor, some additional anionic binding sites for agonist structures must be present on the α-receptor surface so that interactions with these sites strongly enhance the reactivity of the EEDQ target site by way of an induced conformational change in the receptor (Figure 2). Independent evidence for the presence of at least two anionic sites on the α-receptor was provided by the following observations: (a) the bisalkylating agent I was recently shown to act as a very potent irreversible blocker of the α-receptor (59), this being the first time that a bisquaternary "curare analog" is found to display high affinity for this receptor system, and (b) very low concentrations of the alkylating agent DPA, which have no influence on the tissue response to NE, will nevertheless markedly alter the chemical characteristics of phenoxybenzamine action, receptor recovery being strongly accelerated when DPA is initially present on the surface (33). This also suggests that DPA alkylates an accessory anionic site and as a result, the receptor conformation is altered in a manner which renders the phenoxybenzamine–receptor bond much more liabile (alternatively, the DPA receptor species may expose a different active site to phenoxybenzamine). It is of considerable significance then that like the AChE protoreceptor chain and the end plate receptor, the adrenergic α-receptor should also possess more than one anionic site capable of interacting with adrenergic amines and other modifiers so that conformational changes may be induced as can be readily revealed by the chemical accessibility and reactivity of other specific sites. One is tempted to conclude that these three receptor systems are biophysically related. This conclusion may be more sensible than it appears since it accounts rather well for the puzzling fact that drugs (mostly receptor antagonists) do not discriminate too well between the ACh- and the catecholamine α-receptors. These new advances certainly offer more realistic guidelines than the older models in the general area of structure–activity relationships (*see below*).

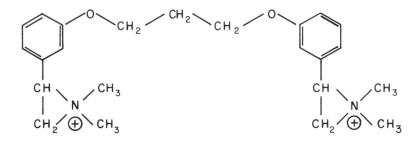

The β-receptor. That the enzyme adenyl cyclase is intimately associated with biogenic amine and peptide hormone action on β-receptors is now firmly established, and there is no doubt that cyclic AMP is the mediator responsible for the adaptive responses of a variety of target cells (*60, 61*). Evidence has also accumulated that cyclase is under the influence of regulatory subunits or discriminators endowed with tissue-dependent specificities (*60, 62*). A role for calcium, possibly as a second messenger of signal reception, at the membrane level has been demonstrated (*52*). We have recently shown that brain adenylcyclase may be calcium dependent, although it suffers inhibition at high concentrations (*63*). Hence, it appears that calcium is probably an essential component of all the receptor systems for neurotransmitters. In the light of these new developments, it becomes more and more evident that the earlier visualizations of a direct interaction of catecholamines with cyclase-bound ATP as a model for β-receptor activation (*2, 50, 64*) may not be applicable since regulatory subunits probably constitute the sites of binding and presumably the receptors themselves. Consequently, structure–activity relationships among β-receptor antagonists are no longer readily interpretable in terms of the older models although it remains to be proved that antagonists interact with the agonist binding sites themselves. In view of our finding that exo-binding predominates in other systems, it

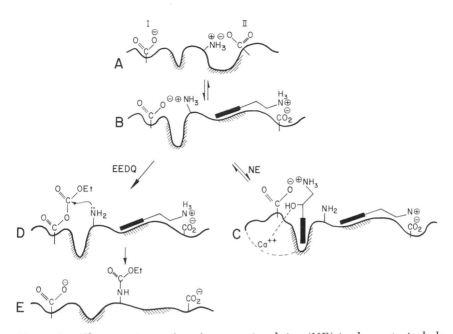

Figure 2. The receptor surface for norepinephrine (NE) is shown to include two anionic sites (A); phenethylamines and related structures (including histamine) interact at Site II and thus induce a conformation change (B) favoring NE binding at Site I, which in turn leads by way of another conformation change to the active, spurred state of the receptor (C). In the B state, the reaction at Site I with EEDQ is facilitated by the increased proximity of a surface nucleophile (–NH₂) to the mixed anhydride intermediate (D → E). Carbamylation of this nucleophile as in E leads to irreversible inactivation of the receptor.

appears likely that the same conceivably applies to β-receptor antagonists; otherwise Fisher's lock-and-key fit principle would be meaningless since both agonists and antagonists would have to share identical binding sites. Because β-receptors are mainly concerned with activation and inhibition of adaptive metabolic responses rather than with the direct generation of action potentials, it is probable that those biophysical parameters which intervene uniquely in neurotransmitter actions on excitable membranes may not be applicable to the β-receptors. This could account for the fact that most non-discriminating drugs which are known to inhibit the responses of excitable membranes have little, if any, effect on the β-receptors. Recently, however, it has been claimed that certain antidepressants (which are potentiators of adrenergic amines) influence the urinary levels of cyclic AMP by a mechanism presumably involving cyclic AMP-phosphodiesterase inhibition (65, 66). However, it is difficult to see how the accumulated brain cyclic AMP could traverse the cell membranes, the blood–brain barrier, the liver and kidneys among other tissues, and appear in the urine as brain cyclic AMP which has escaped the action of phosphodiesterase as a result of antidepressant inhibition of the latter.

The firm conclusion is reached that the catecholamine binding surfaces of the α- and β-receptors are different since most antagonists of the former do not inhibit the latter. It will be interesting to see whether molecular manipulations of the cyclic AMP structure will lead to new useful drugs. The prospects may appear good since cyclic AMP is involved in glycogenolysis, lipolysis, steroidogenesis, membrane permeability, translation, transcription, and as an activator of specific protein kinases (67). This latter property suggests that it may be involved at some metabolic stage in the phenomenon of memory fixation. In view of the sensitivity of various β-receptors to peptide hormones, much more attention may have to be devoted to the synthesis of peptide agonists and antagonists since improved specificity of action may be expected.

The Theory of Sequential Control Sites

In a projected paper, a comprehensive discussion of the nature and role of what we tentatively define as sequential control sites on receptor surfaces (and some regulatory enzymes) will be presented. We shall here be concerned only with those general aspects which are especially relevant to the problem of structure–activity relationships among drugs.

Recent evidence summarized and integrated above makes it clear that at least three receptor systems for cationic neurotransmitters include on their exposed surfaces several anionic binding sites where conformational changes may be initiated or blocked. These findings are at variance with the previous idea that only one active center is responsible for the observed effects induced by neurotransmitters. The systems studied include the motor end plate receptor and the putative protoreceptor chain of AChE, which both carry at least four drug-binding anionic sites per active unit, and the NE receptor, which carries at least two (and probably more such sites, in view of its apparent biophysical kinship to the other two systems). In any event, the exact number of anionic sites is not critical with regard to the basic mechanistic implications. The first question which comes to mind is: why should there be several topographically distinct anionic sites for neurotransmitters when only one should be necessary to nucleate the spurred physical state of these receptors? Considerations of a biophysical nature may provide the basis of an answer to this question. First, it can be agreed that the velocity of nerve impulse transmission across the synaptic gap should occur at the maximum speed attainable, which ideally would require the transmitter to travel at a rate approaching that of diffusion-controlled processes. Hence, the transmitter should be minimally hindered by the natural diffusion barriers to its key sites of action on the post-synaptic receptor surface. Near the receptor surface the problem of timing and efficiency of productive captures can be handled simply by reducing the dimensionality in which diffusion takes place, from three-dimensional to two-dimensional surface diffusion, a fundamental process which has been given a solid quantitative theoretical basis by Adam and Delbrück (68). These authors pointed out that "in the intermediate range of distances of a few microns a new principle may be involved in that the diffusing molecules reach their destination area not directly by free diffusion in three-dimensional space but by subdividing the diffusion process into successive stages of lower spatial dimensionality." Accordingly, if the effector molecule sticks loosely to some sites, diffusion along the surface will be favored (Figure 3) so that the catch at some other key sites will be significantly improved, a consequence of considerable evolutionary advantage for synaptic membrane surfaces and their receptors since shorter reaction times and economic use of low transmitter concentrations are ensured. Bücher (60) has pointed out that surface diffusion may well contribute to the high turnover numbers of membrane-bound enzymes, and the concept was indeed applied even earlier by Trurnit (70) to the system AChE–ACh. It is apparent then that a network comprising several anionic sites on the protoreceptor chain of AChE may contribute enormously to the high rate of catch at any one site, provided that the cationic molecules do not interact too strongly with certain anionic sites as they occur on the resting state of the receptor surface. For this to happen, a lower degree of complementarity of the natural effector or substrate with certain sites may be necessary; otherwise surface displacements might become too sluggish. It may be convenient then to speak of sequential control sites as a natural means of handling the problem of timing and efficiency in the productive catch of nucleators on the surface (Figure 3).

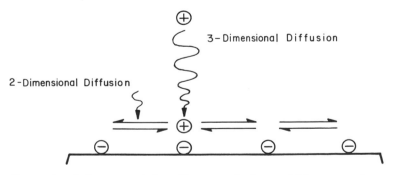

Figure 3.   Schematic of the efficiency of effector (+) capture by a surface carrying multiple anionic sites. Transfer from one site to the other involves two-dimensional translocations, thus leading to a much improved efficiency and timing of catch at any given site.

Well-developed sequential control sites, where conformational changes can be induced, should be especially prevalent among receptor surfaces for neurotransmitters in view of the rapidity with which interneuronal communications must be established in the CNS as an example.

In principle, for effective nucleation and optimum stabilization of the spurred state of the receptors, only one strategic anionic site may need interact with the nucleator, but it seems much more probable that weaker interactions with some control sites may contribute in a cooperative manner to the stability of the spurred state. The immediate environment of the anionic sites will obviously differ from one site to another, and their respective chemical reactivity will be altered by conformational changes, thus providing an explanation for the recent observations (summarized above) with EEDQ (58), curarizing agents (42), and adrenergic α-blockers of the alkylating variety (33). In addition, and most importantly, the sequential control site model allows the prediction that high concentrations of nucleators may saturate some unoccupied sites as they occur in the spurred state of the receptor. This would cause the latter to suffer conformational blockade or freezing (Figure 4), as would be reflected, for instance, in the phenomena of desensitization, tachyphylaxis, etc. Indeed, an excess of ACh will induce "curarization" of the end plate membrane, as would be expected if additional ACh molecules saturate the control sites of the receptor when in the spurred or activated state.

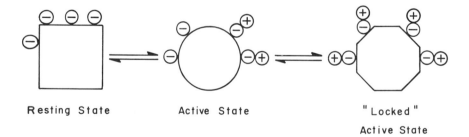

Resting State   Active State   "Locked"
                                             Active State

Figure 4. Schematic of a formal conformational equilibrium between the resting and active state of the excitable membrane receptor of the motor end plate. In the latter state two strategic sites are occupied, and two control sites are free; when saturation of the latter is enforced by an excess of effector molecules, the active state is changed to a more stable "frozen" conformation, leading to prolonged depolarization of the membrane.

Topographical Symmetry *vs*. Molecular Quasi-Symmetry. The microscopic environment of each sequential control site will obviously have its own characteristics, and in view of the postulated lower complementarity of the neurotransmitter for these sequential control sites, the structural requirements for antagonist binding may be much less rigorous than at strategic sites, and strong binding should be favored when the drug

structure is stereoelectronically compatible with the microenvironment of
any one of the control sites. Hence, many structures bearing only a modest analogy (if any at all) to the neurotransmitters may preferably
interact strongly with the control sites rather than the strategic ones where
the neurotransmitter achieves a "lock-and-key fit." Consequently, the
antagonists will perturb the receptor conformation, and if cooperativity
is also achieved, very high potencies may occasionally be observed.
Assuming that a drug can interact with more than one control area at a
time, the receptor conformation may be changed or stabilized more
effectively since a greater degree of over-all complementarity would be
achieved. Of the multitude of orientations which an effector such as
ACh can assume at any two vicinal sequential sites, there exist two where
the molecules will be arranged in tail-to-tail fashion (Figure 5). This is
what would obtain, for instance, if displacement from one site to another
neighboring site is accomplished through a 180° rotational motion. For
this to happen, the two adjacent control areas where the molecules are
interacting might be topographically enantiomeric or possess opposing
physical chiralities. Accordingly, effector molecules possessing suitable

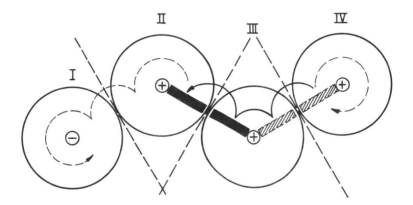

*Figure 5.   Schematic of sequential control sites on the surfaces of the
motor end plate receptor and the protoreceptor chain of acetylcholinesterase. Each circle encompasses an area sufficiently large to accommodate one molecule of acetylcholine. The arrows represent the short-
est possible paths of surface displacements from one site to the other.
In two positions of the effector, a tail-to-tail arrangement is possible
when two molecules are bound on two vicinal binding areas. This
raises the possibility that the two adjacent areas might possess suitable
elements of topographical symmetry or dissymmetry (the planes being
represented by dotted lines). The prediction may then be allowed that
symmetrical, doubly charged effectors (such as succinyldicholine) might
display complementarity with two areas at a time. Hence, each half
of the effector molecule could bear a mirror image relationship to the
other (meso configurations) for optimal interaction with two adjacent
areas at a time (see text and Figure 6).*

elements of symmetry might allow for simultaneous quasi-complemental interactions with two control areas. This may encourage tighter and more selective binding, as well as increased potency if the control sites act cooperatively in the stabilization of a given receptor conformation. The following observations offer substantial support for this topographical theory. Succinyldicholine, a symmetrical molecule resulting from the tail-to-tail fusion of two ACh molecules, is one of the most potent and best known depolarizers of the motor end plate membrane as well as the most effective conformation modifier of the anionic protoreceptor chain of AChE. The postulated topographically enantiomeric relation between the adjacent control areas (Figure 6) involved in the binding of this

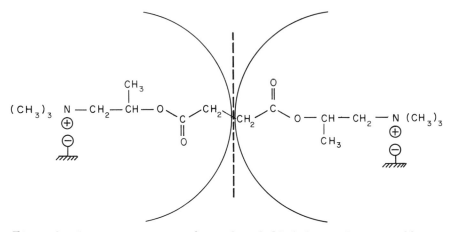

Figure 6.   Interaction of succinyl-β,β'-dimethyldicholine with two neighboring anionic areas. If the latter display a topographical plane of symmetry or dissymmetry (dotted line), the meso isomer should interact optimally, but not the L,L- *or* D,D-*enantiomers. This model agrees with experiment (see text).*

effector is supported by the fact that, whereas the D,D- and L,L-succinyl-β,β'-dimethyldocholine are essentially inactive in both systems, the meso isomer is fairly active (about one-third the activity of succinyldicholine) both at the receptor and enzyme levels (unpublished results) (Figure 6). Moreover, an impressive number of potent curarizing agents are either symmetrical or quasi-symmetrical molecules (such as the toxiferins, tubocurarine, etc). However, as noted above, some of the conformationally sensitive control sites may be less demanding than the strategic site(s) from the stereoelectronic standpoint, and, accordingly, ion–ion interactions [which supply most of the binding energy (7)] with molecules displaying lower degrees of symmetry will also be allowed, which explains why such a vast number of bisquaternary ions are known to possess curarizing activity to some degree. A corollary of considerable importance is that any receptor system which, like the motor end plate receptor or the protoreceptor chain of AChE, is capable of interacting with similarly diverse drug structures may also possess sequential control binding sites where conformational perturbations of one kind or another may be induced. Accordingly, at least two other receptor systems would also include such sites: the adrenergic α-receptor, for which concrete evidence was already given for the presence of accessory sites on its surface, and the analgesic receptor, which is known to respond to as wide a variety of structural types as the curare receptor.

For the neurotransmitter norepinephrine, symmetry considerations similar to those applied above to the succinyldicholine binding sites allow the prediction that quasi-symmetrically disposed binding areas for aromatic rings may be present on the receptor surface (Figure 7), and if the conformational and electronic properties of the drug are compatible with the detailed topography, unproductive physical states may be readily induced in the receptor. The sequential control areas being quasi-symmetrically disposed, the basis of an explanation for the well-established

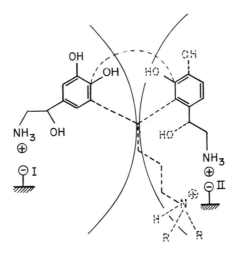

Figure 7. Schematic of the receptor surface for norepinephrine (NE). Site II is selective for phenethylamine patterns (including histamine and serotonin), and Site I for catecholamines. Hence, the vicinal control areas include aromatic binding sites, possibly separated by a plane of topographical dissymmetry. Interactions at Site II cause a conformational change which enhances the EEDQ reaction at Site I (see Figure 2). The spatial arrangement of the aromatic ring binding areas could well fit the structural pattern of the quasi-symmetrical "diphenylmethane" series of drugs (dotted lines).

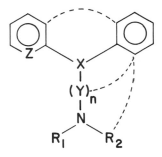

Figure 8. General structure-type, based on the "magic" diphenylmethane pattern of symmetrical skeleton as found in many drugs affecting cholinergic, adrenergic, and histaminergic receptors

recurrence of the "magic" diphenylmethane pattern in a wide variety of drugs may be at hand (Figure 8). Among drugs currently in use which are based on the diphenylmethane pattern, one finds antidepressants, antihistamines, neuroleptics, stimulants, sympatholytics, parasympatholytics, analgesics, etc. Because of the less specific nature of some of the control sites, many of these drugs are not receptor specific. Specificity may be achieved only by capitalizing on the subtle conformational and topographical differences which must distinguish one receptor surface from the other. Concrete model evidence for this view will be published elsewhere. Suffice it to say that this is what is most probably accomplished when the medicinal chemist introduces conformational restrictions (such as bridging) in the diphenylmethane skeleton or when he slightly alters symmetry by incorporating ring substituents (Figure 7). One area of research which appears not to have been explored would be the designing of novel symmetrical or quasi-symmetrical molecules based on the fusion of catecholamine-like rings in various tail-to-tail patterns in the manner successfully applied to curarizing agents. Indeed, we have already applied the principle successfully in the case of the potent symmetrical bisalkylating adrenergic blocker (I) (59) described above.

Finally, one of the most perverse concatenations of receptor properties is found in the area of narcotic analgesics and their antagonists. No theory of structure–activity relationships has survived very long in this field, although recently some interesting studies of the subtle configurational specificity of the receptor have been initiated by Portoghese (71). The only point which may be worth emphasizing at this time is that the extreme conformational diversity of drugs acting at this level is strongly reminiscent of the broad adaptability of the motor end plate receptor. This parallelism suggests that the analgesic receptor may similarly include several sequential control sites on its surface where the principle of topographical quasi-symmetry may be operative (indeed, several strong analgesics belong to the diphenylmethane pattern of symmetrical skeleton). Some practical implications of this concept in the design of novel classes of potential analgesics are rather obvious. With regard to the molecular basis of narcotic-analgesic and narcotic-antagonist actions, the possibility of an analogy with depolarizer and non-depolarizer actions on the motor end plate receptor may deserve consideration. At the moment, it may be worthwhile considering the hypothesis that narcotic analgesics might produce a prolonged, perhaps cooperative perturbation or distortion of the spurred physical state of receptors in the manner which characterizes depolarizers of the end plate membrane whereas narcotic antagonists may stabilize the resting physical state of the receptor, by analogy with tubocurarine-like agents which block their receptor without membrane depolarization. This could account for the fact that certain narcotic antagonists can also display analgesic activity since the receptor would also be blocked, albeit by a different molecular mechanism conducive to a different membrane configuration. If this were true, physical dependence on morphinoids might be linked to membrane collapse by way of a prolonged "depolarization" type of receptor conformational change. In any event, the sequential control site theory for neurotransmitters readily accounts for the occurrence of morphine-like activity in several types of loosely related classes of structures. Finally, it may be worthwhile considering the possibility that certain mental deficiencies or aberrations may be linked, not necessarily to alterations in neurotransmitter availability, but to inborn or acquired defects in the sequential control sites. This would obviously be reflected in a less effective rate of catch by the sensitive membranes and decreased effectiveness of interneuronal communications.

Acknowledgments

The research of the past few years on which this presentation is in part based was generously supported by the National Research Council of Canada, the Defence Research Board of Canada, and Bristol Laboratories. The skillful collaboration of V. DiTullio, J-L. Lavoie, H. Tani, Y-H Tsai, E. Wülfert, I. Macdonald, B. Lippert, and D. Godin, and M. DiTullio, made this research possible.

Literature Cited

(1) Belleau, B., *Can. J. Biochem.* (1958) **36,** 731.
(2) Belleau, B., in "Adrenergic Mechanisms," CIBA Foundation Symposium, J. R. Vane, G. E. W. Wolstenholme and M. O'Connor, Eds., p. 223, Churchill, London, 1960.

(3) Kauzmann, W., *Advan. Protein Chem.* (1959) **14**, 1.
(4) Baker, B. R., "Design of Active-Site-Directed Irreversible Enzyme Inhibitors," Wiley, New York, 1967.
(5) Belleau, B., Lacasse, G., *J. Med. Chem.* (1964) **7**, 768.
(6) Hansch, C., *Accounts Chem. Res.* (1969) **2**, 232.
(7) Belleau, B., Lavoie, J.-L., *Can. J. Biochem.* (1968) **46**, 1397.
(8) Lumry, R., Rajender, S., *Biopolymers* (1970) **9**, 1125.
(9) Belleau, B., *J. Med. Chem.* (1964) **7**, 776.
(10) Belleau, B., *Ann. N.Y. Acad. Sci.* (1967) **144**, 705.
(11) Belleau, B., DiTullio, V., *J. Amer. Chem. Soc.* (1970) **92**, 6320.
(12) Ariëns, E. J., in "Molecular Pharmacology," E. J. Ariëns, Ed., Vol. I, Academic, New York, 1964.
(13) Higman, H. B., Podleski, T. R., Bartels, E., *Biochim. Biophys. Acta* (1963) **75**, 187.
(14) Koshland, D. E., Jr., Nemethy, G., Filmer, D., *Biochemistry* (1966) **5**, 365.
(15) Monod, J., Wyman, J., Changeux, J.-P., *J. Mol. Biol.* (1965) **12**, 88.
(16) Changeux, J.-P., Thiéry, J., Tung, Y., Kittel, C., *Proc. Nat. Acad. Sci. U.S.* (1967) **57**, 335.
(17) Strässler, S., Kittel, C., *Phys. Rev.* (1965) **139**, A758.
(18) Conway, A., Koshland, D. E., *Biochemistry* (1968) **7**, 4011.
(19) Hamilton, C. L., McConnell, H. M., in "Structural Chemistry and Molecular Biology," A. Rich and N. Davidson, Eds., p. 115, Freeman, San Francisco, 1968.
(20) Hill, T. L., Yid-der Chen, *Proc. Nat. Acad. Sci. U.S.* (1970) **66**, 189.
(21) Giacommetti, G., in "Structural Chemistry and Molecular Biology," A. Rich and N. Davidson, Eds., p. 67, Freeman, San Francisco, 1968.
(22) Bartels, E., *Biochem. Pharmacol.* (1968) **17**, 945.
(23) Nomura, M., *Proc. Nat. Acad. Sci. U.S.* (1964) **52**, 1514.
(24) Karlin, A., *J. Gen. Physiol.* (1969) **54**, 245.
(25) Moran, J. F., Triggle, D. J., in "Fundamental Concepts in Drug-Receptor Interactions," J. F. Danielli, J. F. Moran, and D. J. Triggle, Eds., p. 113, Academic, New York, 1970.
(26) O'Brien, R. D., Gilmour, L. P., *Proc. Nat. Acad. Sci. U.S.* (1969) **63**, 496.
(27) Belleau, B., in "Fundamental Concepts in Drug-Receptor Interactions," J. F. Danielli, J. F. Moran, and D. J. Triggle, Eds., p. 121, Academic, New York, 1970.
(28) Karlin, A., Winnik, M., *Proc. Nat. Acad. Sci. U.S.* (1969) **60**, 668.
(29) Karlin, A., *Proc. Internat. Symp. Cholinergic Mechanisms CNS*, Skokloster, Sweden, Feb. 1970.
(30) Csillik, B., Savay, G., *Nature* (1963) **198**, 399.
(31) Nakamura, T., Namba, T., Grob, D., *J. Histochem. Cytochem.* (1967) **15**, 276.
(32) Tazieff-Depierre, F., Lièvremont, M. M., Gzajka, M., *Compt. rend. Acad. Sci. (Paris)* (1968) **267**, 2383.
(33) Moran, J. F., Triggle, D. J., *Life Sciences* (1970).
(34) Belleau, B., in "Physico-Chemical Aspects of Drug Action," E. J. Ariëns, Ed., p. 207, Pergamon, Oxford, 1968.
(35) Belleau, B., Tani, H., Lie, F., *J. Amer. Chem. Soc.* (1965) **87**, 2283.
(36) Belleau, B., DiTullio, V., *Can. J. Biochem.*, in press.
(37) Belleau, B., Tani, H., *Mol. Pharmacol.* (1966) **2**, 411.
(38) Purdie, J. E., *Biochim. Biophys. Acta* (1969) **185**, 122.
(39) Purdie, J. E., McIvor, R. A., *Biochim. Biophys. Acta* (1966) **128**, 590.
(40) Kitz, R., Wilson, I. B., *J. Biol. Chem.* (1963) **238**, 745.
(41) Belleau, B., in "Advances in Drug Research," N. J. Harper and A. B. Simmonds, Eds., Vol. 2, p. 89, Academic, London, 1965.
(42) Belleau, B., DiTullio, V., Tsai, Y.-H., *Mol. Pharmacol.* (1970) **6**, 41.

(43) Leuzinger, W., in "Cholinergic Ligand Interactions," D. J. Triggle, E. A. Barnard, and J. F. Moran, Eds., Academic, New York, in press.

(44) Leuzinger, W., Goldberg, M., Cauvin, E., *J. Mol. Biol.* (1969) **40**, 217.

(45) Rang, H. P., Ritter, J. M., *Mol. Pharmacol.* (1969) **5**, 394.

(46) DiTullio, V., Belleau, B., in preparation.

(47) Karlin, A., *Biochim. Biophys. Acta* (1967) **139**, 358.

(48) Beckett, A. H., *Ann. N.Y. Acad. Sci.* (1967) **144**, 675.

(49) Archer, S., Wylie, D. W., Harris, L. S., Lewis, T. R., Schulenberg, J. W., Bell, M. R., Hallnig, R. K., Arnold, A., *J. Amer. Chem. Soc.* (1962) **84**, 1306.

(50) Bloom, B. M., Goldman, J. M., in "Advances in Drug, Research," N. J. Harper and A. B. Simmonds, Eds., Vol. 3, p. 121, Academic, London, 1966.

(51) Hillarp, N. Å., Högberg, B., Nilson, B., *Nature* (1955) **176**, 1032.

(52) Nagata, N., Rasmussen, H., *Proc. Nat. Acad. Sci. U.S.* (1970) **65**, 368.

(53) Belleau, B., Martel, R., Lacasse, G., Ménard, M., Weinberg, N. L., Perron, Y. G., *J. Amer. Chem. Soc.* (1968) **90**, 823.

(54) Belleau, B., DiTullio, V., Godin, D., *Biochim. Pharmacol.* (1969) **18**, 1039.

(55) Martel, R., Berman, R., Belleau, B., *Can. J. Physiol. Pharmacol.* (1969) **47**, 909.

(56) Belleau, B., *Ann. N.Y. Acad. Sci.* (1967) **139**, 580.

(57) Tuttle, R. R., Moran, N. C., *J. Pharmac. Exptl. Therap.* (1969) **169**, 255.

(58) Kalsner, S., *Life Sciences* (1970).

(59) Belleau, B., Tani, H., *Can. J. Pharm. Sci.* (1969) **4**, 14.

(60) Bär, H. P., Hechter, O., *Proc. Nat. Acad. Sci. U.S.* (1969) **63**, 350.

(61) Sutherland, E. W., Robison, G. A., *Pharmacol. Rev.* (1966) **18**, 145.

(62) Robison, G. A., Butcher, R. W., Sutherland, E. W., *Ann. N.Y. Acad. Sci.* (1967) **139**, 703.

(63) Macdonald, I. A., Ph.D. Thesis, University of Ottawa (1971).

(64) Belleau, B., *Pharmacol. Rev.* (1966) **18** (I), 131.

(65) Paul, M. I., Ditzin, B. R., Janowski, D. S., *Lancet* (Jan. 10, 1970) 88.

(66) Abdulla, Y. H., Hamada, K., *Lancet* (Feb. 21, 1970) 378.

(67) Kuo, J. F., Greengard, P., *Proc. Nat. Acad. Sci. U.S.* (1969) **64**, 1349.

(68) Adam, G., Delbrück, M., in "Structural Chemistry and Molecular Biology," A. Rich and N. Davidson, Eds., p. 198, Freeman, San Francisco, 1968.

(69) Bücher, T., *Advan. Enzymol.* (1953) **14**, 1.

(70) Trurnit, H. J., *Fortschr. Chem. organ. Naturst.* (1945) **4**, 347.

(71) Portoghese, P. S., *J. Med. Chem.* (1965) **8**, 609.

RECEIVED November 5, 1970.

7

The Biological Knowledge Gap

J. J. BURNS

Hoffmann-La Roche Inc., Nutley, N. J. 07110

New drug development—so rapid during the past 20 years—has slowed because advances in biological science have failed to keep pace with those in medicinal chemistry. Despite successes cited in psychotherapeutic and anti-inflammatory drug development, further progress in these areas is hampered by inadequate knowledge of fundamental disease processes and of the mechanism of action of existing drugs. Where more adequate knowledge exists, as in gout and Parkinson's disease, important new drugs have been developed recently. Others can be expected from basic research in drug metabolism and molecular biology now under way in the pharmaceutical industry. However, to avoid unnecessary delay in introducing future drugs, universities, government, and industry must cooperate in formulating criteria for evaluating drug safety and efficacy.

The last 20 years have seen the rapid development of new drugs, largely because of the advances in medicinal chemistry discussed in this volume. Future development, however, will be more difficult. While medicinal chemistry has advanced by finding new methods for synthesizing complicated molecules and isolating and identifying the active substances from plants, bacteria, and mammals, our biologic knowledge has failed to keep pace. We lack basic knowledge of drug action and of disease processes in man, and this lack is certain to delay future advances, especially in treating diseases such as cancer, congenital disease, and viral infections. Even when new drugs are developed, their introduction is often delayed because medical opinions differ on what constitutes valid safety and efficacy data. In short, we are confronted by a widening biological knowledge gap.

Progress in Developing Psychotherapeutic Agents

The rapid development of psychotherapeutic agents and their success in treating mental and emotional disorders was one of the more significant achievements of the pharmaceutical industry in the last two decades. Since clinicians first recognized neuroleptic, antidepressant, and tranquilizing effects of certain drugs, laboratory scientists have sought to understand their psychopharmacology and to develop techniques for discovering improved drugs. These scientists devised behavioral, electrophysiological, and biochemical concepts and techniques and, indeed, have obtained a wealth of information on how such drugs interact with biological systems. Behavioral pharmacology techniques have advanced to the point where they now form the hard core of the pharmacological profile of neuroleptics and tranquilizers. Still, we lack much important information in this area.

One of the most challenging problems has been the search for ways to recognize drugs useful in depression. Since attempts to develop animal models of depression by using drugs to depress the central nervous system have proved less than successful, other approaches have been tried; for example, empirical techniques have been used to evaluate the ability of potential antidepressant agents to antagonize tetrabenazine and reserpine, to potentiate amphetamine or cocaine, and to block the uptake of norepinephrine, yet the limitations of such techniques have become increasingly obvious. They are useful for predicting activity in closely analogous compounds within a chemical class known to be clinically effective, but they are much less useful in predicting such activity in a new chemical class. Admittedly, the evidence that some antidepressants decrease norepinephrine uptake is conceptually appealing, but whether this can predict antidepressant activity has yet to be demonstrated.

We have been more successful in identifying and developing effective neuroleptics (chloropromazine-like drugs) or tranquilizers (meprobamate-like, and chlordiazepoxide-like drugs). Our success has been largely the result of new techniques in behavioral pharmacology. For example, inhibition of conditioned avoidance behavior is generally accepted as a good predictor of chlorpromazine- or haloperidol-like antipsychotic activity. However, once again, compounds different from the established, clinically effective chemical series have failed to produce the effects predicted on the basis of this test. Obviously, we will need greater understanding if we are to identify new and unrelated chemicals with improved therapeutic properties.

There is a great deal of enthusiasm and increasing confidence in the value of anticonflict properties of tranquilizers in animals for predicting anti-anxiety properties in man. To date, the correlation is indeed impressive and appears reliable. Anti-aggressive activity, a predominant property of many neuroleptic and tranquilizing agents, also seems to have predictive value.

Further research in psychopharmaceuticals is obviously important, but our interests should be focused on the areas of greatest medical need. One such area is schizophrenia. No matter how effective today's drugs are, more effective ones will be required.

Moreover, research is needed in new areas, such as learning and memory. Drugs to enhance the performance of patients with mental retardation, senility, and other mental deficiencies would clearly constitute a major contribution. Fortunately, sufficient knowledge exists to begin meaningful research. We can measure learning and memory performance, and certain drugs do enhance such performance. We also have evidence of the possible role of macromolecules in learning-memory functions. Now we need to elucidate further the relationship between animal behavior and intellectual functions in man and also the relationships of relevant neurobiochemical and neurophysiological functions. The task of investigating drugs that may enhance such functions is formidable because clinically effective standards do not exist. These are the challenges we face.

Animal Models for Evaluating Anti-Inflammatory Drugs

In man, arthritis produces pain, swelling, redness, and increased temperature of joints. In animals, the same symptoms can be produced as part of an inflammatory process in which membrane permeability increases leading to cellular destruction. This inflammation, induced by such substances as phenylquinone, carrageenin, and yeast, can be partially prevented by anti-inflammatory drugs, such as aspirin and phenylbutazone. Screening with these tests, scientists were able to select indomethacin and mefanamic acid from large groups of compounds. However, with these same tests they identified many other compounds, which they later had to discard as false positives or producers of toxic effects, particularly ulcerogenic effects.

A more recent model of inflammation is the killed Mycobacterium adjuvant arthritis test. Besides an acute inflammatory phase, it produces a secondary phase characterized by induction of an inflammatory lesion at sites distant from the initial lesion and also by the development of biochemical alterations measured by changes in blood fibrinogen, mucopolysaccharides and α-globulin. These distant changes may be mediated by the kinin systems, such as bradykinin. This new model is affected by most drugs active in the human arthritis and promises better predictive value than earlier models, which measured primarily the acute phases. It permits measuring in man and animals such biochemical parameters as inflammation units related to the α-globulins. Such measurements may

increase our understanding of the arthritic process and give better pre-
dictability for new classes of compounds.

After promising compounds are identified in animals, formidable
problems of drug absorption, blood levels, ulcerogenic activity, and liver
toxicity must be solved. A huge effort has been mounted by major pharmaceutical houses in the synthesis of anti-inflammatory compounds, evaluation by current animal models, extended pharmacological examination,
toxicity studies, pharmacodynamic studies, and the subjective screening
in arthritic patients. So far, this costly effort has not been very productive; no drug has been found to be superior to aspirin in efficacy and
safety for long-term use, yet there is room for much improvement. No
drug cures arthritis. No drug affects the immunoligic aspects of the human
disease, and meaningful animal models are almost nonexistent. The fact
that many screening tests are unreliable indicators of drug efficacy in man
presents a problem in interpretation. Screening results must be considered carefully before deciding to begin the vast effort required to complete
the development of a new drug. If a pharmacologist should discover an
active compound tomorrow, six years or more might elapse before it could
be introduced to the medical profession.

Deficient Knowledge of Drug Action and Disease Processes

The search for new drugs would be greatly facilitated if we knew
more about currently used drugs. In fact, we know surprisingly little
about the mechanism of action of such widely used drugs as aspirin,
barbiturates, the phenothiazines, morphine, and anti-inflammatory agents
—phenylbutazone and indomethacin. If, for example, we knew how
phenylbutazone exerts its therapeutic effect in rheumatoid arthritis, we
could develop a more rational screening program.

We also need to know more about the disease to be treated. Just
having suitable animal models of human disease helps by furnishing more
reliable screening tests. Lack of such models has hindered arthritis research, and the availability of animal models has contributed to our
limited success in hypertension and hyperlipemia research.

An example of the value of understanding the nature of the disease
is the considerable progress made in gout therapy. Gout is characterized
by an overproduction of uric acid, which accumulates in the body, resulting in a painful arthritic condition. Drugs, such as probenecid and sulfin-
pyrazone, reduce uric acid levels by promoting its excretion in the urine.
However, these drugs are less effective in gouty patients with impaired
renal function. For such patients the development of allopurinol, which
inhibits the synthesis of uric acid, has offered an effective new therapy.
Allopurinol acts by inhibiting xanthine oxidase, the key enzyme for con-

verting xanthine through hypoxanthine to uric acid. The xanthine precursors are excreted more rapidly than uric acid, and thus they do not accumulate (1).

Another example is levodopa, a promising drug for Parkinson's disease. It was made possible because of our considerable knowledge of the metabolism and biological action of levodopa and catecholamines in general. Parkinsonism patients have lowered levels of dopamine in specific areas of the brain. But since dopamine does not penetrate into the brain to any appreciable extent, it was necessary to administer its precursor, levodopa, to correct the deficiency. Subsequently, Cotzias (2) contributed to the successful treatment of Parkinsonism by showing that large doses of levodopa were most effective.

Advances in Drug Metabolism and Molecular Biology

Drug metabolism studies have grown increasingly important. A common approach in many laboratories is to ask whether a new drug is active in its own right or whether it owes its activity and side effects to one or more metabolites. This approach has resulted in improved drugs for the treatment of rheumatoid arthritis, gout, mental depression, and schistosomiasis. Also, increased knowledge of drug metabolism has furnished clues to the synthesis of compounds with more desirable absorption, excretion, metabolism, and tissue distribution characteristics.

Drug metabolism studies have been revolutionized by physical chemical techniques such as mass spectrometry and nuclear magnetic resonance. They make possible metabolism studies in a few weeks that previously would have taken months or years. Pharmaceutical laboratories have set up extensive programs in drug metabolism research, which should establish a basis for the future drug development.

The past decade will surely be remembered for the notable advances in molecular biology. Much information is now becoming available: the steps in the expression of genetic information, the intricate details of transcription and translation, and the mechanisms whereby DNA directs protein synthesis. All this will surely help solve some of our current problems, but we need much more information. Only by understanding biochemical changes accompanying viral infection can we rationally search for antiviral drugs. Only by understanding how knowledge is stored and recalled in the central nervous system and whether macromolecules are involved in the memory process can we systematically seek drugs to alter learning and memory. In the foreseeable future, striking advances can be expected in treating those genetic defects in which specific proteins are missing or so altered as to produce a metabolic lesion.

To achieve these advances, pharmaceutical firms have increasingly emphasized research in molecular biology. Hoffmann-La Roche has set up the Roche Institute of Molecular Biology with a staff of 200, including 70 at the doctorate level (3, 4). These scientists have freedom to select basic research problems based solely on scientific merit. They have access to all the firm's modern facilities and can collaborate if they wish with company scientists on problems that might be impossible to solve with the limited facilities and staff of the usual academic institution.

The Need for Safety and Efficacy Criteria

An important gap exists in our knowledge of the best means to evaluate the safety and efficacy of drugs. Often we discover a compound with potentially valuable therapeutic effects in animals only to have its use in human disease limited by toxicity. Or perhaps the drug must be abandoned because the clinical investigator cannot establish its efficacy in man. Species differ greatly: a drug may act one way in the dog, another way in the rat, and still another way in man. How then can we extrapolate pharmacological and toxicological data from animal to man? Recent studies show that metabolic differencies explain many of the variations in species response. Thus, using drug metabolism data we can, with more certainty, infer drug action in man from pharmacological-toxicological studies in animals.

To evaluate the safety of a compound, it must be given to animals for extended periods—periods as long as one to two years in rodents and, in some instances, even longer in dogs. Recent research shows that the metabolism of many drugs is accelerated markedly after repeated administration, and this may lead to less toxicity with continued dosage. Such information bears importantly on the interpretation and design of chronic toxicity tests.

Determining the significance of malformations produced in animals with high doses of a new drug poses difficult problems (5). An overreaction to the thalidomide disaster has fostered an attempt to ensure complete safety by animal experimentation. This admittedly is an impossible goal; under certain circumstances, even such commonly used drugs as aspirin cause malformations in rats and other animals. Clearly, more research is necessary to establish better protocols for these studies and their interpretation.

In recent years people have become concerned about the possibility of genetic damage caused by drugs as well as pesticides, food ingredients and additives, industrial chemicals, and other substances in the environment (6, 7). At present, no one can predict the risk to future human generations based on chemical mutagenic tests in bacteria, molds, fruit flies, and human cells in tissue culture. A conference on "Evaluation of Mutagenic Effects of Chemicals" held Nov. 4–6, 1970 in Washington, D. C., was sponsored by the Drug Research Board of the National Academy of Sciences–National Research Council, together with the Environmental Mutagen Society, the National Institute of General Medical Sciences, Food and Drug Administration, and the Pharmaceutical Manufacturers Association Foundation. The participants in this conference evaluated varying approaches to mutagenic testing and considered new areas of research (8).

Public concern has focused on the possible carcinogenic effects of drugs and other chemicals. Long-term chronic toxicity studies in a variety of species have been started in the hope of minimizing potential risk of cancer in man. However, the results of such studies are difficult, sometimes impossible, to interpret. Yet their economic impact can be enormous, as shown by the withdrawal of cyclamates when bladder cancer was observed in a limited number of rodents. Inevitably drugs will be affected too; already the safety of certain oral contraceptives has been questioned because of possible carcinogenic effects in the breasts of dogs after extended use.

Immunologic effects of drugs remain unpredictable based on animal test data, despite intensive research effort. The pharmaceutical industry has reason for concern; the rare occurrence of blood dyscrasia, even with a needed drug, can seriously limit its use. Years of work on chloramphenicol, for example, have failed to discover why it depresses the bone marrow in some individuals. Nor have scientists learned to predict such severe skin reactions as exfoliative dermatitis from experimental studies. Fortunately, progress in predicting penicillin sensitivity justifies a degree of optimism that similar progress can be made with other drugs.

No discussion of the biological knowledge gap would be complete without mentioning drug abuse. This is one of the most critical problems of our time, yet our understanding of the pharmacology of abuse is almost totally deficient. Why do some individuals abuse narcotics, LSD, marijuana, or amphetamines? How can we predict, based on animal tests, the abuse potential of a new compound? Right now we can only infer abuse potential for compounds related chemically or pharmacologically to drugs with known abuse potential. What is the mechanism of tolerance and addiction? Perhaps there is an immunological basis for morphine and heroin tolerence. Perhaps induction of drug metabolizing enzymes in liver microsomes may explain tolerance to some barbiturates. More research is required to answer these questions.

A major problem in therapy is individual differences in drug response apparently controlled by genetic factors (9). What is a safe dose for one patient may be either ineffective or toxic in another because of faster or slower metabolic transformation. Patients may receive several drugs simultaneously which poses the question of drug interactions (*10*). A variety of drug interactions have been reported, including the ability of one drug to stimulate or inhibit the metabolism of another, interference with renal mechanisms, displacement of drugs that bind to plasma proteins, and interference with intestinal absorption. Almost certainly, investigation of genetic factors and drug interaction will help explain adverse reactions and lead to improved drug safety.

The Work of Government and Industry Groups

In recent years the World Health Organization has published several reports on the principles of safety evaluation (*11*) as has the Committee on Problems of Drug Safety of the National Academy of Sciences–National Research Council (*12*). The committee has studied the question of how much metabolic data is useful at each stage in the investigation of a new drug and surveyed the status and future needs for drug safety research. It has also attempted to familiarize pharmacologists, biochemists, and medicinal chemists with the theoretical and practical aspects of drug metabolism studies. It has held symposiums to review advances in developmental pharmacology, immunopharmacology, mechanism of drug oxidation, chemical mutagenesis, adverse drug reactions reporting systems, and an application of newer physical techniques for drug metabolism study.

Through program project and center grants and through contracts with pharmaceutical firms, the Pharmacology-Toxicology Program of the National Institute of General Medical Sciences has investigated many questions concerned with drug safety. These program and center grants speed the study of drug safety in man by grouping together first-rate scientists in pharmacology, medicinal chemistry and the basic sciences. The Pharmaceutical Manufacturers Association Foundation has also furnished grants to many universities to study mechanisms of drug toxicity.

Government and industry organizations have considered what constitutes adequate clinical efficacy as well as safety—especially the difficult problem of efficacy data for anticonvulsant, analgesic, and psychopharmacologic agents. Particularly noteworthy is the effort of a combined Task Force of the American College of Neuropsychopharmacology and the National Institute of Mental Health to establish principles for evaluating psychotropic drugs. Recently, the Pharmaceutical Manufacturers Association set up panels to formulate efficacy guidelines for several therapeutic classes. The Drug Efficacy Study of the National Academy of Sciences has pinpointed many of the problems in this field, furthering future clinical drug investigations.

Conclusion

Obviously many constraints are operating against the development of new drugs. Among the most important is deficient basic knowledge of drug action and of disease processes. To help remedy these deficiencies, pharmaceutical firms have begun basic research into cancer, viral diseases, organ transplants, and a host of degenerative conditions. However, basic research will require ever-increasing financial commitments over long periods before important new drugs will become available to the medical profession.

Introduction of new drugs is often delayed by differences of opinion on what constitutes valid safety and efficacy data. In many instances, confusion is caused by difficulties in interpreting animal toxicity findings and inadequate criteria for safety and efficacy of a new drug in man. To prevent unnecessarily delayed drug introductions, the academic community together with the Food and Drug Administration and the pharmaceutical industry should work together to establish valid guidelines. Such cooperation will be particularly required when current basic research yields potent new drugs for evaluation.

Scientists have become concerned about the cutbacks in research grant programs of the National Institutes of Health and the National Science Foundation. Equally important is a continuing generous support for predoctoral and postdoctoral training programs, as well as training programs for pharmacology, medicinal chemistry, and related disciplines. Otherwise, advances in the pharmaceutical sciences may be seriously impaired by the lack of appropriately trained researchers.

Literature Cited

(1) Elion, B., Kovensky, A., Hitchings, G. H., Metz, E., Rundles, R. W., "Metabolic Studies of Allopurinol, An Inhibitor of Xanthine Oxidase," *Biochem. Pharmacol.* (1966) **15,** 863–880.
(2) Cotzias, G. C., Papavasiliou, P. S., Gellene, R., "Modification of Parkinsonism—Chronic Treatment with L-Dopa," *New Eng. J. Med.* (1969) **280** (7), 382–383.
(3) Greenberg, D. S., "Molecular Biology—Drug Firm to Establish New Research Center," *Sci.* (1967) **157,** 408–409.
(4) Hoffmann-La Roche Pioneering Innovation, The Roche Institute of Molecular Biology, *Congressional Record* (1967) **113** (129), H10558.
(5) "Principles for the Testing of Drugs for Teratogenicity," *WHO Tech. Rept. Ser.* (1967) **364,** 5–18.
(6) Sanders, H. J., "Part I. Chemical Mutagens—The Road to Genetic Disaster?," *Chem. Eng. News* (May 19, 1969) **47,** 51–71.
(7) Sanders, H. J., "Part II. Chemical Mutagens—An Expanding Roster of Suspects," *Chem. Eng. News* (June 2, 1969) **47,** 54–68.
(8) Harris, M., "Mutagenicity of Chemicals and Drugs," *Sci.* (1971) **171,** 51–52.

(9) "Pharmacogenetics," B. N. La Du, W. Kalow, Eds., *Ann. N. Y. Acad. Sci.*
      (1968) **151** (2).
(10) "Symposium on Clincal Effects of Interaction Between Drugs," *Proc. Roy.
      Soc. Med.* (1965) **58** (11) Pt. 2.
(11) "Principles for Pre-Clinical Testing of Drug Safety," *WHO Tech. Rept.
      Ser.* (1966) **341.**
(12) Report of the Committee on Problems of Drug Safety, Drug Research
      Board, National Academy of Sciences–National Research Council,
      "Application of Metabolic Data to Drug Safety Evaluation," *Clin.
      Pharmacol. Ther.* (1969) **6** (5) 607–634.

RECEIVED November 5, 1970.

8

The Rate of Contemporary Drug Discovery

BARRY M. BLOOM

Medical Research Laboratories, Pfizer Pharmaceuticals, Groton, Conn. 06340

While the rate at which new single entity drug products received regulatory approval and were introduced in the United States during the period 1941–1970 increased continually until the early 1960's, it has declined sharply since. An analysis by drug category, comparing periods immediately preceding and following passage of the 1962 Drug Law Amendments, identifies some reasons for the decline that appear to be attributable to the evolving U.S. regulatory climate. One particularly vexing observation is that while certain types of drugs, notably central nervous system agents, antibiotics, and cancer drugs continue to gain regulatory approval, vitally needed types of agents for other important medical problems of our time, such as cardiovascular and pulmonary diseases, are notably absent among newly introduced drug products.

In trying to understand the mechanism of a process, chemists often find it enlightening to analyze the rates involved. In like fashion, new insights into the nature of contemporary drug discovery might be obtained if we could learn about the rate at which that process has occurred in recent years. There has been much discussion recently about a decline in the rate at which new drugs are being discovered and made available for medical use. This paper assesses the rate of new drug product introduction over the last 30 years, a period which corresponds essentially to the entire modern era of drug research.

The approach is to analyze a list of the basic new agents introduced to medical practice in the U.S. since 1941, using the DeHaen "New Product Survey" and "Non-Proprietary Name Index" as primary source materials (*1*). The DeHaen lists, which contain many kinds of new drug products, have been culled according to a set of exclusion rules we have devised to make them a more meaningful index of the rate of *bona fide* drug discovery.

According to these rules, a drug product was included in our edited list only if it was, at the time of market introduction, a new, single chemical entity intended for human therapeutic use, that did not fall into any of the following, excluded categories: biologicals such as vaccines; diagnostic aids; hospital solutions; non-absorbed high molecular weight compounds; impure extracts of natural origin; new uses and/or formulations of previously marketed drugs; new single components included in previously marketed mixtures; and new salts of previously marketed drugs. Although new salts have been excluded, our edited list does include new esters and other covalently bonded derivatives of previously marketed drugs.

The inherent limitations of this approach are readily apparent. Because it is the only form in which comprehensive data are available to us, we have had to use dates of U.S. new product introductions as an index of the rate at which new drugs are being discovered throughout the world. The justification for assuming that there is a correlation between the time when a drug is first discovered and the date when it is introduced in the U.S. market derives from the consideration that, in all likelihood, the sponsors of any significant new drug today will be strongly motivated to make it available commercially in the United States as soon as possible. Recognizing that the time period from discovery to U.S. market introduction is likely to differ significantly from case to case, we have sought to minimize this potential source of error by restricting the analyses to comparisons involving periods of no less than five years.

Any effort to determine which drug products deserve to be on a list restricted to new, single chemical entities is bound to lead to a few questionable judgments, and the simple exclusion rules we used are no exception. However, the number of debatable cases in this study is too small to cause any serious concern.

We have not attempted to distinguish the differing degrees of innovation that individual discoveries represent. We treat an unimposing molecular modification of a well-established therapeutic principle as if it were entirely equivalent to the discovery of penicillin G or cortisone. Attempts to assess comparative degrees of innovation and medical significance objectively are so difficult that despite the potential value of such judgments in a study like this one, efforts to do so must remain outside the scope of this paper.

Analyses of Data

We have analyzed our edited list to see if it supports the widely held conclusion that the rate of new product introduction has slowed significantly of late. Table I gives clear evidence that this is true. We have carried our analysis through August 1970 and broken the 30-year period under study into five-year segments.

Table I.   Rate of New Product Introductions By Category

Five-Year Period	Average Number of Basic New Agents Introduced Per Year
1941–45	10
1946–50	18
1951–55	31
1956–60	39
1961–65	20
1966–70 (through August)	12

The rate that prevailed during the war years (1941-45) increased steadily to a maximum during the last half of the 1950's, when new entities were being introduced at an average rate of almost 40 per year. There was a sharp decline in 1962, coinciding with the passage of the Kefauver-Harris Amendments to the Food and Drugs Act late that year. The net effect was a decrease by half of the rate of new product introductions during the period 1961-65 in comparison with the previous period. The rate declined further, by almost half again, in the present five-year period, reaching a low in 1969, when only seven compounds appear on the list. (On the other hand, 11 basic new agents gained U.S. regulatory approval during the first eight months of 1970).

Next, we compared the productivity of each five-year period to determine whether any factors that might be responsible for inducing important changes in the rate of emergence of new products were discernible. Although the conclusions will hardly prove surprising, they do offer a means of enhancing our perspective on the evolution of the modern drug discovery effort.

Going back to the first five-year period—1941-45—the over-all level of research activity was significantly lower than that of today. Much of the technology required to support operations of the efficiency and sophistication that are now commonplace was not yet available. The New Drug Application had already come into existence a few years earlier, in 1938, following the elixir of sulfanilamide tragedy, and certification had begun —first, with insulin in 1941 and subsequently with penicillin in 1945. In addition, there were the many complications that the war itself introduced. Despite all of this, the research effort of the period proved remarkably productive. These were the exciting years when American medicine first gained the use of antibiotics like penicillin and streptomycin, and the first of the improved sulfa drugs.

Research at this time was highly eclectic. Chemists were applying an unprecedented effort to probing, emulating, and exploiting nature. Research on vitamins, amino acids, and other nutritional factors was highly productive. Efforts to improve upon such hormones as epinephrine, estradiol, and testosterone were beginning to bear fruit. Molecular modification, which some consider a relatively new form of research endeavor, was already a well-practiced art, and the prevailing standard of therapy that scientists sought to supersede was often pretty low. Even at this early time, improved analogs of more than a dozen different major classes of drugs were beginning to be developed and marketed, including the barbiturate hypnotics, analgesics, antipyretics, local anesthetics, muscle relaxants, pressor amines, mercurial diuretics, xanthines, parasympathomimetic drugs, sex hormones, sulfonamide antibacterials, and antimalarials.

This kind of productivity brought about growth in drug research organizations, and the increased level of research activity was almost certainly a contributing factor during the ensuing period (1946–50), when major breakthroughs occurred in an almost constant stream. Widespread screening of fermentation broths, prompted by the dramatic success of penicillin G, produced, in rapid succession, the first three broad-spectrum antibiotics (chlortetracycline, chloramphenicol, and oxytetracycline). Hormone research, exploiting a growing base of knowledge about steroid chemistry, suddenly yielded rich dividends with the demonstration of the medical importance of cortisone. There were notable successes in both the search for improved analogs of established medicinals and the discovery of entirely new drug classes and prototypes. The first antihistamines appeared, as did the first synthetic anticholinergic drugs. Isoproterenol was made available to medical practice, as were the forebears of nitrofuran antibacterials, nitrogen mustards, adrenergic, and ganglionic blocking agents, among others.

Each new research triumph followed close upon the heels of the last. The number of important goals for discovery research recognizable to medicinal chemists and pharmacologists virtually doubled within a few short years, and it is hardly difficult to appreciate, in retrospect, how these exhilarating achievements set the stage for the peak rate of product introduction that occurred about a decade later.

The next five-year period (1951–55) saw a continuing parade of important new antibiotics produced directly by fermentation, such as penicillin V, neomycin, polymyxin, and the medium-spectrum macrolides. The massive chemical effort mounted in the corticosteroid field, following recognition of the medical importance of cortisone, quickly led to greatly improved compounds, as first hydrocortisone and then prednisolone, a triumph of analog research, became available in commercial quantities, helped by a major infusion of new technology, the development of practical microbiological methods for effecting 11-oxygenation of the steroid nucleus. Compelling evidence that one could create valuable synthetic modifications in the antibiotic field also appeared with the synthesis of tetracycline by hydrogenolysis of chlortetracycline. Perhaps we tend, now, to take some of these achievements for granted, but the path to successful discovery in these fields was anything but clear at the time. How many scientists would have accurately predicted in the early 1950's that knowledge of the relatively simple structure of the antibiotic, chloromycetin, would not lead to the discovery of a single significant analog, while deciphering the nature of oxytetracycline would ultimately allow chemical modification of that complex, multifunctional molecule to afford a number of medically useful new drugs?

Meanwhile, the era of tranquilizer therapy was dawning as successful isolation of crystalline reserpine facilitated the discovery of its unique effects on mental function, while more or less concurrently, astute clinical research revealed the then unique psychotherapeutic properties of chlorpromazine.

Still other important and innovative new drugs were introduced during the same period, including the antihypertensive hydralazine, the anti-inflammatory drug phenylbutazone, the carbonic anhydrase inhibitor/diuretic acetazolamide, and isoniazid for the treatment of tuberculosis.

However, the period of peak productivity (1955–60) still lay ahead. In retrospect, it is apparent that breakthrough discoveries, capable of creating entirely new fields of research, were no longer occurring frequently, although introduction of the first oral contraceptive was yet to come (1957). Instead, among the new products introduced during this prolific period an unusually high percentage of drugs represented major improvements over the then existing standards of therapy. Valuable new antibiotics, both direct fermentation products, and important synthetic modifications like the macrolide esters and the first penicillinase-resistant penicillins appeared. In addition to "the pill," steroid research provided a specific antagonist to the hormone, aldosterone, and superior new topical corticosteroids. Useful new tranquilizers, including chlordiazepoxide, appeared, along with a profusion of drugs for treating mental depression: imipramine and various monoamine oxidase inhibitors. Research toward novel sulfonamide derivatives, a process that had begun 20 years earlier, reached its culmination with the introduction of two important new prototype drugs: the diuretic chlorthiazide and the hypoglycemic drug tolbutamide; a host of other innovative products also appeared at this time, including the antihypertensive drug guanethidine and the antidiabetic agent phenformin.

Then the trend shifted rather abruptly. During the succeeding period (1961–65) the average yearly rate of new product introductions dropped by half. What happened in the midst of a period of unprecedented productivity to bring about such a sharp decline? The decline set in at just about the time of the thalidomide tragedy and the passage of legislation requiring that product efficacy, as well as safety, be demonstrated to the satisfaction of FDA.

But what actually happened? We set about to try to answer this question by comparing the rate of new product introductions by drug category, for the five-year periods immediately preceding (1958–62) and following (1963–67) establishment of the new FDA regulations. It is readily demonstrable, as shown by Table II, that in various well-established drug categories, where a number of adequately useful agents already existed, the development of new products to the point of obtaining FDA marketing approval either ceased altogether or declined sharply following introduction of the new regulations.

Table II. Pre- and Post-1962 Drug Law Amendments

Product Category	Period	
	1957–62	*1963–67*
Antihistamines	9	0
Antitussives	4	0
Antispasmodics	7	2
Muscle relaxants/antiparkinson drugs	8	0
Thiazide-type diuretics	10	2
Sulfonamide antibacterials	5	0
Antiobesity drugs	4	1
Vorticosteroids (systemic and topical)	14	3
Antinauseants	3	1
Totals	64	9

Since the same phenomenon occurred in a number of other, minor classifications that we have not attempted to tabulate, appreciably more than half of the decline in the rate of new product introductions that occurred after passage of the 1962 amendments, came about in this manner.

The trend in three other, major drug categories was somewhat different, however (Table III). In the variegated category, then relatively

Table III. Pre- and Post-1962 Drug Law Amendments

Product Category		Period		
		1957–62		*1963–67*
Psychotherapeutic drugs		25		11
tranquilizers	16		7	
psychostimulants	9		4	
Antibiotics (antibacterial, antifungal)		13		10
Cancer chemotherapy		5		5
Totals		43		26

new, comprising the different types of psychotherapeutic drugs, there was a fall off in new product introductions, but not nearly to the extent observed with the more exhaustively researched classes of drugs tabulated above.

There was virtually no decline in the introduction of new antibiotics. This was partly caused by the emergence of a number of important new semisynthetic β-lactam and tetracycline compounds. Research in the penicillin and cephalosporin fields had been profoundly stimulated by the development a few years earlier of the first practical method for preparing large quantities of 6-aminopenicillanic acid, and this technological breakthrough, along with some brilliant new cephalosporin chemistry, affected the 1962–66 period to a degree that helped offset any constraining influence the new regulations might have had. In fact, the introduction of important semisynthetic β-lactam products like ampicillin and cephalothin in 1963–64 has undoubtedly stimulated a high level of research activity in those fields throughout the decade and on into the 1970's.

With the cancer chemotherapeutic agents, we are probably seeing the cumulative effect of a joint effort on the part of government, universities, and the pharmaceutical industry to curb this dread disease. Because drugs of this type tend, unfortunately, to have a rather narrow range of usefulness, a large number of them are developed. The trend toward introducing more new products in this category has continued to the present, and during 1969 no less than three of the seven new drugs marketed in the U.S. were for treating various forms of cancer.

Aside from a few situations like these, the rate of new product introduction in this country has declined substantially during the 1960's. An analysis of the list of new drugs introduced in the U.S. between 1966 and the present certainly underscores this conclusion. Of the 58 basic new agents made available during this most recent five-year period, no less than 41 (71%) were for treating central nervous system indications (20), infectious diseases (12) or cancer (9). More striking still, and certainly more vexing, is the fact that during this most recent half-decade a total of only seven new drugs were introduced for treating the host of other important chronic diseases that plague modern man, diseases like hypertension, angina pectoris, atherosclerosis, diabetes, emphysema, and rheumatoid arthritis. Although the period did see the introduction of two noteworthy lipid-regulating drugs, two valuable diuretics, a β-adrenergic blocking agent approved for treating cardiac arrhythmias, and a novel agent for the treatment of gout, not one new drug for treating high blood pressure obtained U.S. regulatory clearance. Nor has one (other than some diuretics) since 1963. Not one new single entity bronchodilator product has come onto the U.S. market since 1961. (A mucolytic

agent introduced in 1963 is the only recent single entity pulmonary drug.)
Not one new non-steroidal agent for the treatment of rheumatoid arthritis
has been made available since 1965.

Prospects for the Future

One could reach the rather questionable conclusion that the process
of discovery of significant new agents in these classes has ground to a
halt, but a perusal of the current world medical literature reveals that
potentially important new drugs have been discovered recently in each
of these classes, and several of these new drugs are already available to
physicians elsewhere in the world. This makes all but unavoidable the
strong inference that current U.S. regulatory attitudes governing the
demonstration of clinical efficacy and safety required for NDA approval
have proved so inordinately demanding and burdensome as to seriously
impede drug development and stifle productivity.

Carl Djerassi, who helped pioneer oral contraceptive drugs, has repeatedly stated in the most convincing terms that this is precisely what
has already happened in the field of fertility control research (2).

The present analysis offers other evidence that regulatory factors are
contributing importantly to the slowdown. Can it be entirely fortuitous
that new antibiotics, tranquilizers, and cancer drugs continue to gain
FDA approval with some regularity, while new products for the treatment
of important, chronic metabolic diseases are conspicuous only by their
absence? Those familiar with clinical pharmacology are well aware that
the difficulty of establishing efficacy and safety of a new antibacterial
drug is in no way comparable with the corresponding task involving an
agent for the treatment of a disease like angina pectoris, for example.
Propranolol, the only new single entity cardiovascular drug to reach the
U.S. market during the last three years, has yet to be approved for use
in the treatment of angina, its main application for several years now in
other medically sophisticated countries like the United Kingdom. Perhaps
what recent events suggest is that burdensome regulations may be relatively tolerable in the technically easier fields, but prove to be the "straw
that breaks the camel's back" in the more demanding fields.

We clearly have much to worry about with regard to the effect of the
present regulatory climate on the process of translating new drug discoveries into products that can be made available to our health care
system. However, it is appropriate to ask also about the likely impact of
the current regulations upon the process of discovery itself. This is an
issue that defies rigorous analysis, but one can reasonably speculate that
in a self-stimulating process of the sort this study clearly suggests drug
discovery research to be, any factor, such as restrictive regulations, which

decreases the rate at which vital new information flows from the clinic back to the laboratory will have a profound depressant effect on the rate of discovery. Since we do not know how long it should take for an important negative influence of this sort to exert its full effect on slowing down the rate of discovery of innovative new drugs, one can only hope (and pray) that we have already seen the worst of it.

James Shannon, former head of NIH, has reminded us recently that the great and substantial drug innovations of the 1940's and 1950's were made under a more "laissez faire" attitude of regulatory law (3). An analysis of the sort undertaken in this paper helps one appreciate how rapidly benefits of dramatic magnitude accrued to society from drug research during that period. At the same time, it generates a certain pessimism about the future, by making so clearly evident the profound negative impact on research productivity that restrictive regulatory attitudes have already had in this country during the brief period since 1962. Joseph Cooper of American University, writing on "The Sociology of Innovation in Medicine," points out that "all progress tends to be inhibited by spontaneously arising negative forces which . . . eventually offset or kill the progress with which they are associated" (4). One can only hope that society will realize quickly that it is to its own great detriment to fail to place into proper perspective the problems of benefit and risk inevitably associated with the development and use of new drugs. As this study so clearly reveals, recent progress in making new drugs available for treating the important chronic diseases of mankind has been pitifully slow. Society can ill afford to legislate away one of the most important sources of its own well being.

Literature Cited

(1) Paul deHaen, Inc., 11 W. 42nd Street, New York, N. Y. 10036.
(2) Djerassi, C., *Science* (1969) **166**, 468; (1970) **169**, 941.
(3) Shannon, J. A., M.D., "The Economics of Drug Innovation," p. 83, The American University Center for the Study of Private Enterprise, Washington, D. C.
(4) Cooper J. D., *Proc. Roy. Soc. Med.* (1969) **62**, 48.

RECEIVED November 5, 1970.

Discussion

Leland Chinn (to S. Morris Kupchan): The development of chemo-therapeutic agents from plant sources in the past was based mainly on folklore and general screening programs. Could this approach be made more efficient and intellectually more appealing by devoting a greater effort to understanding the function which these agents serve in the plants themselves? For example, what role does reserpine play in the plant that would correlate with its antihypertensive effect in animals? What is the function of digitalis in the plant that would justify its use as a cardiotonic agent?

Dr. Kupchan: I think it would be fascinating, just as a study in basic science, to know what reserpine does in rauwolfia and digitalis does in foxglove, but I'm not sure just how much this would carry over to the role these agents play in animal tissues. We have had some experience in this regard, in collaborative efforts with plant physiologists and plant pathologists to answer the question as to what some complex natural products may be doing in the plant. In general, it appears that plant biologists are somewhat less advanced than animal biologists in experi-mental approaches to mechanism of action. So, in response to your ques-tion, it would be most interesting to learn more about the function of complex plant-derived compounds, but I doubt that this approach would constitute a more effective pathway to discovery of new natural products with noteworthy biological activity in animals.

Glenn Ullyot (to Dr. Kupchan): The logistics of supply of adequate quantities of plant material is a major factor in seeking drugs from plant sources. Time delays, expense of collecting, and problems of identifica-tion must be faced. What has been your experience with these practical considerations?

Dr. Kupchan: Actually, we've been very fortunate. We have enjoyed the close collaboration with the group under Robert E. Perdue, Jr., at the United States Department of Agriculture. While there certainly have been delays and the logistics problems have been considerable, they've not been overwhelming, by any means. Indeed, the plant kingdom offers a relatively accessible source of compounds. Certainly, plant-derived compounds are less accessible than synthetic products, but they are vastly more accessible than, for instance, products from marine sources.

185

H. C. Caldwell (to Lloyd Conover): Please discuss penicillin allergic-type reactions in the cephalosporins. Is there a crossover, and what is the prognosis for allergy-free cephalosporins?

Dr. Conover: I'd like to introduce my comments with the introductory phrase, "It is my impression that . . . ," rather than claim to speak from the fullness of precise knowledge. There may be someone here who can amplify what I say or possibly correct me. It's my impression that the allergic effects which follow administration of β-lactam antibiotics are caused by the formation of a covalent bond between the antibiotic or its degradation product and serum protein or tissue protein. This penicilloyl or cephalosporoyl protein is recognized by the body as foreign (*i.e.*, antigenic), and antibodies are formed.

There are really two factors to be considered. First, the capability of a particular drug to cause the event which I just described, and secondly the capability of a drug administered to a person in which this process has taken place to be immediately recognized as antigenic and to elicit an anaphylactic reaction. A number of different chemical reactions have been associated with this phenomenon. One of them is simple acylation of protein by the β-lactam. Inasmuch as the mechanism of action of both the penicillins and cephalosporins is also thought to involve acylation by the β-lactam, I think that it is very unlikely that there will ever be a β-lactam antibiotic which is active and which will not in some patients form antigenic material by this same mechanism. It is my impression that cephalosporins have a lesser tendency to sensitize than some penicillins and that not all penicillin-sensitive people react to a given cephalosporin. The differences are probably quantitative and will never be qualitative.

Barry M. Bloom: I should like to address a question to Dr. Biel. John, as the spokesman for organic synthesis on our panel, you gave several examples of rationales that have guided synthesis efforts to successful drug discovery, but I recall relatively little comment about total unabashedly empirical approaches to exploiting the fruits of the organic chemist's labor. This question is really a request to tell it like it is. What percentage of successful drug discoveries among synthetic compounds do you suppose is attributable to people whe are just synthesizing interesting structures and making them available for biological evaluation in various screening programs without any particularly significant underlying rationale?

John Biel: A very good statistical analysis was done during the days of the Army program on incapacitating drugs, and those programs that were based on blind screening of chemicals yielded about three active compounds in 10,000 while mission-oriented type drug research produced probably 10 active compounds per 3000.

Dr. Bloom: This is really an interesting question to a lot of us, I think. Morris, would you like to comment on it?

Dr. Kupchan: I would suggest modification of John Biel's otherwise very beautiful slide concerning "rational drug design" in the discovery of new drugs. Specifically, a clear distinction should be drawn between the limited past contributions of rational drug design to the discovery of new structural prototypes, and, in contrast, the extensive contributions to the molecular modification of prototype drugs. A critical review of the literature reveals that the vast majority of prototype drugs in various areas have come from systematic screening and/or fortuitous and serendipitous discovery rather than from rational design from first principles. Wouldn't you agree, John, that, in fact, rational drug design has played a far greater role in the molecular modification of prototypes than in the discovery of new prototypes?

Dr. Biel: I think that serendipity has to be planned. Unless you have a research person who is primed to make a discovery, he will not make a discovery. There are other factors that play into the hands of serendipity; that's one item I had to leave out because of the pressure of time, but a drug discovery is really something relative. The term discovery is relative in the sense that other disciplines have to be ready to recognize the discovery.

I think Librium and Valium are prefect examples of that thesis; had they been discovered 20 to 30 years earlier, neither the medical, cultural, nor sociological climate would have been ready to stamp this finding as a major discovery. The concept of treating anxiety became really fashionable after the world war. It was the acceptance by the medical profession and the admission by the patient that he is anxious that contributed to the discovery of anti-anxiety drugs.

So in answer to Dr. Kupchan's question, I think there are many factors that need to be integrated for a person to become intuitive. You're not just intuitive because you're born that way, but it does require a knowledge of a certain number of facts that need to be integrated into making a discovery.

Dr. Bloom: Chet, do you have a comment on this question?

Chester Cavallito: As with many differences of opinion, the differences are more semantically based than issue based. What do we mean by rational? I don't believe your question has been answered satisfactorily because we're not all using the term rational in the same sense.

Dr. Bloom: On the assumption that some of you in the audience may feel quite strongly on the subject, is there anyone else who would like to make a brief comment?

Saul Neidleman: I think in one sense the two distinguished panelists have been comparing peaches and apples. It is one thing to talk about

10,000 pure compounds and quite another thing to talk about 300 fermentation broths or 300 plant extracts where you really don't know how many compounds are involved. I would suggest that you could, by making appropriate mixtures of 10,000 compounds, be able to work the statistics to your advantage to make it look as though random screening is better than rational screening. I would agree that it is more a semantic difficulty than anything else. You have to define precisely what it is you're testing—precisely what it is you're looking at—or else the questions and answers have relatively little meaning.

James McFarland (to William Purcell): There is an air of mysticism in the use of molecular orbital parameters. Do you feel that these parameters relate to biological processes that we are already familiar with or do they perhaps relate to something we don't yet understand about how drugs act? If it is the former, would you elaborate on how we might interpret successful correlations with such terms as "highest occupied molecular orbital," "lowest unoccupied molecular orbital," and "frontier orbital"?

Dr. Purcell: Actually, there is a black box around the molecular orbital calculations. This is why I purposely threw the whole thing together this afternoon to try to make it clear that there shouldn't be this distinction, in my mind anyway, between a calculated parameter and one which is measured. With regard to the correlations and their meaning, if one suspects that electron-donating properties are important, one might look for correlations with the energies of the highest occupied molecular orbitals. And I don't think it makes any difference whether you measure this polarographically or whether you calculate it from molecular orbital calculations. If the parameter is there and it is significant and it is a factor in the biological process, I think it is quite legitimate to correlate it. You have to rely on statistics to determine whether there is a correlation or not.

I had a question the other day, "You know what I'd like to do, I'd like to see a Hansch analysis on a series of compounds and then I'd like to see some molecular orbital calculations on the same series." The point is that you don't compare this type of correlation with that type of correlation in this sense. Rather I think it is more important to look at a particular model and then use whatever techniques you need to get the parameters that go into that model, whether you measure the dipole moment or whether you calculate it from wavefunctions or whether you take the charge densities from pK measurements or whether you calculate the charge density. It is not the Hansch model $vs.$ molecular orbitals. That makes no sense to me. Rather it is using molecular orbital calculations to get at fundamental properties of the molecules—the same way that you would get at them if you measured the infrared absorption of the carbonyl to get at the stretch frequency and then use that datum if it has any meaning in the model for the correlation.

Dr. Bloom: In view of the way that we have solicited questions for the panel, it is obvious that the audience hasn't had much of a chance to submit anything with regard to the last few papers, but let me invite comments or questions from the floor with regard to Dr. Burns's paper. Are there any questions for John?

Dr. Ullyot: John, you talked about setting up the institute in which you're going into the investigation of basic biology. Do you think that in itself will lay the basis for rational design of drugs, or is it a source of knowledge of biological systems which we can control and influence and use in seeking new drugs?

John J. Burns: The first thing I should say is that the drug development procedure should have proper balance. We hear a lot about basic *vs.* applied research, and it is very hard for me to define what is basic and what is applied. What is basic today may be applied tomorrow, or vice-versa. It would be a serious mistake to go overboard on any one specific type of approach. There are certain things which we find most exciting, and the fact that we find them most exciting perhaps means that they should be most productive. My own feeling on the subject is that if one is going to have a broadly based drug development program, one must have a good balance between basic and applied research.

The question of random screening came up earlier. When I first went into industry I was very skeptical about random screening. I thought it a waste of time and effort to make thousands of compounds and then to screen them by thousands and thousands of tests. There must be a better way, or to use a better term, a more rational way of finding a new drug. But I think it would be a mistake on the part of any drug development organization to do away with random screening. One doesn't have to justify random screening because it has certainly given us leads, but to make it pay, you have to have good biologists, and they need a proper scientific environment to carry out their work.

In the old days at the NIH they would say "now why don't we set up drug testing facilities for medicinal chemists who happen to be synthesizing compounds under NIH grants so that we can get together a lot of biological data so we'll know what these compounds are doing." I always thought this would be a waste of time because to make random screening work, you must have the necessary pharmacological back-up. If a compound shows an interesting pharmacologic effect in an animal, you have to have good biologists around to study it. Furthermore, you must have good feedback to the chemists. If you don't have good feedback, biologists-to-chemists, and chemists-to-biologists, and have them in a position where they can talk to each other, you're not going to have the proper environment.

Getting to your question about the development of an Institute, there are a lot of things we don't know, and in order to know these things, we're going to have to take a relatively long range approach. I mentioned in my presentation the question of looking for a new drug for virus disease, but if you look at the effort which has gone into viral research over the past 20 years and the product of this effort, it's rather discouraging. One of our problems is that we don't know enough about the question of viral replication, how chemicals may interfere with penetration of virus into cells, etc. What we need is a program which allows a balance between basic research (in the sense of a molecular biology approach) and applied research along with good chemists and good biologists, who are in a position to do the necessary evaluation.

Dr. Cavallito (to Dr. Burns): We've heard a great deal about molecular biology in the last decade. When I read the journals, I find it hard to distinguish this from nucleic acid chemistry. I am wondering, John, if you could tell us what is your concept of molecular biology, which perhaps is broader than nucleic acid chemistry, and how that differs from what was termed biochemistry 15 or 20 years ago?

Dr. Burns: The term "molecular biology" was coined a number of years back. Institutes of molecular biology have been set up in various universities and new departments of molecular biology in medical schools. The major emphasis in molecular biology is on nucleic acid research, although more broadly it is the study of biological processes at a molecular level, and I would certainly not try to distinguish that from biochemistry.

A. A. Larsen: I sometimes regard the issue of biological knowledge as a cop-out. From what John Biel has said earlier, there are many examples of drugs which were discovered before we were fully aware of the details of their mechanism. There is perhaps a link between the suggested biological gap and the situation Barry just mentioned regarding the great effort necessary to get a medicament through the FDA. I have known biologists, who if given the chance, would go away for 20 years to investigate one chemical in one particular biological system.

Question from the floor (to Bernard R. Belleau): In connection with three-dimensional molecule structure, if one obtains data using x-ray crystallography or some other tool, can you apply these data directly to systems where the drug is used in solution or *in vivo*? Do the conformations, interatomic distances, and bond angles under such conditions correspond to the crystalline state?

Dr. Belleau: There are a number of examples wherein the tertiary structure is known through x-ray crystallography, and it appears that in

solution the active site at least seems to retain many of the same properties. However, there is also opposite evidence that in solution interactions
with the solvent will modify the structure appreciably. Now the big
question always arises when working with pure enzymes or pure proteins as models: are you not further from reality the purer your substances
are? When we are using an enzyme in solution, we have evidence that
its specificity will depend upon its state of aggregation. This will also
differ when it is attached say to a membrane. There are changes which
occur that are quite serious, and this is a field for future research. We
are just beginning to appreciate the magnitude of the problem.

Paul Craig (to Dr. Purcell): To continue along the same line, is not
what we just said even doubly true for quantum mechanical calculations,
which in essence calculate a molecule in isolation?

Dr. Purcell: There's no argument about that. I won't try to defend
the work that Kier is doing. If he were here, I'm sure he'd have something
to say about it. His point is that in doing these calculations you have to
start somewhere, and you start with an isolated molecule, and you recognize that that molecule is in quite a different environment in the biological system, but that's in bold face type at the beginning—there's no
attempt to say you're doing the calculation in a biological environment.

Dr. Cavallito: I want to ask a question of our chairman relative to
his very fine closing presentation. Between 1938 and 1962 the FDA
officially had the statutory basis for requiring evidence of safety. However, those individuals who dealt with the FDA are quite acquainted
with the fact that about 1960, in other words two years before the 1962
amendments, there was an implied request for evidence of efficacy on
the basis of the argument that safety in the absence of efficacy was
meaningless. Now let's project that into our present state. The '62 statute
specifically did not give the FDA authority to request comparative efficacy. However, there are some grumblings that perhaps we are beginning
to see the beginning of this kind of requirement. Do you have any comments on that and what that would do to the drug innovation process?

Dr. Bloom: You put it euphemistically, in my opinion. I think there
are a number of familiar examples that are hard to interpret in other
ways than that the FDA is beginning to concern itself with matters of
relative efficacy.

Frank Weisenborn: In Dr. Biel's discussion of the rational approach,
I still don't think anyone has really said how it is or put it all together.
I think it is a mixture of rationality and hope in that in many fields of
medicinal chemistry we look for the sophisticated organic chemist to
build a new heterocyclic molecule because we want to build a broad
protection in terms of a patentable area, and then we look for an experienced medicinal chemist to attach the appropriate side chains. It is a

mixture of rationality and hope, but we do look more towards the economic side than was expressed by members of the panel.

John Fried: It's difficult to add anything really significant to the very excellent thesis presented by Dr. Bloom about the rate of contemporary drug discovery, but one point might be made which makes his analysis even more worrisome. If one considers that the rate of drug discovery has decreased by a factor of 3 and expenditures have gone up by at least a factor of 2, the average cost of development of a new drug has increased by approximately a factor of 6. Now if one extends this analysis, the time may not be too far away before pharmaceutical companies decide that their return on investment for funds spent in research are such that those funds might very well be spent elsewhere. This is obviously a most unfortunate conclusion, but it is somthing that needs to be borne in mind when we talk about drug discovery.

Dr. Bloom: This is certainly an important comment, and I'm sure, John, you would direct people's attention in this regard to the recent article by Carl Djerassi in *Science* which offers some startling time and cost projections for the development of new oral contraceptive agents.

John Topliss: I'd like to comment on your excellent presentation. While I certainly agree with the thrust of your conclusions, I wonder if you perhaps side-stepped one part of the analysis which admittedly is very difficult but which would have made your conclusions a little more rigorous. One should try to estimate the individual worth of the drug discoveries which you mentioned only in terms of numbers. In one period you had, I think, 39 new entities, but we all know in that period many of them were relatively minor modifications. One really has to estimate what each drug adds to the total value of therapy in that area in order to make a fair comparison of the impact on medicine as a whole. Perhaps one might come up with the same sort of answers in this more rigorous analysis, but perhaps the results might not have looked so impressive in terms of the changes which have taken place.

Dr. Bloom: As far as I'm concerned your comments are fairly taken. I do think, however, that my main thesis would not be disproved by an analysis of that sort. Our efforts so far stimulate me to want to try to do exactly the sort of thing that you're talking about, but I have watched others try, and I've tried a little bit myself. So far, I just don't see a way to do the analysis objectively. It's worth thinking about, and I hope others will attempt such an analysis themselves.

Robert Cox: Just a comment, Barry, on your remarks and those of Chet Cavallito regarding the present attitude of the FDA toward New Drug Applications. I certainly agree that there is the implication of relative efficacy, not just efficacy per se in some NAS–NRC recommendations and subsequent FDA decisions. I think that the FDA is often making judgments based upon comparative therapeutic ratios and is moving toward rejection of some NDA submissions if such cannot be justified *via* a more attractive therapeutic ratio than that of products already marketed for pertinent indications.

Dr. Bloom: Dr. Ullyot, do you want to comment on that?

Dr. Ullyot: On the next panel we'll have an FDA man here, and I hope some of these questions will be raised then. Perhaps it is a little unfair to go into these questions very extensively without giving him a chance to hear them. I'd really like to have him comment as a representative of the FDA.

Dr. Bloom: Dr. Conover, what do the results of your questionnaire or any other information that you may have suggest with regard to the present level of research activity directed to finding new antibiotics and fermentation broths? Has this kind of research declined in the last 10 years and will it decline in the future?

Dr. Conover: One of the illustrations that I presented carried cumulative totals through 1965, and to that point the total number of new antibiotics reported for a five-year period had continued to increase. Dr. Perlman of Wisconsin has a summary which extends, I think, to 1968. This makes it appear that there has been a levelling off, but at a much higher level than that of the 1940's and 1950's. The total number of new antibiotic entities reported has not dropped to a level that is low compared with the period when important discoveries were being made at a much faster rate. I would like to think that by broadening the target, as I tried to suggest in my talk, activities directed toward finding drugs of more different kinds from microbiological sources will increase.

Dr. Bloom: We will close by asking Dr. Burns to respond to a question from Dr. Laughlin: "Modern drugs aim to increase the level of well being of individual organisms, especially those who could not otherwise function or survive in their environment. Is this goal truly consistent with the best interests of future members of the species?"

Dr. Burns: Briefly, I think we are faced with certain ethical considerations. If we are able in the next 10, 15, or 20 years to extend life for another 10 or 20 years, or perhaps to allow people to live who normally would die now with genetic disease, but perhaps to live in a way that would be incompatible with a good life, are we doing something good? I would say that this is the type of question I would rather see posed to a panel of philosophers, theologians, and medical people.

There is another question which has come up that relates to the FDA, and I would like to comment on it. We get ourselves into trouble if we tend to think that this problem is basically one in getting a new drug approved. There is another very important issue here. When we look at the 1950's there were certain things that we did in the biological testing of new drugs in terms of toxicity, etc., but now we must do much more. It is not just that the FDA is telling us to do these things, but we have to do them because the whole level of medical science has advanced. The doctor is expecting more information on drugs. The medical students are being taught a different kind of pharmacology than they were 10 years ago. The type of information we have to supply on drugs is much more costly, and it is obviously going to have an effect on the development process. It is not just a question of the FDA giving us problems in requiring new tests, but the tests must be done to satisfy our own feelings on what is necessary for adequate biological information on a new drug.

Dr. Bloom: One of the main thrusts, if not the main thrust, of my argument is that anything which serves to impede the rate at which new knowledge is generated in clinical pharmacology is bound in the end to suppress the whole process. So really we're both arguing for the need for more knowledge.

Drugs—The American System

W. CLARKE WESCOE, M.D.

Sterling Drug Inc., 90 Park Ave., New York, N. Y., 10016

The American system of medicines—their discovery, development and use—stems from a history rooted deeply in man's past. Although it shares this history with its international counterparts, the American system is distinct and unique in many ways. Not the least of these is embodied in the extent to which it has become the object of renewed consumer scrutiny and political maneuvering. A plethora of regulations and controls has become the everyday lot of the system—yet, it remains highly creative, enormously productive, thoroughly viable. It continues to serve its public very well.

In this emotional era of discord, discussion, dissent, and demagoguery, in this period of query about all things made and used and ingested, in this age of quest for a better life in a better environment, a concern with drugs used for spectacular therapeutic achievement and abused with devastating results has become an American preoccupation. The discovery of new chemical compounds with important medicinal properties, once heralded with admiration and acclamation, is now, it seems, more often looked upon as a threat to the integrity of the human body, if not to the structure of society. The word drug itself has come to be used nearly always in a pejorative sense; for that reason I retitle this presentation, to put into proper perspective the discussions to follow: "Medicines, The American System."

There is need for a discussion such as this because of the public preoccupation with the discovery, development, and ultimate delivery of medicines. The great disappointment may be that very few other than ourselves will ever be aware that this symposium was held. We may be engaged in another exercise wherein the well informed and the most knowledgeable will be talking only to each other. Nonetheless, I proceed with the glimmer of hope that together we might produce a little light where presently there appears to be only heightening heat and gathering darkness.

The Evolution of Medicines

Man in his search for medicines to ease his pain, hasten his healing, and cure his disease has created an enthralling story. His early quest for medicines settled logically on the living plants which surrounded him: bushes and trees, their roots, their leaves, their bark. By trial, error, and experience he accumulated a substantial knowledge such that by the time a written language appeared a list of useful products could be recited. Such a list of plant materials is found in the Thebes papyrus dating from the period of 1600 B.C. Even without chemical techniques a certain sophistication was established about plant materials, for as early as the fourth century B.C. Theophrastus was able to write about differences in potency dependent upon the parts of the plant used, the age of the plant, the area of its origin, and its manner of preservation. By the first century A.D. the alchemists of Alexandria were able partly to purify substances by distillation and filtration, and Dioscorides developed some crude sensory and physical methods for testing botanicals.

Perhaps the earliest origins of the pharmaceutical industry are to be found in the trade involving the root gatherers and the middle men: the druggists and the alchemists, well established by Galen's day. From him came a classification of plant materials and, additionally, a long series of complicated plant-based prescriptions for various therapeutic indications.

The specificity and purity of products were as important then as they are now. To assure uniformity, the Middle Eastern civilizations required that medicinal materials be produced by druggists under the supervision of a governmental functionary. The concern of the reputable druggists, pharmacists, and apothecaries of the Western world was expressed by the publication of a formulary in Florence in 1498. Thus, by the beginning of the 16th century both the framework and the principles of our present system had been introduced: commerce, purity of product, self-regulation, integrity, and governmental supervision.

With Paracelsus in the 16th century came the input of innovation, creativity and investigation. Through him came the introduction into medicine of opium and the metals mercury, sulfur, antimony, and iron. The first medicines from the New World, cinchona and ipecac, were introduced into Europe in the early 17th century. In the 18th century came the introduction of digitalis therapy by Withering and the remarkable discovery of the value of vaccination by Jenner.

The 19th century produced the application of true scientific principles to man's search for drugs. Analytical methods were developed to determine the chemical and physical purity of compounds, and the principles of biological assay were introduced. With the contributions of Pasteur and Ehrlich, the foundations were laid for chemotherapy. Semmelweis, Holmes, and Lister began controlled clinical experimentation and introduced the principles of antisepsis. The general anesthetics— ether and chloroform—were adopted into surgical practice. Finally, the contributions of Ehrlich thoroughly established synthetic organic chemistry as a rich source of new medicines.

Three other aspects of the system as we know it today were also introduced in the 19th century. Regulatory legislation was adopted by the British Parliament in 1875. Advertising, complete with product claims, appeared—directed both to the physician and the public, but primarily to the latter. There also arose determined complaints about the cost of medicines, centered on the discovery and marketing of Salvarsan.

The developments of the 20th century defy detailing here. Suffice it to say that in this century came the discoveries of barbiturates, of hormones (and their chemical synthesis), of antibacterials and antibiotics, of oral diuretics, of better analgesics, and of a host of other compounds. Finally, the physician was provided with medications not only for the treatment of symptoms but often for the underlying cause of disease itself.

It might seem that man's search for drugs has transcended all his other quests. Certainly, it has always been one of his intense preoccupations. Perhaps it is all best summarized by the words of Sir William Osler who said, in many speeches to diverse audiences, that the single characteristic separating man from the lower animals is his intense desire to take medicines. To which thought I might add, in the light of history, man's determination to discover new medicines.

The Origin of Pharmaceuticals

In the recitation of history there is always the risk that the surviving relatives of an individual become incensed by the omission of his name. The same risk is run when one attempts retrospectively to compare the contributions of various countries to modern therapy. As is the case with individual credit, where the significant contribution of one man is almost always the culmination of the works of many, there is no national science which clearly stands out above others. All science is international; all science depends upon the collective contributions of many. Discovery is most often the result of superb timing and surpassing good fortune. At the risk, therefore, of precipitating a mild international crisis, let me attempt to assign national contributions to pharmaceutical progress in the 10 categories into which pharmaceutical research effort is most usually classified.

In the field of central nervous system pharmacology the contributions generally have been European. The mild analgesic agents, aspirin and phenacetin, were synthesized in Germany, as was the first local anesthetic agent (procaine), and the original derivatives of barbituric acid as well as the acid itself. Meperidine likewise came from Germany although its usefulness as an analgesic was developed in the United States. Insofar as the newer tranquillizers, depressants, and antidepressants are concerned the contribution is shared among many: Switzerland, Germany, the United States, England, and France.

Anti-infectives and antibiotics have been contributed in large measure by Germany, England, and the United States. The landmark contribution of medicines affecting neoplasms and the endocrine systems can be attributed primarily to the United States and Canada. Medicines affecting the digestive and genitourinary systems were derived from the United States and Germany. Respiratory agents, including antihistamines, can be attributed to France, the United States, Germany, and England. Vitamin therapy has been enhanced by workers from the Netherlands, England, and the United States. Cardiovascular medicines, of which there are many, can be attributed to England, the United States, Switzerland, and Germany. Dermatologicals and biologicals are difficult to classify because of their large numbers. Diagnostic agents, particularly radiopaque substances, have been contributed by the United States, Germany, and the Scandinavian countries.

What a resume of the last 75 years indicates is that most contributions are likely to be derived from highly developed, technological societies, possessed of superb universities. They result, more often than not, from a complex interplay between education, industry, and institutes for research. History indicates even more clearly that major discoveries emanate from those countries in which the pharmaceutical industry is highly developed and exceptionally research oriented. One is led to the inevitable conclusion that many, if not most, significant contributions will continue to come from the research efforts of well-funded, competently staffed industrial laboratories—that without such laboratories, progress will be slow and advances fewer.

The American System

Our domestic system is still evolving. It began with frontier medicine, with practitioners of widely varying educational backgrounds and professional skills. The horse-and-buggy doctor provided more pastoral therapy than he did meaningful medication. Armed with few specifics, he laid on his hands, he comforted, and he cared as best he could for surgical emergencies.

A considerable part of the development of the American system can be related to homeopathy, a type of practice which flourished in this country well into the 20th century. It was homeopathy that established the concepts of close observation of symptomatology, of medicinal therapy for all ailments, and of specific responses to medication. It was homeopathy as well that contributed in large measure to polypharmacy, and it was polypharmacy that gave birth to the American pharmaceutical industry. The industry has its roots in the production and distribution of proprietary medicines and nostrums by physicians and pharmacists possessed of business acumen. Those early founders of the industry are immortalized in the names of many of the leading companies today.

The early days of the American system were characterized by overstatement of therapeutic value, most often expressed in unconscionable advertising to the general public. Those days might best be described as the era of gullibility characterized by outlandish claims, an overtrust in them on the part of the public, and a lack of concern for quality of product.

As a result of these excesses, Congress passed the Food and Drugs Act of 1906, the first major American drug legislation. That act dealt primarily with the important matters of adulteration and misbranding. The extent of governmental authority encompassed by it was exceedingly limited, but it presaged a continuing governmental concern with medicines.

It is of more than passing note that the law was written simultaneously with the expression of great concern over the quality of American medical education. Literally, the development of the system proceeded hand in hand with the establishment of medical education as a university discipline, and the development of medical practice as a science as well as an art.

The blatancy of pharmaceutical advertising and the lack of effective products led to an overreaction to drug therapy: therapeutic nihilism gained an ascendancy. In the early days of this century primary interest was centered in the classification of disease. Clinical pathology achieved a new status, and medicines were largely ignored save for the less than a dozen considered useful in treatment by the sophisticated physician.

A leap forward was accomplished by the system when the industry turned to a research orientation and developed research laboratories. Originally, the industrial research laboratories were staffed with difficulty in respect to those trained in the basic medical sciences. There was a time when membership in the American Society for Pharmacology and Experimental Therapeutics was denied to those employed by industry and removed from those who left universities to join industrial laboratories. This artificial split among scientists was healed, but its echoes are still heard occasionally.

The American system, in its finest sense, operates with industrial and academic laboratories acting in close cooperation. Individuals based in universities frequently serve as paid consultants to industry and perform research underwritten by grants from individual companies. These grants sometimes support specific projects but often provide unrestricted funds for basic research. In this warm, symbiotic relationship rests the greatest strength of the American system.

Pharmaceutical Research

Drug discovery begins in the chemical laboratory with the synthesis of new compounds. These are screened in biological model systems for specific pharmacologic activity; from the results of this preliminary screening, active candidates are selected for more thorough testing. When especially attractive candidates are identified, investigations are enlarged to include metabolic studies, the development of analytical methods, toxicology in several species, and finally, carefully controlled clinical studies. When the occasional winner is produced, as ascertained from careful clinical investigation, all of the data are brought together for submission to the Food and Drug Administration in support of a request for a New Drug Application (NDA). Finally, agreement is reached with the Food and Drug Administration with respect to labeling, therapeutic claims, precautions, adverse reactions that might be anticipated, dosage, and administration.

The actors involved in this complex drama are numerous. They range from chemists, biologists, technicians, pathologists, and clinical pharmacologists in industrial laboratories to biologists, chemists, and physicians in academic laboratories and clinics, to administrative biologists and physicians in the Federal agency and government research institutes, to clinical pharmacologists in non-university hospitals, to clinicians in the private practice of medicine. If the actors are numerous, the outpourings of data are even more so. The final summarization of data for an NDA is encyclopedic in content and volume.

It is remarkable that a system so highly diversified functions so well. Although there are creaks here and rumblings there, sometimes ominous signs of friction among the moving parts, the system is manageable, although the processes are slow. That it does function so well is a tribute to the dedication and intelligence of those who play the major roles—the scientists in industry and universities and government who strive together to resolve differences and obliterate difficulties.

It takes little imagination to realize that a system so diversified, whose production is so complicated by necessarily rigid standards, must be of enormous dimension. Because of its dimension, it is difficult to ascertain with accuracy the actual dollar investment. Excluding governmental funds, the closest approximation to actual expenditures can be derived from the data compiled by the Pharmaceutical Manufacturers Association

(*1*), based upon figures supplied by 71 member firms whose annual expenditures range from less than $1 to more than $20 million. In 1969, the latest year available, these data reveal an industry operating expenditure on research and development of $549 million. For 1970, budgeted expenditures for research were at the level of $624 million, an increase of nearly 14% over the previous year. Of specific interest is the fact that 98.8% of those expenditures were financed by the industry itself.

Of the total operating expenditures in 1969, 88.6% was spent within the industry, 9.7% was spent outside the industry (for consultants, research institutions, medical schools, hospitals), and 1.7% was spent on government contracts.

The research installations of the industry in 1969 employed 20,230 personnel of whom 10,345 were scientific and professional staff and 9,885 were technicians and supporting staff. Of the total, 3,775 held doctoral degrees.

With respect to other industries, the pharmaceutical industry stands high in the amount of dollars expended for research; with respect to its own dollars expended and lack of support from governmental contracts it stands highest. Beyond that, the industry's allocation of 18% of its own funds to innovative, fundamental research is the highest ratio reported for any industry in the United States, according to the National Science Foundation.

One strength of the American system, beyond the collaboration between industry and academic institutions of high quality, rests in the competition between laboratories, a hallmark of the free enterprise system. Although it is difficult to assign ultimate credit for discoveries, it is safe to say that the industrial laboratories make a significant contribution to science. They stand now as the prime developers of new medicinals, a fact pointed out by Sir Derrick Dunlop (*2*) in a statement made in 1967: "Of the seventy most valuable drugs introduced to medicine in this century since the discovery of aspirin in 1899, sixty were discovered and developed by scientists in the laboratories of industry."

All systems have their unusual characteristics, and this one is no exception. One of these is the high ratio of expenditures on research and development to sales. In 1969 the industry expended on research 11.1% of the dollars generated by sales (*1*), approximately five times the average percentage of all other industry.

The research orientation of the pharmaceutical industry, demonstrated by its heavy investment, is dictated not only by the striving to bring new and improved products to the market for the benefit of man, but also by the fact that medicinal products tend to rapid obsolescence. Conceivably, this tendency may lessen in the future. That it has been a factor in the past cannot be denied.

What was true in the past about discovery, however, will undoubtedly continue into the future. That truth is, a great many compounds
must be synthesized to find one that is safe, efficacious, and useful. In
1967, for instance, almost 176,000 compounds were tested by pharmaceutical laboratories. Of those, only 1,375 were active enough and sufficiently safe to warrant testing in humans. For each compound reaching
the market, 7,000 were screened and underwent preliminary testing (3).

To put this another way, and in a more global context, in the decade
1958–1968 there were 300 new basic drug entities introduced to physicians. In that same decade expenditures made for research and development exceeded $3 billion (4). On the average, then, an expenditure of
$10 million was required per entity before $1 was generated in sales.
Although it is not statistically fair to make such a comparison, note that
$549 million were expended on research and development in 1969, and
only nine new chemical entities were released to the market (5).

This peculiarity of rising research expenditures and declining introductions of medicines serves to point out that developmental research
will continue to be increasingly more costly. Involved in these costs are
the relatively new required investigations relating to bio-availability, metabolism, drug interactions, and analytical procedures. All of this indicates that the likelihood of the price of prescription drugs falling significantly is remote at best if the pharmaceutical industry is to survive as
an economically viable enterprise. Indeed, any other industry would be
considering substantial price increases in similar circumstances.

Yet, despite these facts, the "high cost" of medicines, often confused
with other health care costs, continues to be a matter of great concern
to the public. What the public does not comprehend is the remarkable
stability of medicinal prices in a highly inflationary economy. The Bureau
of Labor Statistics' data have been largely ignored: they show on a base
of 1957–1959 as 100, a rise in the cost of living index by 1969 to nearly
128 and a concomitant decline in the retail cost of prescription drugs to
an index of only 89 (6). No prices are complained about as much as are
those for medicines, yet no greater benefit is derived from any other
products.

For perspective, in 1969 the average charge for a prescription was
$3.68 (7), considerably less than the price of a carton of cigarettes, or an
evening meal in an average restaurant.

Generics, Patents, and Advertising

Pertinent to this discussion are the matters of generic prescribing
and the compulsory licensing of patents, whereby the results of one company's costly research could be shared by others who had made no invest-

ment. It appears now that the inequity of this situation is becoming well appreciated. Further, scientific evaluation has indicated the pitfalls inherent in the use of generic drugs. Price cannot be the only consideration. The words of John Ruskin put the matter of price in proper context: "It's unwise to pay too much, but it's worse to pay too little. When you pay too much, you lose a little money. When you pay too little, you sometimes lose everything, because the thing you bought was incapable of doing the thing it was bought to do. The common law of business balance prohibits paying a little and getting a lot—it can't be done."

Finally, as a characteristic of the system, we deal with an unique situation in which the sales effort is directed not toward the consumer but toward a professional who makes a choice for him. A great deal of controversy has centered about the promotion of ethical medicines. There are those who believe that little advertising of ethical medicines should be done; there are those who believe that there should be none. Some physicians request and appreciate direct mail materials while others ask to be removed from mailing lists. Ethical medical advertising should be looked upon as educational material, as indeed I look upon it. It is foolhardy to believe that busy physicians will read enough of the scientific literature or attend sufficient postgraduate courses to keep alert to advances in therapeutics. Ethical advertising is restrained to the point of dullness; it is primarily informational. Without it, the benefits of some medication might be denied to some patients. It is true that "full many a rose is born to blush unseen"; there is no reason for a significant medicinal discovery to be kept secret or merely to hope that a physician will stumble upon it as he reads the literature. To do that would be foolhardy on the part of the industry and inimical to the best interests of medicine and patients alike.

The Impact of a Changing Society

Remarkable changes in society in the past 10 years have had great impact upon the system; perhaps the greatest has been wrought by a tremendous improvement in the mechanisms of communications. From a society relatively uninvolved in world affairs because it felt remote from them, we have turned into a society deeply involved because we are catapulted into the midst of events by the miracle of instant communications with pictures. We see a war being fought half-way round the world as we sit in our lounge chairs; we observe riots in distant cities of our own and other lands while they are still in progress.

Instant communication leads to instant involvement and instant concern. It also leads to lack of contemplation and lack of thought; rather, it leads to emotional responses and a desire for instant reaction. In a fast moving world it is logical to think that all processes should be speeded up and all things should be improved in a matter of hours. It looks and seems so simple that the logical tendency is to forget that complexities exist.

In an exceedingly complex world we see a yearning for a return to the simple life, a withdrawal on the part of some of our young from the realities of life. For many of the young, a simple, uncomplicated, unregulated existence seems the ideal. At the same time, we have entered into a decade of concern that prompts new complexities, more regulation, and more governmental supervision.

All of this leads to a society characterized by contentiousness. There is today, in many instances, no thought for reasoned discussion; there is, instead, the presentation of non-negotiable demands, the mouthing of convenient catchphrases. This is a time when many plead for the federal government to step in with centralized regulatory authority over broad new areas—the environment, consumer products, health—and a time when there is a determined thrust for the decentralization of much other authority. There are those who believe that participatory democracy can work for large social structures as it once worked in the small town meeting. This is the day of "power to the people" even if the people do not fully understand the ramifications of problems. "Right on" is the thrust even if "on to where" has not been defined. We exist and we persist in a plethora of paradoxes. Frustration is the mode of the day.

Finally, we live in a society where the producer of any medical product has become subject to enormous liability. Fears are raised deliberately in the minds of many by sensational, one-sided reporting, to the point where one hesitates to take any medicine. The basic tenet of pharmacology, that any medicine is inherently a toxin, is forgotten. In a society raised to the highest peak by science, in a society which is the best educated in all of history, the present tendency appears to be toward non-science and irrationality. Man appears to be descending from the cerebral to the mid-brain level, controlled by his gut feelings rather than by his intellect.

There is little wonder then that we have a drug-conscious society where medicines developed for therapeutic advances are abused and where drugs for which there is no rational or therapeutic use are taken in ever increasing quantities by the weak, the poorly informed, the mentally disturbed, and the constitutionally inadequate. Inevitably, the pharmaceutical industry is blamed for these shortcomings of society because it happens to be the most visible target in an era when many (public and political) refuse to discriminate between medical use and drug abuse.

The pharmaceutical industry has experienced this "target" phenomenon before. The extent of governmental authority was broadly increased with the enactment of the Food, Drug and Cosmetic Act of 1938 which provided the important governmental power to rule upon the safety of medicines before they were allowed to reach the market. Tremendous advances were made in the 1940's and 1950's in the introduction of new, safe and effective medicines, and the industry experienced remarkable growth. It might be said, however, that the industry became carried away by its own growth and successes. Without question it resorted, in many instances, more to salesmanship than to a concern for what was best for the patient and the practice of medicine. As a consequence, it entered (even engendered) an era of distrust, which, retrospectively, signalled the real beginning of the new times of discord and dissent in which we live.

During the Congressional hearings on the Food, Drug, and Cosmetic Act, the pharmaceutical industry was unfortunately unequal to the task of presenting its story of magnificent achievement. Rather than a positive approach, it adopted a defensive stance. As a result of the hearings, the act was amended substantially; the amendments extended governmental authority to manufacturing practices, and more important, to the establishment of efficacy before a new product could be marketed.

No one could complain about these purposes. The regret to be voiced is that these developments resulted from one-sided, acrimonious hearings from which the industry has never fully recovered in the matter of public confidence. Great accomplishments were down-graded; ridicule was the order of the day.

The Drug Evaluation Study

Just now we are beginning to see the ultimate results of some of these changes as the Food and Drug Administration begins to implement the findings of panels appointed by the Drug Research Board of the National Academy of Sciences–National Research Council to pass upon the efficacy of marketed drugs. As the findings of these panels are revealed, the impression is most often given that a substantial group of all-knowing men, with broad clinical experience, have studied in depth all the data pertaining to the drugs in question and have reached from those studies a rational, scientific decision. Let me dissent from that impression, at the risk of provoking anger from some, but hopefully, considered thought on the part of others.

I have great respect for scientists. I have lived with them all my adult life. I consider myself to be one of them. My experience indicates that none of them is all-knowing, that each of them is subject to as many biases and prejudices as is the layman. The impression given that the National Academy (incidentally, a very narrowly drawn group) has made decisions is erroneous; rather, small groups of appointed academic experts have prepared reports. Few if any of them, were Academy members themselves. The Academy itself did not review their findings, and, certainly, the Academy released no reports. Dominant chairmen could exert great influence on the conclusions of these reports.

As one reads the actual reports, one cannot fail to conclude that in many instances the panels were recommending changes in information provided to physicians and not considering (or recommending) that their comments would remove medicines from the market place. Yet the latter is exactly what has happened. Further, one gains the impression that often their opinion, rather than fact, ruled the day—an opinion that was substituted, without debate, for the cumulative, years-long opinion of many clinicians. No one would desire the discontinuation of ineffective medicines more than I would, but I question arbitrary disdain for lengthy clinical experience, and I fear what appears to be the present thrust: the establishment of a single product for a single therapeutic indication. I believe choice should and must be allowed the clinician in selecting medicines for his patient.

The withholding of a medication that has achieved clinical acceptance on the basis of clinical observations over many years is as important an action as the introduction of a new compound. In the current actions following upon the drug evaluation reports, millions of clinical observations have been rejected or ignored. This is in remarkable contrast to the situation as it relates to adverse reactions, where a single report, often unsubstantiated, is accepted with finality.

There has been in the last decade a great preoccupation with untoward reactions, an inevitable resultant of the use of medicines. Package inserts read like horror studies, for every possible reaction must be included, no matter how remote the occurrence might have been, or how little connection it might have had with the medicine in question. If there is any great need today it is for a scientific evaluation of adverse reactions. The costly scientific substantiation of safety and efficacy so reasonably requested stands in stark contrast to the unscientific evaluation of adverse effect reporting (8).

We have had a recent personal experience in respect to pentazocine. After receiving reports concerning indiscriminate use of the compound, we made determined efforts to obtain body fluid samples for analysis from those suspected of such use. In more than half the instances where pentazocine had been implicated, analyses revealed neither the parent compound nor its metabolites. Rather, analyses revealed the presence of other compounds known to be abused. We are certain that if similar efforts were made the same would be found in respect to other drugs.

Medicines and the Political Arena

Our past decade has seen the emergence of additional political figures with an intense interest in medicinal affairs, many more than was
once the case. Inevitably, then, politics intrudes into the regulation of
American medicinals in a way not comparable elsewhere in the world.

Federal administrators are subjected to the surveillance of committees
sometimes to the extent that it would appear difficult for them to carry
out their responsibilities. A considerable amount of their time is spent
in hearings, time that could be spent more profitably in the administration
of their agencies.

Congressional hearings on important subjects are often held on short
notice. The witnesses to be heard are selected by committee members
and, often, under the guise of lack of time, many with substantive pres-
entations are not heard at all. Hearings tend to be contrived and one-
sided; what purport to be democratic processes at times resemble the
worst of totalitarian exercises.

A few members of Congress strive for the appearance of having
virtue entirely on their side. They have no compunction about investigating any subject—save that of their own operations. An interesting
comment was quoted in the *New York Times Magazine* of July 19th, 1970
in that regard, from a member of Congress who was explaining why no
public hearings were held by the Ethics Committee: "I think the committee has plenty of power. I don't think we should have a setup where
every crackpot in the area can for political reasons or otherwise come in
and try to get some headlines at the expense of a Congressman. They
would do it. You must know that." Apparently, there is recognized a
difference in "crackpots" and a difference in gaining headlines at someone
else's expense or having them result from one's own purported actions.

Surprisingly and detrimentally, in a time when medicines of greater
specificity as well as potency became available, there was a thrust in
medical schools to shorten the curriculum in pharmacology or to spread
its teaching among many people not trained in the discipline. Pharmacologists object, but there is a much louder voice from family practice,
from sociologists and from medical students who seem ready to enter
the profession without a really basic knowledge of what a quality practice
of medicine is all about.

These medical students come from the student groups that have
railed against "the establishment" until they have convinced themselves
that such a group exists. They should learn what the so-called "establishment" does to those the students consider members of it. They are unaware, for instance, that governmental agencies do to corporations what
they would not dare do to individuals. They are unaware that to achieve

a hearing, a corporation first has to present evidence that it can win the hearing. They are unaware that in many of our industry-government relations the indication is clear that the English principle of innocent until proven guilty has been abandoned. They are unaware that presently there are being proposed wide-ranging statutes that would make Federal agencies the lawmakers, the prosecutors, the juries and the judges.

International Regulations

Perhaps one of the most dramatic changes in the last decade has been the "internationalization" of medicinal controls. No longer is each nation operating entirely independently. The World Health Organization is becoming a more prominent organization; a great deal of data are shared between governments. A governmental decision in one country today is very likely to be repeated promptly in many others. Much of this is for the good; what has to be assured is that national prejudices will not be substituted for scientific accuracy.

Because there is this tendency toward the rapid sharing of data between governments and because some companies from the United States market new products abroad, it is appropriate to describe the systems as they exist elsewhere.

The drug registration system in Britain is less complex and much less costly than that of the United States although it is certainly no less effective and no less protective of the consumer. The British system is much less formal, less bureaucratic, and operates on a level of much more mutual respect than ours. It is relatively new in principle of operation but appears to work effectively. Under that system a request is made of the registration authority to carry out clinical trials after the careful laboratory studies have been made. The request is accompanied by full data on animal studies, including teratology, and on tolerance studies performed on human volunteers. When permission is given, the clinical trials are performed and, when complete, are submitted to the Committee on Safety of Drugs (Scowen Committee) with a request for permission to market. The Committee either approves, requests further studies, or disapproves. In the event that formula changes and changes in dosage forms are required after that time, these too are submitted to the Committee just as is the case with an NDA supplement in this country.

The system in France is a very rigid one, albeit a less bureaucratic one. A *visa* expert must be used, usually an academician who is an acknowledged expert in the field of disease for which the medicine is intended. The company seeks out such a *visa* expert; there is apparently little concern about possible conflict of interest in this system and apparently a trust in both parties by the government authorities. When a *visa* expert has agreed to serve, all the preliminary data are submitted to him: animal studies, toxicology, and clinical studies. Ordinarily, he will then perform some animal or chemical studies himself. Approval can be sought for only one dosage form at a time, and all tests must be performed on the same batch of drug. If the *visa* expert approves, he indicates that fact to the government, and marketing can proceed. For a new dosage form, all work must be repeated.

At present the Scandinavian countries are in the process of reconciling their system among themselves. Denmark, Finland, and Norway now have systems like that of Britain. In Sweden, however, a protocol must be submitted to the Health Ministry for each clinical study to be undertaken. Such a protocol must contain all animal work, including toxicology and, specifically, perinatal toxicology in at least one species. The Health Ministry finally evaluates the evidence after the protocols have been completed and, if it approves, grants permission to market.

The Future

The American system has matured through successive eras: gullibility, nihilism, scientific discovery, and distrust. Through the maturing process great changes have occurred, and changes will continue to be made. What concerns the American public is that these changes occur in an atmosphere of trust and mutual confidence created by statesmen (not demagogues) and industrial leaders (not tycoons), with a single-minded concern for the public good. There is no reason why industry and government cannot work together toward this end; indeed, preliminary moves toward this end are in progress. What is required is integrity and fairness of mind in all involved, such that equitable decisions can be reached.

Reasonable change for the public good should be sought. Unreasonable suggestions for change should be opposed. Single standards, equitably administered, should be the rule. Pedantry should not stand in the way of efficient discovery; bureaucracy should not stand in the path of therapeutic progress. Our hope is that we enter upon a new era—an era of trust—trust earned and deserved, an era where rationality guided by intellect serves for the public, not the political, good.

Literature Cited

(1) "Annual Survey Report," Pharmaceutical Manufacturers Association, Washington, D. C., Dec. 1970.
(2) Address before the American College of Clinical Pharmacology and Chemotherapy, Atlantic City, N. J., April 28, 1967.
(3) "Commentaries," p. 5, Pharmaceutical Manufacturers Association, Washington, D. C., Feb. 1969.

(4) Douglas, James M., *Financial Analysts J.* (Sept./Oct. 1970) 115.
(5) deHaen, Paul, "New Products Parade," January 1971, page 1.
(6) "Social Security Bulletin," pp. 44–5, U. S. Department of Health, Education and Welfare, Social Security Administration, March 1970.
(7) *Amer. Druggist* (April 6, 1970).
(8) Roth, Catherine H., Trout, Monroe E., *Hospital Formulary Management* (1970) **5**, 13.

RECEIVED November 5, 1970.

10

Research and Development in the
Pharmaceutical Industry

C. W. PETTINGA[1]

Eli Lilly & Co., Indianapolis, Ind. 46206

In recent years, research and development costs in the drug industry have increased rapidly as sophisticated chemical and pharmacological techniques have required expensive equipment and specialized training. Today, emphasis in research is on mechanisms of drug action, safety and toxicology, problems of the validity of animal testing, and problems in pharmaceutical and control procedures. Working under increased government regulation and public scrutiny, the pharmaceutical industry faces increased complexity of new drug applications and evaluation of existing drugs and must rely on statistical research when the public demands scientifically impossible absolutes in effectiveness and safety. The industry, striving with all available technology and thoroughness to provide the best therapeutic agents, must have the cooperation of the medical profession and patients to achieve this goal.

In his excellent review (*1*), W. C. Wescoe has recounted some of the history of drugs and the pharmaceutical industry in the United States. His key points are:

(1) The development of the drug industry as we know it today has substantially occurred only in the last 50 years.

(2) The most rapid development, accompanied by the greatest number of changing circumstances, has taken place in the last few years. Eli Lilly & Co., for example, is 94 years old; yet, in terms of growth, it took 75 years to reach the first $100 million sales level, 14 years to reach $200 million, 4 years to attain $300 million, only 2 years for $400 million, and a little more than 1 year for $500 million. Stated in another way, the number of years required to advance $100 million in sales declined rapidly from 75 to 14 to 4 to 2 to a little more than 1.

[1] Present address: Elizabeth Arden, Inc., 3 East 54th St., New York, N. Y. 10022.

211

Other business parameters changed swiftly in a similar fashion. During the last 10 years, while sales grew 200%, the number of employees nearly doubled; earnings per share increased more than 300%; R & D expenditures are more than 2½ times what they were. The drug industry as a whole is growing rapidly and changing rapidly. In recent years increased sales have provided the financial base for ever-increasing research and development (R & D) expenditures. Are these expenditures generating the new technology and products that can provide a broader base for projecting increasing sales dollars during the next decade?

The question is not answered easily. However, at this time, there is little or no evidence that the drug industry plans to curtail research and development spending in the 1970's. In fact, the present level of recruiting supports the general belief that 1971 R & D expenditures again will increase for the total pharmaceutical industry.

It is a well recognized fact that the so-called research productivity within the drug industry is changing. Each year the Pharmaceutical Manufacturers' Association publishes the total dollar expenditures for R & D submitted by its member firms (2). If this total figure is divided by the number of new products introduced during that year, one can arrive at the average cost for R & D per product. During the last 10 years this cost has risen about 20- or 30-fold (a value which may vary within that range since there are different ways of defining a new product). The average cost of researching and developing a significant new product is now rapidly approaching $50 million dollars.

These escalating expenditures are a factor of prime significance not only for R & D management but also for total company management. It is a matter that should concern the public at large and especially those who have research experience and technical training.

It will help us to understand the reasons for the rapid increase in R & D costs per product entity if we go back to Dr. Wescoe's historical viewpoint. Sophisticated broad-scale research is relatively new, but its beginnings are rooted in a number of disciplines: botanical science, pharmacognosy, analytical chemistry, and other basic pharmaceutical sciences. Organic chemistry, biochemistry, and pharmacology were not introduced to the industry until the 1920's and 1930's. Even at that time chemistry was rather unsophisticated, and pharmacological techniques were rudimentary. Not until the 1940's and 1950's did we see the introduction of modern pharmacology with its complex intrumentation and electronic sensing. Only in the last 10 or 20 years has organic chemistry broadly applied such devices as infra-red spectrometry, nuclear magnetic resonance, mass spectrometry, and x-ray diffraction apparatus. Previously, the identification of the structure of an antibiotic often required 10 to 20 man-years of work. Compare this commitment of time and effort with the achievements of the late 1960's, when it was possible to elucidate fully the structure of an antibiotic by x-ray diffraction sometimes in as short a period as 30 days—1/12th of a man year.

However, modern equipment and modern technology, although they speed progress, are extremely expensive. The investment of a quarter of a million dollars in equipment alone for one physical chemistry lab is not at all unusual.

The installation, use, and maintenance of such equipment require scientists with an unusual degree of specialized training. Modern drug metabolism procedures enable us to select for pharmacology and toxicology studies those species of animals whose metabolic patterns most nearly resemble those of human beings. After all, our knowledge of the safety and efficacy of a drug substance is of paramount importance for man. The appropriate selection of a species for pharmacology testing and for safety evaluation can be done critically only if we have a model system which is valid. We must be able to extrapolate knowledge gained in animals to the area of clinical pharmacology and clinical medicine if our lengthy animal experiments are to have any real meaning.

It is often said that drug research is more difficult today than it was 25 years ago because of the greater complexity of the medical problems being studied. In part this is true; in part it is false. For example, in the early 1920's the usefulness of insulin in treating diabetes was discovered by Banting and Best. For nearly 50 years diabetics have been able to lead active and useful lives of relatively normal duration as a result of this discovery. If one critically reviews the literature of diabetes today, looking for an explanation of the mechanism of action of insulin, one cannot help but be astonished that after 50 years we have really achieved very little in a true understanding of the disease itself, but we do know a great deal more about insulin's role in carbohydrate and lipid metabolism. We do not know why certain inherited characteristics can lead to a predisposition to the disease. We cannot explain why some diabetics appear to have adequate stores of insulin in their pancreas. The interrelationships of insulin, glucagon, other hormones, and the central nervous system are poorly understood. No one has explained satisfactorily the regulation of insulin synthesis within the islet cells or its release into the blood stream when food is ingested. Although useful clinical entities for the treatment of diabetes have been found, the ways in which these drug substances act are still largely unexplained.

Much the same can be said for antibiotics. Although some 30 different antibiotic substances are available for the treatment and prophylaxis of infectious bacterial disease, the role of natural factors and their interrelationship with the antibacterial action of antibiotics are not completely understood. Only small beginnings have been made in the true understanding of the relationships between infectious agents and how this relationship can be modified favorably by the use of antibiotics. In no way do I wish to minimize the importance of present drugs in maintaining health in treating disease, and in alleviating pain. Today's modern physician has many powerful physiological substances without which his practice would be severely hampered. We can predict with certainty that 10 to 20 years from now many other useful agents will be added to the physician's armamentarium against disease and suffering. The physiological systems in which these drugs operate and the way in which they exert their influence will in all likelihood remain the subject of considerable study for decades to come. Today, more than at any time during the last 50 years scientists are engaged in carbohydrate and lipid research. From this research should come new knowledge leading to better therapy and, hopefully, prevention of diabetes.

We have already alluded to the increased demand for the knowledge of safety and toxicity factors and of the mechanisms of drug actions. As new technology becomes available to pharmacologists, biochemists, and biologists, their natural curiosity, plus the demands of the physicians to know how drugs operate and exert their influence, have led to further studies of the mechanisms of drug actions. In addition, many studies are aimed at demonstrating the safety of both new and old medicinal substances. The discovery that thalidomide, an extremely useful drug, was dangerous because it caused abnormal development of the fetus when taken in the early part of pregnancy did more than any other single factor to stimulate renewed interest in animal toxicology studies. I am convinced that the demonstration by Lenz in Germany (3) and others that thalidomide caused phocomelia, was the prime mover in getting Congress to pass the 1962 Amendments to the Food and Drugs Act.

Inserts in the packages of many widely used drugs carry statements such as: "Not recommended in pregnancy," "In women of child-bearing age weigh potential benefits against possible fetal hazards," or, "The safety of 'X' for use in pregnancy has not been established; therefore, this drug should be used in pregnant patients only when, in the judgment of the physician, its use is deemed essential to the welfare of the patient."

Today all new drugs are subjected to teratology studies to indicate their safety in pregnant females. However, when our studies on a new drug are complete, we can be reasonably certain only that the incidence of abnormal mice, rats, rabbits, or other animal species is not increased above the normal incidence, even though the drug is administered in high doses to the animal mother before, as well as after, conception, and during the full-term of pregnancy. We can likewise be quite certain about the lack of effects on the new born when the drug is administered to the lactating female, but, we cannot say with certainty that the drug will be safe in human beings when administered during pregnancy.

It is imperative that scientists, physicians, and the lay public, as well as our legislative bodies, be made aware that no amount of testing in animals can guarantee the safety of a medicine in all human beings. A complete lack of side effects in animals does not *prove* safety in man. Similarly, the appearance of abnormal offspring in the litters of animals given drugs during pregnancy does not necessarily mean that these substances will be unsafe when taken by pregnant women. However, no one can ever recommend that pregnant women make the heroic experiment of testing substances that produce phocomelia in animals.

In addition to the growth in scope and complexity of the physical, chemical, and biological sciences in industrial pharmaceutical research we have seen a renewed interest in pharmaceutical research, including product formulation, efficacy standards, new regulations governing good manufacturing practices, and better control procedures to ensure the quality of drugs for domestic and foreign markets.

It is inappropriate to dwell at length on the new standards for detecting bacteria in parenteral products and products designed for oral or topical medication. More people than ever before are at work in American industries, government laboratories, and academic circles reviewing drug standards. Under study are such subjects as bio-availability of drugs and methods for detecting not only the amount of active ingredients present in pharmaceutical preparations but also the presence of trace impurities. The latter may either negate the desired drug action or may cause unwanted side effects.

Government Regulation

Perhaps the greatest single change that has occurred within our industry has been in the area of government regulation and public scrutiny of our total operations. For years the pharmaceutical industry felt that its obligation consisted solely of relating to the professional members of the health professions: physicians, dentists, pharmacists, and nurses. Little or no attempt was made to make our industry understood by the man in the street, by the legislator in the state capitol, or by the Congressman in Washington. By and large, we felt we had only one public— the physicians and medical personnel who used our products to treat patients. Although a few articles appeared in the popular press in a vein similar to Paul DeKruif's "Microbe Hunters" (4), there was little understanding of the drug industry. People did not know how drug research was carried out; they had little idea how drugs were distributed or how they were made available through the chain of distribution, including wholesalers, drug stores, and hospital pharmacists.

The Kefauver hearings in 1960 did much to change this total situation. The pharmaceutical industry and the safety and efficacy of drugs have been, and will continue to be, the subject of conversation over bridge tables, by news commentators, and in the daily press. Senators and congressmen will continue to hold hearings because the public is interested in health and people are concerned with the safety and efficacy of the drug substances prescribed by their physicians. The Food and Drug Administration has formulated its requirements for the safety and effectiveness of new drug substances (5), which have greatly increased the complexity and scope of the investigations now required for a new drug application. For example, in the mid-1950's less than 100 patients were needed for clinical testing to secure FDA approval of a new antibiotic. Today, however, no drug manufacturer would submit a new drug application to the FDA unless several hundreds or even thousands of cases were studied in detail, and all the results were carefully correlated. This does not necessarily mean that in all cases the FDA receives better information today than it did 15 years ago. Twenty-five well documented, thoroughly studied cases may give almost as full an understanding of the clinical effectiveness and safety of an antibiotic as several hundred cases that appear to be less well studied and repititious. However, the facts of the matter are such that volumes of information must be collected, correlated, and indexed.

Several hundreds of pounds of documents covering the chemical and physical properties of an experimental substance and its behavior in animals must be prepared for submission to Washington. Clinical pharmacology and clinical experience obtained with a new drug substance in many centers of research must be correlated, reviewed, and summarized. This information is reviewed not only by the sponsoring company's scientists but also by outside investigators. It is finally reviewed exhaustively by the FDA. Following approval, the companies must continue at regular intervals to submit additional reports to the FDA on all experiments in animals and in human beings to support the continuation of FDA approval to distribute a product in interstate commerce. The industry and I believe that modern technology and our modern society demand that as much information as possible to made available not only to the FDA but to medical investigators and to physicians regarding the safety and efficacy of therapeutic agents sold in the United States today. We support completely the general purpose and objectives of the FDA.

However, we must remember that in the biological sciences and in the medical sciences, especially within the general area of biological sciences, there are very few absolutes. Biologists all tell us that variation is the usual event rather than the unusual event. This is why statistical research and the use of statistics is so important in all biological science.

For this reason the microbiologists use millions of organisms in a microbiological assay. It is the reason why precise measurements of the growth response of a new nutritional agent must be measured in more than one hog or in more than one beef animal.

The presence of certain unusual genetic characteristics within the human race, the concommitant use of other drugs, and all of the factors which make each patient an individual require that medicine be practiced by men with professional judgment. I know of no drugs that are absolutely safe or absolutely effective. For example, combinations of estrogens and progestins, as found in modern birth control products, are virtually 100% effective. However, if these agents are given to 100 normal married women who are fertile, about one pregnancy will occur each year that these 100 women are on therapy. There has been much publicity and much attention paid to the conception rate in women who are on the pill. Noted medical research men have argued with the pregnancy rate—0.6/100 woman years; 1.0; or 1.3. These small differences turn out to be of little consequence to the biologists who prefer to view the numbers as 98.7; 99.0; or 99.4% effective.

Of course, it is little comfort to the woman who wanted to avoid pregnancy when her doctor tells her she is the 1 in 100 who has conceived. The public has been led to believe that modern medical science and effective drug regulation, coupled with the good practice of medicine, will guarantee absolute effectiveness and absolute safety. This cannot be true.

Recently, the National Academy of Sciences–National Research Council reports (6) on the effectiveness and safety of certain drug substances have been demanding considerable attention—and work—within the FDA, within the industry, and within medical circles. Certain products have been found to be of questionable value, even though they have long had a time-honored place in American medicine. As an individual, and as a scientist I can generally agree with most if not all of the conclusions contained in the presently published reports rendered by those scientists and medical people who made up the *ad hoc* committees appointed by the NAS–NRC. Many of the antibiotic combinations which the FDA has now found to be of lesser importance in the physicians' armamentarium are indeed products whose function can be performed perhaps even better by newer, safer, more effective products. However, the combination of penicillin and procaine penicillin, which does provide a long acting dosage form of this time-honored drug, and is still very effective and very safe, in my opinion ought not to have been questioned by the FDA. I applaud, however, the FDA's recent decision to ask industry to supply new additional evidence in one year.

Quite frankly, I do fear the tendency within Americans is to look for a quick, ready, pat answer to all of our problems. As scientists, we know that our biggest job is critically to define the problem before we begin to seek answers. One must be certain of his facts before judgment is rendered, and even then one must be prepared to alter his decision if new facts emerge. For example, a few years ago it was decided that the installation and subsequent use of seat belts in automobiles would significantly reduce deaths and personal injuries in accidents. Later, it was decided that shoulder harnesses would further reduce the toll. Hence, these safety devices are now mandatory in automobiles sold in the United States. Although my sample is small, I have statistics on the drivers who wear and those who do not wear shoulder harnesses in all cars that are equipped with head rests (which became mandatory about a year after shoulder harnesses were required). On a recent trip I asked my children to conduct this survey because my personal observations indicated less than 10% of the drivers I observed were wearing shoulder harnesses. This survey was also carried out on a trip from Indianapolis to Chicago. We found that about 7% of the drivers were actually wearing shoulder harnesses; no shoulder harnesses were worn in the remaining 93% of the cars. I am neither critical of the law nor of shoulder harnesses. The point is that while regulations can force the installation of shoulder harnesses, they cannot ensure their acceptance by drivers.

So, too, with drugs. We can do extensive research; we can exhaustively study the behavior of physiologically active compounds under a variety of circumstances, in a number of different animal species. We can extensively study the clinical behavior of these substances in research hospitals and in academic institutions where medicinal skills are very high, and where intensive laboratory nursing and other aids are available. If, however, the physician does not carefully use the information presented to him, if he misuses the product, or if the patient fails to follow directions, we can expect inordinate increases in product failures and in side effects. It is very important that we, as scientists, as members of the industry, as physicians engaged in medical research and medical practice, and as responsible regulatory officials, look carefully at the total problem, that we attempt to use our best capabilities to weigh fully the balance of risk vs. benefit, and that we do not indulge in either capricious regulation or irresponsible marketing and merchandising practices. I will quickly grant that there may have been examples where drug companies have behaved in a fashion of which none of us can be proud. The main objectives of the pharmaceutical industry within the United States are identical to those of the medical profession and of the public servants who deal with regulatory problems at the FDA. We are all anxious to provide the best possible therapeutic agents wherever they are needed by physicians and patients alike.

If we exercise good judgment, if we make use of all the technology that is available, we can achieve our joint objectives. Although many problems lie ahead of us, these problems are not obstacles to progress but offer us greater opportunities to serve.

Literature Cited

(1) Wesco, W. Clark, ADVAN. CHEM. SER. (1971) **108**, 195.
(2) "Pharmaceutical Manufacturers Association Yearbook, 1969-1970," Washington, D. C., 1970.
(3) Lenz, W., *Deut. Med. Wochenschr.* (1961) **86**, 2555–2556; *Lancet* (1962) **1**, 45.
(4) DeKruif, Paul, "Microbe Hunters," Pocket Books, Inc., New York, 1966.
(5) "Requirements of the U.S. Food, Drug and Cosmetic Act," Food and Drug Administration, U.S. Department of Health, Education, and Welfare, Publ. No. 2, U.S. Government Printing Office, Washington, D. C., 1970.
(6) "Drug Efficacy Study, Final Report of the Commissioner of Foods and Drugs, Food and Drug Administration," U.S. Government Printing Office, Washington, D. C., 1969.

RECEIVED February 8, 1971.

11

Basic Biomedical Research: Its Impact on Drug Discovery

BRIAN F. HOFFMAN, M.D.

Department of Pharmacology, College of Physicians and Surgeons, Columbia University, 630 West 168th St., New York, N. Y.

The interdependence of discovery in biological research and advance in drug development is clear; this fact does not argue, however, for the predictable success of "goal-oriented" research except in special cases. In the past, basic biomedical research and drug development have made contributions of great value to the well being of mankind. If similar contributions are to continue, there must be a national commitment to support both training and research in the biomedical sciences since university resources are no longer sufficient to meet this need. Although government must provide the major financial support for these activities, there are major opportunities for the pharmaceutical industry to contribute to innovative programs and to collaborate with universities in developing ways to evaluate the ultimate consequences of possible developments in biomedical science and therapy.

Many of the advances in our understanding of biology and disease have led to the discovery of new drugs, and further the availability of new, biologically active substances most often has resulted in the acquisition of new understanding of normal and abnormal biology. The best examples are familiar to all; I prefer to avoid assuming a necessary and unique cause-effect relationship between sequential events. Indeed, I am much more impressed by the uncertainty of attributing cause to effect and by the apparent role of chance in many important discoveries.

This does not mean that I have doubts concerning the mutual independence of basic biological research and drug development. It does mean, however, that I would question seriously any plan or system under which a major part of our research and training effort was directed categorically towards certain stated objectives such as the solution of a problem in clinical medicine. I would be equally concerned by any trend in drug development which might seriously limit the discovery of new compounds because they did not have an immediate practical application.

Discovery, both in biological science and drug development, most often results from a complex reaction. This reaction requires more than the identification of a problem and the acquisition of biological data which describe it. The reaction also requires a reason—which may be ambition, curiosity, or a social or economic pressure—a reason to do something about the problem. It also requires the technical ability to do what seems to be indicated or at least the means by which the necessary techniques can be developed. Whether or not necessary new techniques materialize depends not just on the driving force for the reaction but on other complex interactions which include the state of knowledge in a variety of fields and the adequacy of information exchange between them.

While these ingredients may constitute the major reactants and the energy source for discovery, the reaction almost certainly will proceed slowly if at all in the absence of an essential catalyst. This catalyst is the adequately prepared mind or, more ofen, the conjoint action of more than one such mind.

I will describe only one example of the complex chain of events that results in discovery—discovery in drug development, in biological science, and applied therapeutics—to demonstrate both the interdependence of discoveries in biology and drug development and the practical benefit to society which results from the traditional mode of operation of our scientific community.

Isoniazid, one of the most active of the tuberculostatic drugs, was discovered because it had been shown that nicotinamide exerted some tuberculostatic action (1). A deliberate search for more effective but related chemicals revealed that many pyridine derivatives, including congeners of isonicotinic acid, also were active. Further, it was known that the thiosemicarbazones could inhibit the growth of M. tuberculosis. An attempt to synthesize the thiosemicarbazone of isonicotinaldehyde provided, as the first intermediate compound, isonicotinylhydrazine, or isoniazid.

This is an example of the direct interdependence of drug development on basic biomedical research. Knowledge gained from studies on microbial metabolism and knowledge of organic chemistry were used to develop an effective therapeutic agent. Nevertheless, chance also played a role in the sense that the activity of isoniazid was discovered and not overlooked. However, the sequence of discoveries did not stop here.

When isoniazid and its isopropyl derivative, iproniazid, were administered to patients with tubeculosis, both agents caused a marked improvement in mood or sense of well-being. Because there were properly

trained clinical investigators collaborating with basic scientists, it soon
was determined that this effect on mood did not result solely from ame-
lioration of the basic disease but rather reflected a direct effect of the
drugs employed (2). This finding led to the use of these agents in treating
depressed psychiatric patients and a concomitant search for the mechanism by which they modified brain function. Soon it was found that
iproniazid, but not isoniazid, inhibited monoamine oxidases (3). This
discovery led to the synthesis of other inhibitors of MAO and, as an
incidental result, to the introduction into the therapeutic armamentarium
of several antihypertensive agents.

Because of a variety of undesirable effects, the MAO inhibitors actually are of only limited value in treatment of either psychiatric patients
or hypertensives. Also, as we know now, it is likely that many effects of
these drugs result from actions quite independent of their ability to inhibit MAO. The mechanism by which they modify mental function still
is unclear. Nevertheless, the finding that a drug which could inhibit
MAO also modified brain function was quite important since it provided
one of the many bits of information necessary to foster continued interest
in the role of monoamines in the transfer of information in the central
nervous system, and provided one of many tools necessary for studies on
this problem (4). The dogma of electrical transmission across central
synapses was almost unquestioned until neurophysiologists succeeded in
recording postsynaptic potentials from single neurones through intracellular microelectrodes (5)—an experiment that could hardly be described as goal oriented in the sense we now use this term.

This interest in the nature of chemical transmission in the central
nervous system continues to bear fruit. For example, studies on nerve
terminals of postganglionic adrenergic fibers (6) and on the adrenal
medulla had, over a period of many years, provided a fairly clear picture
of the biosynthesis, release, reuptake, and destruction of the adrenergic
transmitter norepinephrine. Other studies had shown that in patients
with classical Parkinson's disease parts of the brain—the substantia nigra
and corpus striatum—contained less dopamine than did normal brains
(7). Dopamine is one of the intermediates in the biosynthesis of norepinephrine from phenylalanine.

Even though the precise role of monoamines in brain function still
is unclear because of many suggestions that they are responsible for certain types of information transfer between cells, the finding of a low
dopamine content was deemed significant. Since dopamine does not enter
the brain from the blood stream, treatment of Parkinson's disease was
attempted with L-dopa—L-dihidroxyphenylanine—the normal biological
precursor of dopamine. The result of this experiment was gratifying in
that L-dopa proved to be an extremely valuable therapeutic agent, far

surpassing others formerly available. Had means not been available to provide L-dopa in suitable amounts and had the pharmaceutical industry been unwilling to invest in the synthesis and experimental use of this compound, the clinical hypothesis resulting from the biological data probably still would await adequate test.

Studies on the metabolism of a microorganism—M. tuberculosis—not only contributed to the treatment of psychiatric disorders and hypertension but also played a role in providing a truly dramatic improvement in the treatment of an extremely important disease of the central nervous system, a disease which afflicts many people and severely limits their ability to function. There are many links in this chain of events, and some can be identified as chemists, biological scientists, or clinicians. Unseen links are the universities, the donors who supported research, the administrators in the pharmaceutical industry, and the patients who volunteered to take new, untried drugs.

Role of Government

How were these links forged, and how did they come to form such a chain? What changes might decrease the likelihood that new discoveries will result from similar sequences? Of paramount importance in this regard is the role of government and government support of research and training. Over the past 25 years governmental support has grown in magnitude and therefore in importance.

For this reason many are distressed by recent changes which have influenced and will continue to influence both basic biological research and drug development. Some of these changes may be described as changes in national policy. Many, quite obviously, are the inevitable and usually random by-products of the life processes of bureaucratic and political entities and the interactions between them. The most important, however, are changes in the attitudes of government and of society.

One often reads that the time has come for government to curtail its support of "pure" research in the biological sciences and emphasize the support of "goal-oriented" projects. Arguments affirm that enough basic biologic information is available to solve many currently pressing medical problems if only it were or could be applied. This argument often includes the statement that not only should support of basic research be curtailed but there should be a change in the pattern of training in the biological sciences and medicine. This change would result in the training of more technologists, who would find the means to apply existing knowledge to human problems, and the training of more physicians, who would immediately make new remedies available to those in need of them. There are as many implications to these statements as there are untested assumptions underlying them.

It is true that government support of basic research and training has been almost unbelievably generous and effective since the end of World War II. It also is true that during this period, and largely as a result of this same support, our knowledge of biology and disease has increased at a phenomenal rate. What is not true is that society has failed to benefit from these activities and from the expenditure of tax dollars made in their support. Parenthetically, what is quite unfair is to neglect the concomitant contributions made by the pharmaceutical industry and

Table I. Additions to the Therapeutic Armamentarium[a]

Therapeutic Use	*Drug or Class*
Antiarrhythmics	Procaine amide, Lidocaine Diphenylhydantoin Propranolol
Arteriosclerosis, Hyperlipidemia	Nicotinic acid Clofibrate Cholestyramine
Diuretics	Carbonic Anhydrase inhibitors Benzothiadiazines Ethacrinic acid Furosamide Aldosterone antagonists
Antineoplastic Agents	Alkylating agents Antimetabolites Antiproliferative agents
Antibiotics	Penicillin Streptomycin Chloramphenicol Erythromycin Nystatin Amphotericin Griseofulvin Bacitracin Polymycin Tetracyclines Neomycin Kanamycin Tyrothricin Cephalosporin Gentamycin Novobiocin

Table I. Continued

Therapeutic Use	Drug or Class
Tuberculostatics	Aminosalicylic acid
	Isoniazid
	Cycloserine
	Viomycin
	Streptomycin
Antimalarials	Chloraquine
	Primaquin
	Chloraguanide
	Pyrimethamine
	Trimethoprim
Heavy metals antagonists	
	Dimercaprol
	Ethylenediamine tetraacetic acid
	Penacillamine
	Deferoxamine
Psychiatric disorders	
	Phenothiazines
	Buterophenones
	Rauwolfia alkaloids
	Benzodiazepines
	MAO inhibitors
	Imipramine
	Amitriptyline
	Lithium salts
Convulsive disorders	Acetylureas
	Oxazolidinediones
	Succinimides

[a] A partial listing

many other components of the private sector of our economy. A simple means of evaluating one aspect of the practical benefits to society of the research and research training during this period is to compare the drugs listed under selected headings in a leading textbook of pharmacology published in 1940 (8) to the same listings in a current text (9). Such a list is provided in Table I. The period in question was one during which biological scientists and the pharmaceutical industry provided more new and effective remedies for important illnesses than during any other period in history. Also, during this time there was an almost parallel improvement in the means available for recognizing and diagnosing diseases and in techniques for treatment which did not depend on drug administration. To say or imply that there has been a failure to translate the new discoveries of biological science into socially useful means for the prevention and treatment of disease is simply to ignore fact. Undoubtedly, there is a need for the delivery of improved health care to a greater number of people. However, in many ways, this problem is almost entirely unrelated to the nature and effectiveness of past governmental support of basic biomedical research.

Equally fallacious is the assumption that the system of government support of biological research would become more effective if the support became more "goal oriented." Under this system, I assume, problems would be identified and rated in terms of relative importance. Also, support would be allocated to solve those problems which appeared to be most important and within the current scope of scientific and technical competence. Allied with this change in the support of research would be the inevitable shift in allocation of funds for research training. Experience has shown that while this idea is not necessarily incorrect, most often it is not applicable to the real world of biological investigation. This is so because in most instances we simply do not have enough basic information to identify the problems to be solved. If we are unable to identify the problem clearly, even the most proficient manager cannot make the other necessary decisions.

The past provides so many examples which support this statement that it is difficult to know which ones to select. However, I will mention a few. One might quite reasonably decide that death due to myocardial infarction constituted a socially important problem. Further, one might assume, as many did several years ago, that inhibition on some aspect of the blood clotting mechanism would prevent or modify the incidence of coronary artery occlusion and thus decrease mortality from myocardial infarction. We all are familiar with the tremendous amount of time and effort devoted to the use of anticoagulants in attempts to modify the course of coronary artery disease and with the negligible results which came from this "goal-oriented" program. All are familiar with the initial enthusiasm for such things as cancer chemotherapy, artificial hearts and, most recently, heart transplants. Each program provides good evidence to support the contention that identification of a problem usually has been made in terms of superficialities. For example, the "problem" in terms of cardiac transplantation, was not a question of the surgical feasibility of the transplantation procedure, the availability of agents which would suppress the immune response of the patient or even the availability for techniques for tissue typing. The problem was much larger, much more subtle and, to me, still only ill defined. Had it not been for the apparent effectiveness of the first successful cardiac transplantation (again the role of chance in discovery) I feel quite certain that the same people who planned for a massive program of cardiac transplantation in this country would have come to quite a different decision.

Obviously, sometimes, "goal-oriented" research can be and has been effective. This happens when both the information necessary to identify the problem and the techniques necessary for its solution not only are available but are known to the proper people. When this happens, the goal often is achieved reasonably expeditiously as was the case in the synthesis of BAL as an antidote to lewisite (10) or the development of PAM as an antidote for the organophosphorous compounds (11). However, the success of attempts to solve limited and clearly defined problems does not argue that similar success can be anticipated when large, poorly understood, and often illdefined problems are set as goals.

Here I will mention only one example. Disturbances of cardiac rhythm are an important medical problem. Quinidine, the d-isomer of quinine, is one of the most effective agents available for the treatment of cardiac arrhythmias. The discovery that quinine, and subsequently quinidine, could be used to treat certain arrhythmias must be attributed to luck. A patient of Wenckebach, a famous Viennese physician, noted in 1912 that when he took quinine for his malaria it also caused his rapid, irregular pulse to become slower and more regular. In 1918 Frey compared several cinchana alkaloids and found that quinidine was more effective in treating atrial fibrillation than quinine. Subsequently, quinidine was found to be effective against many other cardiac arrhythmias.

Since quinidine has many effects on living systems, its use as a therapeutic agent is associated with many toxic or undesirable actions. For years the search for a better agent has continued. Basic scientists identified the actions of quinidine on the heart, and many representatives of the pharmaceutical industry synthesized and evaluated a host of chemicals with similar actions. However, to my knowledge, no clinically superior drug ever resulted. Only recently have we begun to understand why.

It was inappropriate to attempt to improve on quinidine as an antiarrhythmic drug until there was some reliable information on its mechanism of action. This could not be obtained until there was an understanding of the mechanisms responsible for the production of arrhythmias in diseased hearts, and the techniques and information necessary for this understanding still are insufficient. To be more specific, it was incorrect to identify the need to treat cardiac arrhythmias or even a specific disturbance of rhythm as a "problem" and equally incorrect to set the search for a compound exerting some but not all of the actions of quinidine as a "goal."

Although I have strong reservations concerning the ability of government to identify problems and set goals for biomedical research, I do recognize the fact that government must remain involved in support of these activities. Indeed the need for continuing governmental support is greater now than at any time in the past. While at one time it was reasonable for universities to support some fraction of research and research training, changes both in the cost of research and the financial resources of the universities are such that we have become completely dependent on continuing and increasing government participation. The cost of biomedical research increases as a function of its complexity, and this complexity usually increases in proportion to the amount of information available on the problem under study. A larger and longer fraction of the dwindling financial resources of the universities will have to be allocated to meet the ever-pressing need to increase the size of classes and increase the amount of time faculty members devote to teaching. At the same time the income available to the universities is decreasing in relation to necessary expenses. As a result, the ability of the universities to support predoctoral candidates, postdoctoral trainees, and established investigators will decrease until, in the absence of adequate government funding, in many areas these activities sooner or later will cease to exist.

There are other reasons why government support of basic biomedical research and training not only should continue but should be a national commitment. The best people will not enter the long and difficult training programs in biomedical science unless they are reasonably certain that upon completion of their training they will have an opportunity to use their skills and knowledge effectively and productively. Even if it were possible for the universities to continue training programs, in the absence of direct support of research highly competent investigators would be forced to turn to other activities. Some might turn to teaching, but it is not always correct to assume that the best laboratory scientist will be the best teacher. What is essential to attract the best people and to ensure continuing scholarly activity in biomedical science is a reasonable guarantee that the truly competent investigator will be able to devote his life to the studies which seem to him most important, most interesting, and most exciting.

It is not sufficient to guarantee direct governmental support of research in basic biomedical science. There also must be continuing support of training and continuing salary support of qualified investigators.

If one concludes that there will be a continuing need for long term support of basic biomedical research, then one also must ask what should be the nature of this support and how should it be allocated? Although it may be inevitable that government agencies will identify broad areas in biomedical research where, because of real or imagined social pressure, support will be more generous, funds also should be made available in other areas to support research on good ideas. The history of the National Institutes of Health and the National Science Foundation has borne out the lesson learned throughout the centuries by the universities. A reasonable return on an investment is most likely if support is granted to individuals who have demonstrated their ability to identify important problems and work effectively towards their solution. Nevertheless, support also must be made available to the new and untried investigator who has had good training and who has a good idea. Obviously, evaluation of this sort of idea can be made only by the best scientists, who should serve not only on the initial review of applications for research support but also should participate in all subsequent decisions.

The identification of research goals must not preclude the support of good ideas, which are truly rare, or the support of good scientists. This argument is based strongly on the contention that it usually is impossible to identify the particular group of discoveries which will provide the keystone to the solution of a problem. Further, when a solution materializes, the benefits to society often are immeasurable. One only need think of the effect of adequate chemotherapeutic agents on tuberculosis; the tremendous change in the treatment and well-being of the emotionally ill which resulted from the discovery of chlorpromazine and a host of other drugs which modify mood and affect or the immense benefit which resulted from the development of effective means to immunize against poliomyelitis.

While I have more or less described a program of government support similar to the very best parts of past and present National Institutes of Health (NIH) programs, I believe that some changes in the pattern of support should be considered. Obviously the allocation of funds for research training should be completely free of poiltical influence or regional, economic, or other considerations. Funds for the support research training should not be diverted to other types of training such as residency programs. Funds allocated for research should not be used to deliver health services or to develop programs. There probably should be greater flexibility in the support programs at all levels. More important, support of research training probably should be less categorical. In many instances it will probably be necessary to provide the biological scientist of the future with a more varied educational experience than can be derived from our present system. It might be reasonable to develop training programs which would combine offerings in biochemistry and pharmacology or chemistry, pharmacology, and physiology with the admixture taking place either at the predoctoral or postdoctoral level. Programs such as the Medical Scientist Program, which provide M.D. candidates with research training in basic biological science, should be strengthened. Finally, as our understanding of biology and medicine increases, there will be an increasing need for people trained not only in the current biomedical disciplines but also in areas which we cannot yet identify.

I am not insisting that our present system, or systems formerly employed, are ideal. Clearly, means should be developed to provide the basic biological scientist with an understanding and appreciation of the importance of applying the results in his research to socially important problems. This can be done in part by the universities and medical centers, but this requirement presents an opportunity and challenge to the pharmaceutical industry. The effective transfer of information from basic to applied research depends on an understanding on the part of standing on the part of the medical practitioner or the pharmaceutical industry of the possibilities which have been made available by basic research. This sort of understanding can result only if the basic biological scientist is in continuing contact with the various individuals who might apply the results of his research to the solution of practical problems. Obviously, therefore, means should be developed to change the attitudes of all concerned and to foster continuing contact between individuals and groups who ordinarily do not take advantage of the contributions made in disciplines related to their own.

I have no suggestions which are certain to solve these problems. I do have some ideas which might deserve consideration. I am not concerned so much with means to change the attitudes of the basic biomedical scientist. The search for relevance already is a major concern of the young, and this concern only will increase in the future. I am more interested in developing means to foster the exchange of ideas and information. Industry should participate much more in the support of training in all the biomedical sciences and not emphasize so strongly areas of direct interest such as chemistry or clinical pharmacology. It also should contribute to training at both the predoctoral and postdoctoral levels. This contribution need not be only direct financial support, it probably should include the participation of industry personnel and the use of specialized facilities available in industry. In pharmacology, for example, students could benefit greatly from contact with experts in drug development or in clinical evaluation. Industry also should be willing to participate more fully in the support of basic research, as opposed to research which clearly contributes to the evaluation of potential therapeutic agents.

Means should be developed to further the exchange of personnel between industry and the academic institutions. This could be done by developing programs under which members of either group could spend one or two years working as a member of the other. The faculty member might benefit greatly from an opportunity to work full-time in a laboratory where he would have access to the personnel and facilities developed by a pharmaceutical company and, through his presence, might even make some contribution. A member of an industrial research group similarly might benefit from a year or two in a basic science department. Finally, industry could try to make greater use of the members of the basic biomedical science departments in our universities. Several members of such a department, carefully selected because of demonstrated competence and knowledge, might provide invaluable advice at many points during the sequence of steps leading to the introduction of a new drug and likely would serve more effectively in this capacity than the traditional consultant. More important, however, would be the fact that, through such an arrangement, many basic biomedical scientists would be brought into contact with representatives of industry and would learn of new attitudes, problems, and areas of concern.

The system should include a formal mechanism to study the probable and possible long range effects of any possible discovery. For example, if means can be developed to implant artificial hearts in many elderly patients, someone should ask if it is reasonable to do so in terms of cost, actual contribution to the well-being of the patients and possible consequences. If a large fraction of research support is to be allocated to studies on genetic engineering, some part of that support should be made available to evaluate the ultimate psychological, social, and economic effects of success. As we approach the time when more and more becomes possible, the identification of research goals becomes less important than a serious consideration of the consequences of discovery. In this area an effective joint action by industry and academia would be most important and perhaps would contribute to the solution of many of the other problems.

Literature Cited

(1) Fox, H. H., "The Chemical Attack on Tuberculosis," *Trans. N.Y. Acad. Sci.* (1953) **15**, 234–242.

(2) Delay, J., Deniker, P., Harl, J. M., "Utilisation en Therapeutique Psychiatrique d'une Phenothiazine d'Action Centrale Elective," *Ann. Med-psychol.* (1952) **110**, 112–117.

(3) Zeller, A. E., Barsky, J., Fouts, J. R., Kirchheimer, W. F., Van Orden, L. S., "Influence of Isonicotinic Acid Hydrazide (INH) and 1-Isonicotinyl 2-Isopropyl Hydrazide (IIH) on Bacterial and Mammalian Enzymes," *Experientia* (1952) **8**, 349–350.

(4) Brodie, B. B., Shore, P. A., "A Concept for a Role of Serotonin and Norepinephrine as Chemical Mediators in the Brain," *Ann. N.Y. Acad. Sci.* (1957) **66**, 631–642.

(5) Eccles, J. C., "The Physiology of Synapses," Springer-Verlag, Berlin; Academic Press, New York, 1964.

(6) Euler, U. S. von, "Twenty Years of Noradrenaline," *Pharmacol. Rev.* (1966) **18**, 29–38.

(7) Hornykiewicz, O., "Dopamine (3-Hydroxytryptamine) and Brain Function," *Pharmacol. Rev.* (1966) **18**, 925–964.
(8) Goodman, L., Gillman, A., "The Pharmacological Basis of Therapeutics," MacMillan, New York, 1941.
(9) Goodman, L., Gillman, A., "The Pharmacological Basis of Therapeutics," 2nd ed., MacMillan, New York, 1970.
(10) Stocken, L. A., Thompson, R. H. S., "Reactions of British Anti-Lewisite with Arsenic and Other Metals," *Physiol. Rev.* (1949) **29**, 168–194.
(11) Wilson, I. B., Ginsburg, S., "A Powerful Reactivator of Alkylphosphate-Inhibited Acetylcholinesterases," *Biochem. Biophys. Acta* (1955) **18**, 168–170.

RECEIVED November 5, 1970.

12

The Role of the NIH in Health Research

ROBERT W. BERLINER, M.D.

Deputy Director for Science, National Institutes of Health, U. S. Department of Health, Education, and Welfare, Bethesda, Md. 20014

The National Institutes of Health contains 10 research institutes and six research and service divisions. It has also been responsible since 1968 for national development of health manpower and communications. National support for medical research and development rose from about $160 million in fiscal 1950 to almost $2.7 billion in 1970. The Federal share for those years was $73 million and $1.7 billion, of which NIH contributed $28 million (38%) and $872 million (53%). The 1971 budget for the institutes and research divisions, as presented to the Senate, represents an increase of $87 million (9%) over 1970. Departments of chemistry and biochemistry received 1656 NIH research grants totaling $59 million in fiscal 1970. In addition, contracts supported target research programs in cancer chemotherapy ($18 million), pharmacology–toxicology, chemistry communications, and contraceptive development.

Passage of the National Cancer Act in 1937 marked the beginning of the National Institutes of Health (NIH) as it exists today. In creating the National Cancer Institute, Congress established a pattern for a categorical approach to biomedical science. Similar actions by Congress in the postwar period led to the establishment of what are now 10 research institutes within NIH (Figure 1).

Most of these are oriented toward groups of diseases—allergic and infectious, arthritic and metabolic, cardiovascular and pulmonary, neurological, etc.—which are major causes of death or disability in the United States. Three of the institutes, however—the Institute of General Medical Sciences, of Child Health and Human Development, and of Environmental Health Sciences—have roles that cut across categorical lines.

Through a reorganization of the Public Health Service in 1968, NIH is now responsible for developing health manpower and communicating biomedical information as well as for medical research and training.

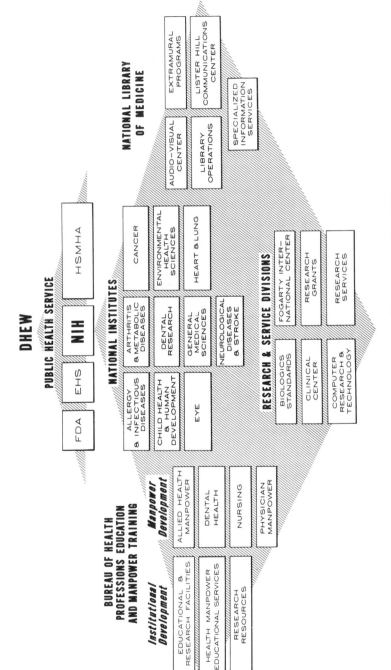

Figure 1.   Breakdown of research institutes within NIH

World War II provided the impetus for a heavy national investment in research. Before the war, medical research represented a very small segment of the budget of academic institutions. Objectives were modest, and the goals were largely those of the individual investigator. Total medical research expenditures for the nation came to about $45 million. Only a small part of this, some $3 million, came from the federal government. Industry accounted for the bulk, some $25 million, while foundations and voluntary health agencies supplied $12 million, and another $5 million came from endowment sources.

Largely because of the success of research in attacking major problems related to the war effort, public attitudes toward federal investments in science and technology underwent a change following the war. Research activities in all sectors began to expand, and sponsorship patterns began to change. Total support for biomedical research and development rose from about $160 million in fiscal 1950 to almost $2.7 billion in 1970. As a proportion of all the nation's R & D, medical research funds increased over this period from about 5.6% to 10%.

The nature of this change is reflected in Figure 2. Between 1947 and 1950 federal support had more than doubled, rising from $27 million to $73 million. By 1955 federal support had exceeded non-federal, though the latter continued to increase. The annual federal expenditure is now about $1.7 billion, representing some 62% of the total. Growth rates for the funds contributed by industry and state governments (the latter not shown separately in the figure) have been roughly equivalent to those of the federal government, but the contributions of private individuals and foundations have been increasing less rapidly.

When we examine the breakdown of federal sponsorship (Figure 3), we find that the major supporter of biomedical research is the Department of Health, Education and Welfare. Twenty years ago the Atomic Energy Commission and the Department of Defense played major roles, contributing respectively 25 and 14% of the total federal support. At present, each of these two agencies, and the Space Agency, accounts for 6 or 7% of the federal sponsorship. The Department of Health, Education and Welfare's share is mainly attributable to NIH, and a considerable part of the non-NIH portion is represented by the National Institute of Mental Health. [The National Institute of Mental Health was included in NIH until it became a separate bureau in 1967.]

Today NIH accounts for about a third of all support for biomedical R & D in the United States. Its role is greater if the focus is put on academic research since little of the industrial investment goes to academic institutions. If, in addition, contributions to research training, and of research training to the conduct of research, are taken into consideration, the NIH role is even larger.

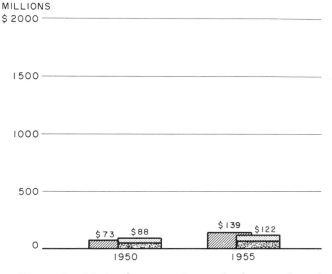

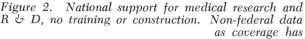

Figure 2. National support for medical research and R & D, no training or construction. Non-federal data as coverage has

The current level of funding by NIH is illustrated in Tables I, II, and III. Table I presents, by organizational component, the estimated obligations for fiscal year 1970 and the administration budget as presented to the Senate Appropriations Committee. The latter figures constitute an increase over the original budget, made in response to the actions of the House of Representatives. This revised administration request would provide a net increase of $123 million, or a little less than 9%. Of this, $87 million is for the institutes and research divisions, including major increases for certain research programs, as indicated in Table II:

(a) The National Cancer Institute, for studies on the relationship between viruses and cancer

(b) The National Heart and Lung Institute, for investigations related to atherosclerosis

(c) The National Institute of Dental Research, for work on the prevention of caries

(d) The National Institute of Child Health and Human Development, for a program on population and family planning

Modest increases are also proposed for the new programs of the Eye Institute and the Institute of Environmental Health Sciences. The other institutes would rise a little above their 1970 levels, which are generally below their 1969 levels. Table III shows the distribution of the increases by activity. $25 million of the increase is for the regular research grant programs. Increases are also proposed for the specialized research centers and, to a lesser extent, for the categorical and general clinical research centers.

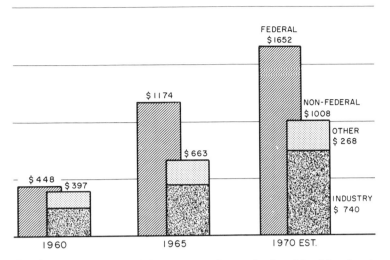

development (1950–1970). Covers only medical and health-related
since 1964 are not strictly comparable with those for prior years,
been improved.

Collaborative reseach and development is a category of work generally carried out through research contracts. The substantial increase in
this category represents emphasis on research in viral oncology and in
family planning and contraceptive technology.

It is appropriate at this point to digress briefly to discuss the goals
of NIH's involvement in the support and conduct of research because
these goals are sometimes misunderstood. In fact, medicinal chemistry
is one field in which something less than ideal communication concerning
goals has resulted in some distrust and dissatisfaction on the part of
advisory groups and investigators who have applied for NIH support.

Research is an activity pursued with many motives and purposes.
In fact, a particular effort may be pursued with different objectives by
the investigator, by his institution, and by the supporting agency:

(a) An investigator may be motivated by his desire to achieve understanding and conceptual mastery; by the pleasure he gets from success
in solving problems; by his aspirations for recognition; by the gratification
he may derive from knowledge that contributes to progress against disease.

(b) An academic institution fosters research because scholarship
requires creation of new knowledge as well as transmission of existing
knowledge.

(c) NIH supports research not, as in the case of the National Science
Foundation, for its contribution to science itself. NIH is not a science
agency; it is a health agency. Science is the means, health the objective.
Congress appropriates funds for NIH to conduct, support, and coordinate
research, to the extent that these activities are relevant to the maintenance

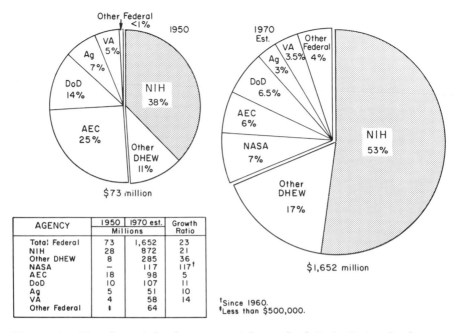

AGENCY	1950	1970 est.	Growth Ratio
	Millions		
Total Federal	73	1,652	23
NIH	28	872	21
Other DHEW	8	285	36
NASA	—	117	117[†]
AEC	18	98	5
DoD	10	107	11
Ag	5	51	10
VA	4	58	14
Other Federal	‡	64	

[†]Since 1960.
[‡]Less than $500,000.

Figure 3. Trends in federal support of biomedical R & D for fiscal years 1950–1970 (obligations in millions of dollars). Covers biomedical research projects, resources, and general support but not training or construction.

of the health of the American people and to the causes, diagnosis, treatment, and prevention of disease.

Consequently, NIH seeks to support, in a broad context, research that will advance its mission. This objective is not necessarily the one pursued by the investigator or his institution. The basic role of the National Advisory Councils, which by law must recommend support of a project before it can receive grant funds, is to ensure the relevance of the scientifically meritorious projects supported to the mission of the institute and to the purpose for which the funds are provided.

Table I. NIH Budget Totals (in millions), FY 1970-71

	Program	1970 Estimate	1971 Rev. Adm. Request	Increase 1971/70
Obligations	Total NIH	$1417	$1540	$123
under	I/D	974	1061	87
new budget	BEMT	414	451	37
authority	NLM	19	20	1
	OD and bldgs.	10	8	−2

Of course, we recognize that progress in health is utterly dependent upon science and that ultimately all science, at least all "natural science," springs from a common base. No research is so fundamental that we can say that it does not have and never will have relevance to health. Nevertheless, we must recognize a level sufficiently remote from biomedical research that its present contributions can have little if any import for the foreseeable future. For example, current work in subatomic particle physics is unlikely to have an early influence, despite the tremendous importance in biomedical research of the atomic physics of a generation ago. Few people would expect the NIH to support work in present-day atomic physics.

On the other hand, as we go up the tree of science we reach branches that often diverge from that of biomedicine. The farther we go out on such pathways, the less likely it is that the findings will contribute significantly to the progress of medical science. Thus it is far more likely that work in fundamental organic chemistry will yield results relevant to the mission of NIH than, say, work on the chemistry of plant hormones, interesting though the latter may be in its own right.

Table II. NIH Budget by Organizational Component (in millions), FY 1970-71

NIH Component	1970 Est. Oblig.	1971 Rev. Adm. Request	Increase 1971/70
Total NIH	$1417	$1540	$123
Total I/D	974	1061	87
NCI	181	207	26
NHLI	161	178	17
NIDR	29	35	6
NIAMD	132	136	4
NINDS	96	100	4
NIAID	98	101	3
NIGMS	148	152	4
NICHD	75	94	19
NEI	24	26	2
NIEHS	18	20	2
DBS	8	9	1
FIC	3	3	0

Returning now to some of the specifics of the NIH role, the data presented indicate that research has become, in the postwar era, a major component of the academic scene. The support of research and the training of scientists influence the stability of many institutions of higher learning across the broad range of their activities.

Table III.   NIH Budget by Program Activities
(in millions), FY 1970-71

Program Activity	1970 Est. Oblig.	1971 Rev. Adm. Request	Increase 1971/70
Total NIH	$1417	$1540	$123
Regular research grant program	435	460	25
noncompeting	313	318	5
competing	122	142	20
Special research grant programs	157	171	14
general research support	50	53	3
specialized research centers	14	21	7
categorical clinical research centers	10	11	1
general clinical research centers	35	38	3
other	48	48	0
Collaborative R & D	127	166	39
Research training programs	179	177	−2
fellowships	47	45	−2
training grants	132	132	0
All other programs	519	566	47

Much research today requires access to large-scale resources, technical skills, and cooperative scientific relationships available only in an institution adequately staffed and administered. To help meet these problems new support programs were devised by NIH in the early 1960's, programs which funded general facilities such as primate centers, general and categorical clinical research centers, and various special resources. Other institutional programs include general research support grants, which enable institutions to strengthen their research capabilities. Today the total funding of such special resources and general research support amounts to $157 million.

Chemistry has long held an important place in all NIH programs. Data compiled for fiscal 1968 show that almost $30 million, or 8% of all NIH grant funds awarded for individual research projects, was allocated to the support of chemistry, while nearly $39 million, or 11%, went to biochemistry (excluding grants awarded by the Bureau of Health Professions Education and Manpower Training and the National Library of Medicine). These figures are inferred from the disciplinary character of the primary review groups that recommended grant support; they are the amounts awarded for applications reviewed by the Study Sections for Biophysics and Biophysical Chemistry (A and B), Biochemistry, Medicinal Chemistry (A and B), and Physiological Chemistry.

Another estimate has been made by summating NIH project grants to departments of chemistry and biochemistry for the years 1967 through 1970. Table IV shows that there were about 1900 awards in fiscal 1967, dropping to 1656 in 1970, while the dollar amounts rose from $60.4 million to $63.2 (1969) and then dropped to $59.3. These figures clearly yield an underestimate of the support of chemistry since it is obvious that neither all chemistry nor all biochemistry are confined to university departments that carry those names. In addition, they do not include a considerable amount of chemistry supported by the contract mechanism.

In recent years, several large targeted programs have developed. The first was in cancer chemotherapy, which was organized in 1955 when Congress asked the National Cancer Institute to undertake a large-scale attempt to find new and better antitumor drugs.

During the first decade, the Institute organized a program that provided sources of new drugs from synthetic and natural products, animal tumor systems for screening the chemicals, extensive animal studies for toxicity and safety of drugs, resources for the study of the action of drugs in animals and man, formulation of drug products, and finally clinical trials—all the familiar activities of any organization for pharmaceutical development.

The work in this field is not competitive with the pharmaceutical industry. Much of the support, in fact, goes to industrial contractors. Rather, the program is an attempt to carry out a coordinated and targeted effort in a field in which the necessarily high risk and heavy investment makes large-scale venture unattractive to industry.

Strong congressional interest in the cancer chemotherapy program led to its rapid expansion. Between 1956 and 1961, contracts increased from about $800,000 to $24 million. Fiscal 1965, in which $29 million was awarded, marked the high point, and subsequent funding has been around $20 million a year. If direct operations and grants as well as contracts are taken into account, the current level of the program is about $50 million.

The systematic search for antitumor drugs involves a variety of efforts. Empirical testing of natural and synthetic products continues, but scientific selection of materials for screening is playing a larger and larger role. Availability of numerous chemicals that cause regression of clinical cancer is beginning to make possible study of the relation of chemical

Table IV. NIH Project Grants to Departments of Chemistry and Biochemistry, FY 1967-1970 (Dollars in millions)

Fiscal Year	Total		Chemistry		Biochemistry	
	Awards	Amount	Awards	Amount	Awards	Amount
1967	1901	$60.4	839	$25.0	1062	$35.3
1968	1826	63.5	816	26.2	1010	37.4
1969	1860	63.2	836	26.2	1024	37.0
1970	1656	59.3	730	24.4	926	34.9

structure to anticancer activity. It is to be hoped that the choice of compounds for introduction into the screen will be increasingly determined by structure–function considerations, so that directed synthesis may gradually displace, or at least heavily supplement, much of the empirical screening.

Major successes in drug control have been mainly in the area of rapidly growing tumors, such as acute lymphocytic leukemia, Burkitt's lymphoma, choriocarcinoma, Wilm's Tumor, and Hodgkin's disease; many of the most highly active anti-cancer drugs, such as methotrexate and vincristine, affect cells only during the division cycle. The types that are poorly responsive to drugs, such as cancers of the lung, breast and colon, are slow growing. It is hypothesized that susceptibility to cancer drugs may be determined by the fraction of cells dividing at any one time. Attempts are being made to extend to the slower growing tumors what has been learned from successful chemotherapy in man.

An activity highly relevant to the subject of this book is the pharmacology–toxicology program of the National Institute of General Medical Sciences. This program provides support for multidisciplinary research and research training on problems related to the use and misuse of drugs. Last year, 64 predoctoral trainees in pharmacology and toxicology earned Ph.D. degrees. This represents about half of the total annual production of pharmacologists in the nation.

The program's effectiveness in providing pharmacologists and toxicologists for academic, industrial, and government positions is indicated in the placement of institute trainees who completed their training in the period 1964–66. Of 186 trainees who finished this program, 108 joined faculties of universities and colleges, including 89 on medical school faculties. Twenty entered government service, 45 entered private industry, and 14 went on to additional training.

The institute is now funding 10 research centers and 10 program projects, multidisciplinary in nature and covering a continuum of research from molecular pharmacology to direct application in man. About half of the institute's annual investment in pharmacology–toxicology, which totals $17 million, is represented by research grants. Research training grants account for a third of the total program, with the remainder divided between fellowships, research contracts, and a small research associates program.

At Tufts University School of Medicine, the institute supports a collaborative drug surveillance program as a model for reporting adverse drug reactions. This project is intended to identify and characterize untoward drug reactions in man by prospective study and to evaluate drug efficacy in a large patient population. The computer-oriented project encompasses a network of 10 hospitals involving 6000 hospitalized patients and more than 60,000 drug orders.

Several activities of the National Library of Medicine relate specifically to drugs and chemicals. In 1965, NIH, the Department of Defense, and the National Science Foundation initiated a program with the Chemical Abstracts Service for development of a national registration system for chemicals. The program was designed to serve as an authoritative source of information on chemicals and drugs. During the next several years, more than one million compounds were entered into the system. Information on both structure and nomenclature, as well as bibliographic data, have been included in the service. The registry enables one to determine whether a given structure or name is on file and to identify other synonyms as well. A new registry number is assigned whenever a new structure is uncovered.

Shortly after this activity was initiated, the National Library of Medicine (NLM) and the Food and Drug Administration (FDA) were given responsibility for providing more specific access to health-related information about drugs and chemicals. It was decided at that time to build a data base from the chemical registry system which would fit the specific requirements of NLM and FDA. A subsidiary project was established with Chemical Abstracts Service as part of the chemical registry contract, which is administered by the National Science Foundation. The data base was built from information available in the files of NLM and FDA and from approximately 40 standard reference sources on drugs and chemicals.

These sources included, among others, the "U. S. Pharmacopoeia" and the "Merck Index." Thus, the common data base would contain compounds known to be of interest to people in the health field, including drugs, antibiotics, hazardous materials, pesticides, nutrients, and food additives as well as "inert" compounds in such substances. Chemical Abstracts Service processed these sources against its registry system and added registrations as well as synonyms as they were found in these standard references. The data were delivered to FDA and NLM in a form suitable for processing in their machine systems.

In addition to the registry numbers, the material in the common data base includes information on molecular structure, official "U. S. Pharmacopoeia" and other names, known synonyms, and codes indicating the sources of information. The data have been worked into the computer systems of both FDA and NLM and have been reproduced in a six-volume Desktop Analysis Tool, which is available from the Clearinghouse for Federal Scientific and Technical Information (Springfield, Va.). The first output of the data base consisted of approximately 30,000 chemical substances and approximately 150,000 names and synonyms.

The National Library of Medicine is using this file as an aid in indexing information on drugs from the world's biomedical literature. The Library's Medical Literature Analysis and Retrieval System (MEDLARS) uses a controlled vocabulary to gain consistency in indexing. In the past, the number of specific drugs and chemicals that could be explicitly identified by this vocabulary was limited to somewhat less than 1000. All other materials have been indexed under more generic chemical class terms and could generally not be listed in *Index Medicus* or retrieved from MEDLARS explicitly.

In a second generation of MEDLARS, which is planned for implementation this fall, it will be possible, with the aid of the data base established through the Chemical Abstracts registry system, to index biomedical publications with many more specific terms and chemicals than has been possible under MEDLARS I. While it is not projected that this extensive listing of chemical compounds be included in *Index Medicus,* it will be possible to provide such listings in other MEDLARS products. Thus a current publication of the Library, the "Toxicology Bibliography," will list the biomedical literature by any desired chemical classification.

A new and rapidly expanding program with a heavy involvement of chemistry is in the field of contraceptive development. This program is administered by the Center for Population Research in the National Institute of Child Health and Human Development. The budget currently being considered by Congress includes, in addition to funds for grants, some $6.5 million for contracts in the contraceptive development program, an increase of more than 60% over funds obligated for this purpose in 1970. The urgency of the problem of population growth and the strong pressures for improved technology for its solution indicate that support in this area will probably continue to increase in the next few years.

Four possible points of attack on the reproductive process have been identified for particular study:
(a) Maturation and fertilizing capacity of spermatozoa
(b) Oviduct function and gamete transport
(c) Biology of the ovum
(d) Corpus luteum function and implantation

Research in these areas may lead to agents that alter normal sperm development or interfere with mechanisms controlling transport of sperm or ova in the oviduct or with the normal composition of oviductal fluids. It may be possible to prevent ovulation, to interfere with ovum development, or to cause early cessation of function of the corpus luteum.

Patentable inventions are frequently among the products of the expenditure of public funds through NIH grants. The aim of the Department's policy is that the results of research supported by grants of public funds be utilized in the manner that will best advance the public interest. To quote from the official regulations and procedures:

The public interest will in general be best served if inventive advances resulting therefrom are made freely available to the Government, to science, to industry, and to the general public.

On the other hand, in some cases it may be advisable to permit a utilization of the patent process in order to foster an adequate commercial development to make a new invention widely available. Moreover, it is recognized that inventions frequently arise in the course of research activities which also receive substantial support from other sources, as well as from the Federal grant. . . . In all these cases the Department has a responsibility to see that the public use of the fruits of the research will not be unduly restricted or denied.

The Assistant Secretary for Health and Scientific Affairs has the power of determination in the disposition of the rights to patentable discoveries arising during work supported by either grants or contracts. It is the intent to see that the involvement of government funds in the discovery does not impede public use of the fruits of the research. Recognizing that commercial development may be desirable, the Government can and does on occasion assign exclusive rights to certain inventions to encourage their development and application.

A number of possible options are available for handling the rights to patentable inventions, and there are a number of models available in the practices of various government agencies. In the chemotherapy program of the National Cancer Institute, there is provision for contractors to obtain patents on drugs developed in the program, provided they are marketed at a reasonable price, in sufficient quantity, and within a reasonable period of time. Another procedure was used by the Department of Transportation in relation to development of the supersonic transport (SST). This provided for the contractor to bear some 10% of the developmental costs and for the government to recover its investment from the profits that would subsequently derive from the development.

While possible arrangements other than those we now use may be worked out for future programs, such as that in the area of contraceptive development, such agreements should encourage industry–government cooperation and at the same time further the public interest. Perhaps sharing of both costs and profits will be the most equitable model.

Clearly, the period of rapid growth has passed, and indeed, it would have been unrealistic to have expected it to continue, even if we had not come into a period of severe fiscal restraints. It is also unlikely that we will ever return to growth rates for medical research as a whole comparable with those that prevailed between 1955 and 1965. Over the last three or four years, as funds have remained relatively stable while research costs have increased continually, there has been a considerable decrease in the effort that NIH funds have been able to support. I am convinced that this represents entirely the pressures of fiscal problems and not any decision to abandon research on health problems. In fact, the department has stated that its policy is to maintain at least the present level of effort, although this has required some modification in the face of fiscal realities. At the same time, the Congress, in its action on last year's budget and more emphatically in its actions to date on this year's, has indicated its strong support for a continued attack on health problems through research.

Despite the general dissatisfaction with the delivery of health care and the manpower available to effect this delivery, neither the manpower nor the resources devoted to health research is large enough to affect seriously health care delivery, even if they were diverted entirely to that purpose. At the same time it must be recognized that the only prospect for an improved product for delivery by an improved delivery system lies in continued growth of knowledge through science.

RECEIVED November 5, 1970.

13

Government Regulations and Drug Development: FDA

JOHN JENNINGS, M.D.

Associate Commissioner for Medical Affairs, Food and Drug Administration,
Public Health Service, Parklawn Building, 5600 Fishers Lane,
Rockville, Md. 20852

*The Food and Drug Administration (FDA), accused of pro-
moting regulations which stifle research and keep good
drugs off the market, replies that the regulations reflect practices that have evolved in the pharmaceutical sciences, and
represent FDA efforts to improve the quality and expedite
the processing of submissions and the introduction of really
new drugs. Studies cited suggest that the cause of decline in
the introduction of new drugs is that research and development by the drug industry have been primarily the improvement of products or processes rather than the discovery of new chemical entities. Industry's approach may
be counter-productive in that scientific expertise has been
devoted to imitative rather than innovative research. An
appeal is made to examine this proposition and to promote
vigorous, imaginative programs of drug research in an effort
to return to the innovative stage.*

The Food and Drug Administration is keeping good drugs off the market. Their regulations are stifling research. The dearth of new drugs
is a direct result of the 1962 efficacy amendments.

These charges (referring to Amendments to the Food, Drug and
Cosmetic Act) are all too familiar to those concerned with the discovery
and development of new drugs. This chapter examines the basis of such
charges and offers a suggestion regarding research and development.

History of the Food and Drug Administration

Since 1906, the year the Food and Drugs Act was passed, the
primary concern of the FDA has been consumer protection. In the area

of drugs, it has meant that proprietary or patent medicines with dangerous habit-forming ingredients and adulterated medicines, a great threat
at the turn of the century, were taken off the market.

In the early days, the FDA was restricted to action after injury had
occurred and the agency had to prove not only cause and effect but also
intent. Then, just as better laws are often born out of tragedy, in 1938
the Congress saw the need for the new Food, Drug and Cosmetic Act
after more than 100 persons had died of taking an untested elixir of
sulfanilamide made with a toxic solvent. The new law required for the
first time that drugs be proved safe before being allowed on the market.
Formal evidence of efficacy was not required, although, as we all know,
the two factors of safety and efficacy cannot really be separated.

In 1962 the Act was further amended to require substantial proof of
efficacy before a drug could be marketed. The hearings leading to the
1962 amendments were first framed in the context of economic considerations. However, the thalidomide tragedy relating to the safety of drugs
changed the complexion of the deliberations and led almost ironically
to the amendments which required a proof of efficacy. Of course, at the
same time, further regulations concerned with safety, including those
governing the investigational use of new drugs and those which provided
for continued surveillance of marketed drugs, were promulgated.

Hence, we are keeping some drugs off the market, but at the same
time, we are helping to speed safe and effective drugs to the market.
Furthermore, we have recently reorganized our agency so that our scientists can perform the most efficient service possible for the American
people.

Today, the professional personnel of the FDA includes approximately
200 physicians, 80 pharmacologists, 100 pharmacists, 900 chemists, and
100 microbiologists. The staff also includes 650 inspectors and supporting
administrative and clerical personnel. The most recent reorganization of
the agency provides for three separate bureaus and the Office of the
Commissioner, constituting the Washington headquarters, and 17 district
offices. Each of the bureaus, the Bureau of Drugs, the Bureau of Foods,
Pesticides, and Product Safety, and the Bureau of Veterinary Medicine,
is sufficient in scientific and regulatory capabilities. In the future, as
more funds and personnel are available, certain subunits of these bureaus
may be elevated in stature to carry out more efficiently the intent of the
law and to provide better consumer protection.

To take the Bureau of Drugs as an example, there is an Office of
Scientific Evaluation with divisions formed along pharmacologic lines
such as the Division of Neuropharmacological Drugs, the Division of
Cardiopulmonary-Renal Drugs, and the Division of Metabolic and Endocrine Drugs; an Office of Compliance; an Office of Pharmaceutical Re-

search and Testing, with divisions such as Drug Biology and Drug Chemistry. and an Office of Scientific Coordination with divisions of Biometry and Epidemiology, Extramural and Clinical Research, and the Center for Drug Information.

The reorganization of the FDA into bureaus on product lines increases its efficiency by delineating clearly the responsibilities of the various units and by coordinating the scientific and regulatory activities relating to the major product categories.

Discussion of FDA responsibilities lead to the question: what part does the Food and Drug Administration play in the discovery and development of drugs? The FDA is basically a regulatory agency whose primary consideration is consumer protection. It administrates several specific acts of Congress—the one of interest here being the Food, Drug and Cosmetic Act, as amended. Its basic requirements are relatively simple and might well serve as a model for future legislation regarding all products. Before a drug is introduced into the market, it must be shown to be safe and proved to be effective. The language of the Act states that the proof of efficacy of a drug must consist of substantial evidence derived from adequate, well-controlled investigations, including clinical investigations, conducted by qualified experts. This requirement, which seems so obvious and simple, after eight years has not yet been completely accepted by all concerned and is the focal point of the criticisms of the FDA as a barrier to drug discovery and development.

The decisions required of FDA scientists fall into two broad categories. One of these concerns is the safety and efficacy of the drug substance as a therapeutic entity. Although the decision that a drug is safe and efficacious is a difficult one and fraught with danger, on the one hand, of prematurely releasing a drug which later proves to be harmful, or on the other hand, of unduly delaying because of excessive caution an agent which would be of benefit in a serious condition, it is nevertheless a decision which is usually made within a reasonable length of time. For one thing, the drug that is truly effective usually attracts supporters and becomes known to investigators and practitioners through scientific journals, and the agency's decision-making process is usually carried on in the light of these public discussions. For another, as scientists and consumers, we in the agency are eager to speed to physicians and patients drugs that are truly safe and effective. The primary cause of the much touted delay in FDA decision-making is beyond all question the poor quality of the data, particularly those of the clinical investigations, submitted to us. Although the quality of the data has improved over recent years, some sponsors still do not recognize that a few carefully conducted studies are much more persuasive than a mass of poorly documented case studies or even carefully documented random clinical reports.

The second type of decision that the Food and Drug Administration must make is one that is at least as important and—unlike the decisions regarding safety and efficacy—must be made repeatedly. This is the surveillance of the quality of drug products on the market. In its approval of a new drug application the FDA approves not a drug substance but a finished dosage form. Indeed, the clinical trials which demonstrate safety and efficacy of the drug must be carried out with the marketed dosage form or with a dosage form that can be established as therapeutically equivalent. Thus, quality control enters early into the approval of a drug for marketing and continues to be of considerable importance until the drug is removed or replaced by newer products.

Arrangements were made with the National Academy of Science (NAS) through its National Research Council (NRC) to undertake responsibility for evaluating drugs marketed between 1938 and 1962, years in which important Amendments to the Food, Drug and Cosmetic Act were enacted. Part of the implementation of the Academy's findings is the approval of abbreviated NDA's (new drug applications) on the basis of labeling which conforms to published requirements, adherence to good manufacturing practices, and demonstration of bioavailability, or another adequate demonstration of drug activity. This is the first step toward assuring the physician and the consumer that chemically identical drugs with identical labeling are therapeutic equivalents.

From time to time the agency has found it necessary to propose changes in, and additions to, the regulations. For the most part they are aimed at clarifying the requirements of the Act as we interpret it, providing consumer protection, dealing with clinical investigations, and expediting the processing of submissions. At the agency, we have not conceived of these functions as constituting any new restriction on the discovery, development, or investigation of drugs. For example, our new requirement of a 30-day delay before beginning clinical trials, after the receipt of an application for trial of a new drug (in the form of an IND or notice of claimed exemption from the restriction on interstate shipment), provides the agency a chance to evaluate the proposed use of the drug in the human subject and to determine whether there are adequate safety data from experiments in animals to warrant the commencement of human studies. Under previous regulations, the investigator could begin clinical trials in humans as soon as he had mailed his notice. Frequently enough to cause real concern, we have found that data from studies in animals were not adequate to support the type of studies that had been undertaken in human beings. We believe that this 30-day delay, with its waiver provision for extraordinary circumstances, constitutes a minor restriction—if any—compared with the potential benefits in the protection of subjects.

Another regulation that has stirred considerable controversy is that which sets forth our criteria for an adequate, well-controlled clinical trial. We are convinced that this regulation merely reflects the practices that have become widely accepted during the evolution of the science of clinical pharmacology. We see in this regulation no restriction beyond that imposed by Congress in its 1962 Amendments to the Act, and by setting forth clearly what is expected, we hope that the data submitted will be improved thus speeding the processing of applications. Our recent approvals of certain new drugs with a smaller volume of data than has often been the case, I believe, show that we are prepared to apply these scientific principles in a reasonable fashion.

Role of the National Research Council

Should the National Research Council be requested to review pending new drug applications? The fact that the law fixes the responsibility for review and approval of new drug applications on the Food and Drug Administration (through delegation from the Secretary of Department of Health, Education, and Welfare) is something that need not be considered as insurmountable since laws can be amended. However, unless the law were amended radically to change the substantial evidence requirement, it is difficult to understand how experts of the Academy could, in satisfaction of the Act, require less rigorous proof than that now demanded by the FDA. We have used consultants from time to time, including panels of the National Academy of Science–National Research Council (NAS–NRC) when confronted by especially knotty problems of safety and efficacy, but when these experts were fully aware of the requirements of the Food, Drug and Cosmetic Act, in every case they applied standards and criteria that were every bit as strict as those of the FDA's own reviewing officers.

If the proposals for review of new drug applications by the National Academy of Sciences–National Research Council, the National Institutes of Health, or other scientific bodies are advanced with the idea of providing more expertise than resides in the FDA, our use of outside experts makes this approach unnecessary—regardless of the requirements for a change in the law.

If these proposals are advanced to separate the approving function from the regulatory function, the two are inseparable from a practical point of view. Our regulatory actions must be based on scientific decisions, and our scientists must be fully aware of our regulatory responsibilities.

Presumably, any such arrangement would leave within the truncated FDA the responsibility for the decision relating to the continued quality of the marketed product. Time after time changes in the status of the marketed product have required the focusing of expertise from all of the disciplines currently represented in the FDA. To remove from the Agency the basic medical expertise (and such an arrangement would result in nearly total removal) would seriously impair consumer protection.

Finally, I firmly believe that rather than dismembering the agency we should continue our efforts, ideally with the support of everyone concerned, to broaden and deepen the expertise resident in the agency, and to make even more effective our employment of scientific expertise wherever it may reside.

Appearance of New Drugs

"Why do we see so few truly new drugs?" One answer offered frequently by industry is represented in the testimony in 1969 by the President of the Pharmaceutical Manufacturers Association, C. Joseph Stetler. He told the Subcommittee on Public Health, Education, and Welfare of the House Interstate and Foreign Commerce Committee: "Without attempting to identify the cause, it is a fact that the number of new drugs, particularly new single chemical entities marketed each year, has drastically decreased since the passage of the 1962 amendments. The impact of that legislation has been felt throughout the industry, particularly in research and development areas." Mr. Stetler went on to cite figures for 1959 and 1968 showing the decline of 72% in new prescription drugs marketed and a decline of 83% for new single chemical entities. While disclaiming any attempt to "identify the cause," Mr. Stetler implied that it arises from "administrative encumbrances" and "important differences in the procedure that must be followed in developing present new drug applications." He said, "Another cause of delay is the general lack of qualified experts within FDA."

The dearth of new drugs is often attributed to the 1962 amendments and the Food and Drug Administration, but it is a fact that the post-World War II peak for approved new drugs came long before the 1962 amendments. In 1955 357 new drug applications (NDA's) were approved. Except for 1959, there has been a steady decline since 1955—with only 70 NDA's approved in 1963 when the Kefauver-Harris Amendments became effective. Thus, there was a sharp decline of approved new drugs before 1963.

Following implementation of the 1962 amendments, the only marked change in the downward curve of the slope was in 1967 when the number of approved NDA's rose to 74, after which it dropped to 56 in 1968, and fell off to 48 in 1969. Fifty-one, however, were approved by the FDA the fiscal year 1969-70 (close to one a week).

Of the 51 new drugs approved in fiscal year 1970, about 20 could be considered "new entities"—*i.e.*, new chemicals not previously marketed in the United States. However, many of these, although technically new entities, represented merely variations on familiar themes and in some cases nothing more than molecular manipulation. The number of new drugs approved in that period that could be considered as significant contributions to the pharmacopoeia is small indeed.

The number of NDA's under review in the FDA at any one time is usually between 100 and 150. Although we hope that some of them, at least, will represent significant contributions to therapeutics, a casual examination leads to the conclusion that the percentage will be about the same as in the recent past.

A look at the drugs in the earlier phases of investigation, the IND stage, does not provide any reason to expect improvement within the near future. About 1000 IND's were submitted in 1963 in response to the 1962 amendments. By 1967 IND submissions had declined to less than 700 but rose again to nearly 1000 in 1969. However, about one-half represented multiple submissions for a few special drugs, notably lithium carbonate and L-dopa. We are currently responsible for a total of 3430 IND's, certainly a large enough number to contain a respectable quantity of significant drugs. Although prognostication is even more dangerous at this early stage of development there are not many real breakthrough drugs in that large volume.

There is no question of the constant down-trend in the innovative significance of the drugs being developed today. The question is: "why should this be, when millions of dollars are poured into research and development (R & D) each year by our drug industry?" Our major firms spend vast amounts of manpower and time budgeted for research and development. Why is it unrewarding in terms of actual medical progress —why is it unrewarding for the consumer, for the patient?

As scientists we must accept the results of scientific studies even when they upset cherished beliefs. Virtually every type of study on the R & D effectiveness of the large laboratories in major industries points to the fact that for several reasons the largest companies will not be the largest contributors in terms of original research and development. Whether we look at a broad, horizontal study of industry in general over a considerable period of time, or a narrow vertical study of any one company, the results are the same.

In a broad study based on extensive research, D. Hamberg (*1*), of the University of Buffalo, has found that "with few exceptions, the large industrial laboratories are likely to be minor sources of major inventions."

He points out that the larger firms are primarily involved with improvement inventions—devoting much research toward bettering the products they already turn out or toward improving the processes of production. This is not to gainsay such improvements or to question the need for such research. The discovery of penicillin would have benefited humanity but little if rapid improvements in technology had not made it available on a massive scale, but if we are looking for original contributions—in other words, new drugs and numbers of new drugs, such as produced the "Golden Age of the Wonder Drug" following World War II— apparently we must look to other than the R & D programs of the large drug firms.

Studies from the turn of the century show the major laboratories contribute a very small percentage of our new important inventions. For instance, W. M. Grosvenor (2) in 1929 found that of 72 major inventions —such as the submarine, the dial telephone, the diesel engine, and calcium carbide—produced between 1889 and 1929, only 12 (or 17%) originated in corporate laboratories.

A study headed by Jewkes (3) and published in 1958, found that of 61 major inventions after 1930 only 20% emanated from the laboratories of large corporations. Such inventions as air-conditioning, automatic transmissions, and the jet engine were the work of independent inventors. In 1962 W. F. Mueller (4) at DuPont, found that between 1920 and 1950 only 28% of their 18 new products originated from their own research. Two of the company's three most commercially important products were completed by their research laboratories by the early 1930s, when their research budget averaged $5 million a year—far less than it is today.

A study in 1965 by William S. Comanor (5), deals with research and technical change solely within the pharmaceutical industry. Comanor's analysis provides "some evidence that in the pharmaceutical industry there are substantial diseconomies of scale in R & D which are associated with large firm size; and that these disadvantages are encountered even by moderately sized firms."

Study after study points out what has and has not come out of massive research efforts, but there is one interesting paper prepared in 1958 by McGraw-Hill (6) that shows what the companies expect from their research. In the survey almost every large company in U.S. industry and commerce was asked: "how soon do you expect your expenditures on R & D to pay off?" Ninety-one percent said within five years, but the history of major inventions shows that most have taken much more time before they were even ready for marketing. So it would seem that major laboratories—although heavily funded and stocked with expertise—are not so much looking to original products as they are to improved products already in the line, which would require a shorter period of development.

Today we have fewer small firms than we had 10 years ago; some of them have passed out of existence, but others have been absorbed into the larger laboratories; hence, we have more talent coming under the umbrella of the large firms—subject to their goals and direction.

What has corporate talent produced? If we return to review some recently approved drugs and confine our attention to a particular category, neuropharmacology, there are three drugs of some clinical importance. Two of these, lithium carbonate and L-dopa, were not the products of the type of research that characterizes the drug industry today. Ketamine, the only other drug in this category of more than passing interest, apparently was the result of a massive screening program which could probably be carried out only in a laboratory of the type we have been discussing. Commercial considerations aside, the efficiency of this approach must be questioned in the light of the failure of this technique to produce anything of real significance in cancer therapy.

The approach to research in industry today—the massive frontal assault on research problems—simply is not proving, and may never prove, to be as effective as the foray of the independent researcher.

The approach taken to research in industry today is actually counterproductive to the goals. Vast resources—in time, in money, in expertise—are being tied up on projects of questionable or little significance to actual medical progress.

Even today a study by Mueller and Tilton (7) does not change the impression that much of our scientific expertise in the field of drugs is being used solely for economic goals—with the occasional happy coincidence of medical progress.

According to these authors:

The bulk of the empirical evidence on the origin of major inventions suggest that the R & D laboratories of large corporations have not been an important source of major inventions. . . . The same communication gap which may keep large firms from financing R & D activity directed toward major inventions may inhibit them from funding the development needed to convert a major invention into a commercially successful product or process innovation. This is particularly likely when the invention is made by small firms or individuals outside the company.

We are confronted with a problem of tremendous importance to us as scientists and as citizens: the steady decline in the discovery and development of significant new drugs. Anything that might help to resolve that problem deserves serious attention. The proposition set forth here, obviously not an original one, should be examined. The studies cited should be either accepted or proved invalid. If they are valid, then isn't it time to consider new approaches to productive, creative research? Isn't it time to consider turning to some of the more research-oriented schools and universities and funding some of their operations independently or setting up small satellite laboratories to conduct basic research autonomous from but funded by the large parent company? Isn't it time to return to the innovative rather than the imitative stage of research and development in the drug field?

Obviously no one knows fully why we see so few new and significant drugs. Scientists must examine the problem scientifically and not settle for easy answers that may put the mind at rest but bring us no closer to a true solution.

Literature Cited

(1) Hamberg, D., "Invention in the Industrial Research Laboratory," *J. Political Econ.* (1963) **71**, 95–115.
(2) Grosvenor, W. M., "The Seeds of Progress," in "Chemical Markets," pp. 23, 24, 26 (1929).
(3) Jewkes, J. Sawers, D., Stillerman, R., "The Sources of Invention," pp. 72–88, Part II, London, 1958.
(4) Mueller, W. F., "The Origins of the Basic Inventions Underlying Du Pont's Major Product and Process Innovations, 1920–1950," in "Universities-National Bureau Conference, The Rate and Direction of Inventive Activity: Economic and Social Factors," pp. 323–346, Princeton, N. J., 1962.
(5) Comanor, W. S., "Research and Technical Change in the Pharmaceutical Industry," *Rev. Econ. Statistics* (1965) **47**, pp. 182–190.
(6) "The Annual McGraw-Hill Research and Development Survey," in "Methodology of Statistics on Research and Development," National Science Foundation, Washington, D. C., 1959.
(7) Mueller, D. C., Tilton, J. E., "Research and Development Costs as a Barrier to Entry," *Can. J. Econ./Rev. Can. Econ.* (1969) **2**, 570–579.

RECEIVED November 5, 1970.

Changing the Economic Image of the Pharmaceutical Industry

FRANCIS J. BLEE

Beach, Widmann & Co., Two Decker Square, Bala-Cynwyd, Pa. 19004

The key economic characteristic distinguishing the drug industry from other industries is the heavy dependence on innovation and the high level of expenditures on research and development. Research and development should be viewed as an investment and capitalized by the industry in all published figures. If research expenditures are capitalized, the return on shareholders' equity of the industry is reduced from 19% to 15%. Comparison with electric utilities demonstrates that a 6–9% reduction in drug industry prices would reduce the industry's return on investment to a level equal to the electric utility industry.

In discussing the economic image of the pharmaceutical industry there is a lack of good economic data on the pharmaceutical industry in general and on the economics of pharmaceutical innovation specifically. This is a fruitful area, however, and deserves greater economic research efforts.

The drug industry can be viewed as the creator and deliverer of an innovative service, the most significant of which is discovery. The actual production, marketing, and distribution of drugs, while a valuable and highly efficient operation, is not much different from proprietary drugs or several other consumer industries. Hence, the production, marketing, and distribution cycle could be performed by many other industries lacking in the creativity which is so essential to the pharmaceutical industry. I believe that the industry has misunderstood its own role, overemphasizing production and distribution and underplaying its most distinctive economic characteristic—*i.e.*, the creative process of discovering and developing new pharmaceutical products.

Pharmaceutical Research

The economics of an innovative pharmaceutical industry have been changing dramatically over the last several decades. In the 1950's, although precise measurements are not available, pharmaceutical research was highly productive and apparently quite profitable. Broad generalizations can be made, centering around the fact that large numbers of new chemicals entities, combination products, and duplicate products were introduced in the decade of the 1950's on research budgets which by today's standards appear to be quite modest. For example, in the seven-year period 1956–1962, prior to the new drug regulations of 1962, the industry introduced an average of 44 new chemical entities per year. This was in an era when one or two years seemed like a long time for development of a new drug product. The time span for developing a new drug product has increased tremendously since the early 1960's with estimates currently ranging from 7–10 years or more. Moreover, owing to the increasing scientific complexity of discovering and developing new drug compounds and a more stringent regulatory climate, the number of new chemical entities introduced by the industry in the seven-year period immediately following the new drug regulations of 1962 fell to an average of 16 new chemical entities per year. The other part of the equation is the amount expended on research in these comparable periods. Between 1956 and 1962 the industry spent approximately $1.3 billion on research, whereas in the 1963–69 period research and development (R & D) expenditures were approximately $2.6 billion. The changing economic climate reflecting rising research costs and fewer new products is obvious. Using a very simple formula of dividing the number of new entities into the research costs for each of these seven-year periods produces a cost per new chemical entity of approximately $4 million in the 1956–62 period and $23 million in the 1963–69 time span (Table I).

Table I. Average R & D Investment per New Chemical Entity[a]

Period	R & D Investment, Millions	Total Number of New Entities[a]	R & D Investment per Entity, Millions	Average Number of Entities per Year
1956–62	$1,270	311	$ 4.1	44
1963–69	2,605	113	23.1	16

[a] Source: R & D investment: Pharmaceutical Manufacturers Association. New chemical entities: (9).

This comparison is subject to oversimplification; for example, how much of the R & D is indeed a quest for completely new compounds, and is a new chemical entity actually a reasonable barometer of R & D productivity? Without attempting to justify these figures or debate the accuracy of specific numbers, it is obvious that there has been tremendous increase in the cost of discovering and developing a new drug product (*1, 2*). It is also obvious that the nine new chemical entities introduced by the industry in 1969 will have to achieve truly significant sales levels to justify a level of approximately $500 million annually being spent on human ethical research and development in the 1968–69 period (*3*).

Erroneous conclusions often seem to have been drawn regarding the industry's true profitability. It is true that the drug industry has generally ranked high among American industries in terms of return on sales and return on investment. However, I believe that the investment as stated in the annual report of the typical drug company understates the actual investment since research and development costs have systematically been written off against profit and do not appear in the investment portion of the balance sheet. The technique of annually amortizing research and development expenditures may be relevant for other industries and is also consistent with conservative accounting practices. However, the resultant balance sheet investment fails to recognize the truly unique dependence of the pharmaceutical industry on research and development and the fact that as a percentage of sales the industry's research investment is larger than any major industry. For example, since industry figures on capital expenditures are not available, we can cite an industry leader, Merck, and point out that in the three year period 1967–69 Merck spent $163 million on research and development compared with $118 million on capital expenditures for plant and equipment. I suggest that it is a truly unique relationship for a firm in any industry to have spent 38% more on research and development than on plant and equipment expenditures, and I suggest that this is fairly typical for most research oriented firms in the drug industry. According to U.S. government figures, the pharmaceutical industry in 1969 had a return on investment of approximately 19%. The significance of capitalizing research and development can be illustrated by the fact that the industry's return on investment can be reduced to 15% using an arbitrary 5-year amortization of R & D expenditures (Table II) (*4*).

Having discussed return on investment, I should consider the risks associated with the anticipated return on pharmaceutical investment. Again because of a lack of available data, we must subjectively observe that the research investment being made by the industry carries a high degree of risk owing to the degree of uncertainty involved in new product research. I believe all would agree that new product research is inherently more risky than the process improvement or cost reduction type research indicative of many other industries. Attempts have been made

Table II.[a]   Drug Industry Return on Shareholder's Equity
Assuming Capitalization of R & D

Year	Begin-ning Equity	R & D Invest-ment	R & D Write-Off	Ending Equity	Profit Before R & D	R & D Write-Off	Profit After R & D	% Return On Equity
A	$49.62	$4.50	$ 0	$49.62	$14.10	$4.50	$ 9.60	19.3%
1	49.62	4.50	0	54.12	14.10	0	14.10	26.1
2	54.12	4.50	.90	57.72	14.10	.90	13.20	22.9
3	57.72	4.50	1.80	60.42	14.10	1.80	12.30	20.4
4	60.42	4.50	2.70	62.22	14.10	2.70	11.40	18.3
5	62.22	4.50	3.60	63.12	14.10	3.60	10.50	16.6
B	$63.12	$4.50	$4.50	$63.12	$14.10	$4.50	$ 9.60	15.2%

Assumptions
- (1) Sales are $100.00 per year
- (2) Pre-tax R & D = 9% of global sales
- (3) 50% tax rate, after tax
  R & D = 4.5% of sales
- (4) Profit after tax = 9.6% of sales
- (5) Unadjusted equity = 49.6% of sales
- (6) Five year write-off of R & D

[a] Source of ratios: (*10, 11*).

to measure the risk of the industry, with no apparent conclusion having been reached (5, 6, 7). The question is whether or not the risk is increasing. As the previous figures indicated, more dollars must be invested in each research project with a consequent larger loss if the project does not come to fruition. In addition, the degree of certainty in achieving a marketable product would also appear to be less than in the past because the scientific obstacles have become more formidable. Since we are dealing with research involving the highly variable human being, there are obviously a tremendous number of unknowns involved in the reaction to various drugs. Perhaps the reason that attempts to measure risk have been unsuccessful is the fact that we may be dealing with uncertainty rather than risk, and the concept of uncertainty may not be susceptible to statistical measurement. It is true that as measured by continued profitability one would have to say that the risks of research have not yet been reflected in greatly reduced profitability or produced any financial crises like that of Penn Central. Nevertheless, we see other indications of intensified risk; for example, the effects of increasing R & D uncertainty may have contributed toward the proposed combination of Schering and Plough.

Role of Patents

To offset the dearth of new product introductions, the industry has generally been compensated through greater longevity of products already on the market. Also, the ability to introduce new products abroad in advance of U.S. clearance has enabled the industry to sustain a faster growth rate in foreign countries than here.

However, during the 1970's, as patents expire on the "wonder drugs" of the 1950's, the profitability of the industry will be under increasing pressure. Hence, we must conclude that drug industry risk will increase further in the future because of (1) patent expirations, (2) generic competition, and (3) the greater threat of product withdrawals inherent in a climate of stringent enforcement by the FDA and consumer protection by all governmental bodies.

An essential part of the economics of innovation in the United States has been the patent system. Patents have been viewed traditionally as a reward for creativity. Recently, drug patents in the United States have come under fire as representing a mechanism which tends to create an artificially high pricing structure by reducing competition (8). In defense of the patent system with regard to pharmaceutical products, we can cite the U. S. drug industry's high level of innovation over the last several decades, whereas in other areas of the world where patents have not existed (the Iron Curtain countries and Italy) innovation has generally not been at a very high level in the drug field. The lack of data makes it difficult to analyze precisely the effect of patents on the drug industry in the United States except in very general and somewhat subjective terms. It would appear that a private enterprise industry could not afford to spend the sums presently being spent on pharmaceutical research without some hope of recouping this investment and also earning an adequate return at least equal to alternative forms of investment. It is also obvious to me that from a public policy standpoint the economic effect of eliminating drug patents or reducing the patent life must be analyzed with respect to expected future return on the present level of research investment and not based on the situation in the late 1950's or early 1960's where returns may have been unusually high.

Regardless of one's position on drug patents it appears that the economics of the research oriented drug industry, with resultant patent protection, has created a climate of product competition rather than price competition. The relative rigidity of drug prices has perhaps engendered as much criticism as the level of prices. If the industry is to answer to charges of excessively high prices, objective economic analysis in depth will be required.

Further, the effect of rising research costs and fewer new product introductions has generally reduced the number of firms which are able and willing to enter the research oriented pharmaceutical industry. It is not possible to determine how many firms have been forestalled from entering the industry because of the high threshold of research expenditures; however, it is obvious that there have been very few new entries into the research oriented part of the industry in the last decade. The difficulty of entry can also be underscored by remembering the number of large chemical companies which have unsuccessfully attempted to enter the drug industry in the last few years. In addition, perhaps the most successful small company in the industry, Marion Labs, rather than attempting to assume the burden of a large research.operation has apparently chosen to develop research contacts through licensing agreements rather than incurring the large fixed costs associated with in-house research.

Promotional Costs

It seems that the industry still continues to suffer from a poor economic image brought on by charges of high prices and a lack of meaningful price competition. Perhaps the Achilles heel of the economic story at the moment is the level of promotional expenditures which at approximately 25% of sales are more than twice the industry's commitment to research. Although the industry must be convinced that this promotional effort is necessary, this category of expenditures .is the most difficult to defend. It also appears that the industry may be burdened with a somewhat outmoded and expensive distribution system. Although we have all heard the arguments justifying pharmaceutical promotion and the present distribution system, it appears that this problem must be attacked on two fronts: (1) every effort must be made through cooperation between manufacturers, wholesalers, and retailers to lower the promotion and distribution bill for the drug industry, and (2) in-depth economic support must be generated to demonstrate the benefits to the consumer of the present marketing–distribution complex.

Returning again to pharmaceutical research, it should be added that the industry has also been widely criticized on the grounds of molecular manipulation, me-tooism, and duplicative programs. Although these charges may have contained some validity in the late 1950's and early 1960's it seems that the problem has been corrected by rising research costs and the knowledge that clinical testing on a me-too product today is just as expensive as on a truly unique compound. It also appears obvious that the introduction of a satisfactory number of unique compounds will be necessary to justify the current level of research expenditures.

The industry has had a fine record from the standpoint of new product innovation and a rather miserable record in explaining the economics of the research oriented pharmaceutical firm. In short, it has spent billions on scientific research but a pitiful amount on economic research, and today it suffers greatly from a lack of meaningful economic information, the type of hard data necessary to convince a government agency.

Because of the generally poor understanding of the industry's economics and the social overtones regarding any aspect of the health industry, it is not surprising that voices call for either the government to assume the entire burden of innovative drug research or for the industry to be treated as a public utility, regulated with regard to profitability and return on investment.

It would appear that there are striking economic differences between the normal concept of a public utility and the drug industry as we know it today. The chief difference centers around the topic of this volume, and that is the fact that the discovery and development process is the most critical factor in the pharmaceutical industry but plays a far less important role in public utilities. Also, the monopoly value of a drug patent which can lose its economic value instantly upon the development of unexpected side effects, or through the introduction of a superior product by a competitor, is considerably different from the relatively absolute monopoly accorded the typical public utility. We must also wonder whether capital can be attracted into the high risk game of new product research under conditions of regulated profitability and return on investment. Indeed, even under present free enterprise conditions, we wonder whether the high costs and risks of doing new product research and the risks of increasing government intervention have not caused substantial sums to be allocated out of pharmaceutical research and invested in diversification opportunities, such as, cosmetics, clinical laboratories, and medical instruments.

Tables III and IV estimate, in a very broad sense, how much of a price reduction it would take to lower the drug industry's return on shareholders' equity to equal the electric utility industry. Using U.S. government figures for the drug industry and the Edison Electric Institute data on electric utilities, I have developed a statistical comparison between the two industries. The financial ratios are quite different with respect to profit margins and capital requirements. For example, the drug industry, often criticized for having high profit margins, realizes about $19 pre-tax profit on each $100 of sales, whereas the electric utility industry realizes about $23 for each $100 of sales. On the other hand, shareholders' equity is $50 for the drug industry compared with $120 for electric utilities on each $100 of sales. Combining the profit and investment figures produces a return on shareholders equity, before taxes, of approximately 37% for the drug industry and 19% for the electric utility industry. Although there would appear to be a considerable spread between the two rates of return, if the drug industry sales level were reduced by just 9%, the resulting return on investment would be equal to the electric utility industry, or approximately 19% before taxes (*see* Table III).

Into the investment base for the drug industry should be incorporated the research and development investment. Using what I consider to be the more realistic return on shareholders' equity for the drug industry, that is, with R & D included in the investment base, it would require only a 6.5% reduction in drug industry prices to lower the return on investment to the same level as the electric utility industry—*i.e.*, 19% (*see* Table IV). When it is realized that out of the 9% or 6.5% savings, depending upon one's preference, that the government takes approximately 50–52% in taxes, the actual saving to society is probably about half of the pre-tax reduction or between 3 and 4.5%. Although these figures are used in an illustrative sense, this comparison underscores my belief that (1) return on investment is the valid ratio when considering relative profitabilities of various industries, (2) with R & D considered as

Table III. Adjustment of Drug Industry Return on Equity to Equal Electric Utilities[a]

	Drug Industry	Electric Utilities
Sales	$100.00	$100.00
Pre-tax profit	$ 18.60	$ 23.10
Shareholder's equity per $100.00 sales	$ 50.00	$120.00
Pre-tax return on shareholder's investment	37.2%	19.3%
Reduce drug industry sales by 9% = $9.00 adjusted sales	$ 91.00	$100.00
Adjusted pre-tax profit	$ 9.60	$ 23.10
Adjusted pre-tax return on equity	19.3%	19.3%

Assumptions
  (1) Sales are $100.00 per year.
  (2) All costs remain constant; therefore, a reduction in sales produces an equivalent reduction in pre-tax profit.

  [a] Source: Drug industry ratios: (*10*).
       Electric utility ratios: (*12*).

Table IV.   Adjustment of Drug Industry Return on Equity to Equal Electric Utilities[a]

Drug Industry Equity Adjusted for R and D

	Drug Industry	*Electric Utilities*
Sales	$100.00	$100.00
Pre-tax profit	$ 18.60	$ 23.10
Shareholder's equity per $100.00 sales *(adjusted for R & D)*	$ 63.00	$120.00
Pre-tax return on Common equity	30.0%	19.3%
Reduce drug industry sales by 6.5% = $6.50		
Adjusted sales	$ 93.50	$100.00
Adjusted pre-tax profit	$ 12.10	$ 23.10
Adjusted pre-tax return on equity	19.3%	19.3%

Assumptions

(1) Sales are $100.00 per year.
(2) All costs remain constant; therefore, a reduction in sales produces an equivalent reduction in pre-tax profit.
(3) Drug industry net return on shareholder's equity = 15.2% = 30.0% pre-tax return, as adjusted for capitalization of R & D, per Table II.

[a] Source: Drug industry ratios: (*10*).
     Electric utility ratios: (*12*).

part of the investment base, it appears that only a modest reduction in the drug industry pricing level will have a rather sharp effect on return on investment, and (3) when viewed in this light, it appears that the relative profitability of the drug industry is not nearly as high as other comparison may have suggested.

Summary

I would urge the development of hard economic analysis, exploring in depth many of the theories which are being advanced with regard to the economics of the drug industry today. Further, I believe a sizeable credibility gap exists today between the industry's concept of its economic structure and the view of the government and the general public. The industry has helped to create this gap by failing to understand its own unique economic characteristics. Industry accounting practices which improperly handle the substantial research and development investment have served to intensify the gap between those in the industry and the view from outside. Future emphasis must be directed toward closing this credibility gap and reorienting economic thinking toward the present and future economic structure of pharmaceutical innovation, relieving society from outdated concepts of the past.

Literature Cited

(1) Clymer ,Harold, "The Changing Costs of Pharmaceutical Innovation," in "The Economics of Drug Innovation," Joseph Cooper, Ed., p. 109, The American University, Washington, D. C., 1969.
(2) Mansfield, Edwin, "Discussion," in "The Economics of Drug Innovation," p. 149.
(3) Mund, Vernon, "The Return on Investment of the Innovative Pharmaceutical Firm," in "The Economics of Drug Innovation," p. 125.
(4) Schulman, Rosalind, "Discussion," in "The Economics of Drug Innovation," p. 213.
(5) Fisher, I., Hall, G., "Risk and Corporate Rates of Return," *The Congressional Record*, U. S. Senate (90), Part 5, pp. 2120–2129.
(6) Markham, Jesse, Conrad, Gordon, *The Congressional Record*, U. S. Senate (90), Part 5, pp. 1674–1678.
(7) Mueller, Willard, *The Congressional Record*, U. S. Senate (90), Part 5, pp. 1809, 1816.
(8) Task Force on Prescription Drugs, *Second Interim Report and Recommendations*, U. S. Department of Health, Education, and Welfare, Washington, D. C., 1968.
(9) DeHaen, Paul, New Drug Parade, Paul DeHaen, New York, 1969.
(10) "Quarterly Financial Report for Manufacturing Corporations," Federal Trade Commission-Securities and Exchange Commission, Washington, D. C., 1969.
(11) "Annual Survey Report, 1968-69," Pharmaceutical Manufacturer's Association, Washington, D. C.
(12) "Statistical Year Book of the Electrical Utility Industry," Edison Electric Institute, New York, 1969.

RECEIVED November 5, 1970.

15

Drugs and the Real World of Medical Practice

GEORGE E. BURKET, JR., M.D.

Medical Arts Center, 349 North Main St., Kingman, Kan. 67069

Two worlds revolve in the field of medicine—the world of drugs and the world of medical practice. They both move in the same direction and with amazing synchronization. Communication between them takes many paths to many areas, and although it is quite complex, it is improving daily. The physician is indebted to the drug industry as well as to research, in public and private institutions, for providing so many new drugs for so many valid uses. Tradenames offer an easy, convenient, and timesaving way to prescribe new drugs. For the future the clinical physician confidently expects more miracle drugs. Arteriosclerotic cardiovascular disease and cancer represent the foremost challenges to pharmaceutical researchers.

In discussing drugs and the real world of medical practice, we must first contemplate the significance of the title. The practice of medicine has always been associated with the use of drugs whether they be termed drugs, concoctions, or potions. History records physicians' compounding prescriptions in an Egyptian society 15 centuries before Christ, and the annals of medicine through more than 2000 years are filled with new remedies for old and new diseases and ailments. Why, then, does the title of this paper suggest a distinct separation between drugs and medical practice? One must trace the pathway of time for the answer. Through the ages drugs have not been the exclusive property of physicians. History records the use of drugs in religious ceremonies, and chemical warfare can be traced to the fifth century B. C. "Truth serums" have been advocated in solving crimes, and thousands of proprietary drugs are used without the advice of a physician.

Looking elsewhere, one also finds that physicians have no exclusive claim to the development of drugs or to the compounding of medication.

As far back as Hippocrates, 2500 years ago, apothecaries prepared prescribed concoctions. Until the dawn of our present scientific era, it was commonplace for friends or relatives to prepare "appropriate medication" (usually based on folklore). Those in family medicine are aware that a certain amount of folklore medicine still remains—*e.g.*, honey and vinegar for arthritis, potato poultices for cellulitis, and spider webs to stop bleeding in a laceration. We now know that many of the crude drugs which were found empirically to be effective long before the modern scientific era actually contained drugs which have been identified and are used today—*e.g.*, quinine from cinchona bark, digitalis from foxglove, and opium from the poppy. In fact, pharmaceutical companies are exploring botanical species around the world in search of basic new drugs which can be synthesized or altered for medicinal purposes (*1*).

Since the civilizations before Christ there has been a division between the physicians who diagnosed and prescribed drugs and those who discovered and compounded them, with the grey area in betweeen in which certain physicians performed equally well. We have then what could be termed two worlds of medicine, worlds which fortunately revolve in the same direction and with amazing synchronization.

Since the beginning of scientific medicine, dating from an indefinite point in the 18th century, these two areas have become increasingly distinct, and with the scientific explosion of the past 30 years, identification seems complete. Medical practice is now involved with new methods of diagnosis, therapeutic techniques, and health care delivery while the drug industry is involved in the development of new chemicals and biologicals and their manufacture—each world stimulating the other and working remarkably well together. Our subject then deals with how some of the products of one world are utilized within the other—the real world of medical practice.

In medical practice the use of drugs and their function have a significance very different from that in the world of strict scientific research and manufacturing. The clinical physician must consider not only the physiologic aspects of therapy but the psychological and social aspects as well (*1*). The pharmaceutical industry seems to be aware of this fact as evidenced by advertising in medical journals. For example one illustration depicts a middle aged man who was able to resume marital relations after taking a coronary dilator. Another ad depicted the curvaceous doll who was able to wear her bikini after her eczema was cleared by a certain unguentum. Still another asked, "How long can she wait?" when referring to a preparation for curing monilial vaginitis. Other illustrations might include, "If he kisses you once, will he kiss you again," and, "Even your best friend won't tell you."

The clinical physician must relate to situations like this every day. Such situations may seem idiotic to the science writer or to those who seek any reason to criticize the pharmaceutical and medical professions, but they are very real concerns to the physician and his patients. If critics or skeptics think that the illustrations in any way affect the judgment of the clinicians, regardless of the physiology involved, the therapeutic results, or possible adverse effects, they are sadly mistaken.

Development and Use of Drugs

The importance in medical practice of function relating to drugs is best outlined by Barber (1) in "Drugs and Society." " 'A drug,' say Goodman and Gilman (2) in their standard textbook on therapeutic pharmacology, 'may be broadly defined as any chemical agent which affects living protoplasm, and few substances would escape inclusion by this definition.' So broad a definition indicates that the problem of definition is still with us. Indeed it is, and all the more so since anything considered to be a drug takes on an important part of its significance from social and psychological meanings attached to it by individuals and by social systems,"

Barber illustrates with a few examples. "A recent dispute between the Food and Drug Administration and a pharmaceutical manufacturer originated in the assertion by the FDA that the product Quell which was being sold as a dietary food was in fact a 'misbranded drug.' " Again, the FDA has held that the ink stain used for diagnosis in fungal infection is a drug. This stain, manufactured by a company producing ink for fountain pens, is essentially no different from the fountain pen ink. Dial soap, because of its antibacterial claims is also classified as a drug. Indeed, any item listed in the United States Pharmacopoeia (U.S.P.) is legally defined by the Food, Drug, and Cosmetic Act as a drug. Included, therefore, as drugs are certain gauze bandages listed in the U. S. P. The social and psychological definitions of materials of all kinds are highly relevant to their being named "drugs." We might even say that nothing is a drug, but naming makes it so.

Dr. Barber concludes, "An adequate definition of a drug will start with the assumption that anything involved in human behavior needs to be considered at the physiological level, the psychological level, and the social level, and particularly needs to consider these three levels in interaction with one another . . ."

These statements illustrate the considerations the physician must give to drugs in medical practice. They also indicate how lengthy this paper might be if this subject were discussed thoroughly and in detail. Instead, let us dwell more specifically on the clinical physician's attitudes concerning subjects of more immediate and mutual interest.

The Pharmaceutical Industry

The pharmaceutical industry holds the highest position of admiration and respect in the opinion of most physicians. The physician views its accomplishments in the past 30 years as something akin to miraculous. Those who have been in clinical medicine for over 30 years remember too well the depressing deaths from pneumonia, puerperal septicemia, meningitis, influenza, typhoid fever, bacterial endocarditis, tuberculosis, tetanus, and complications of syphilis, and we easily recollect the crippling of poliomyelitis, osteomyelitis, and rheumatic fever.

Today all of these and hundreds of other diseases and ailments are controlled or cured by modern drugs. In 1910 quinine, ether, morphine, alcohol, mercury, iodine, digitalis, diphtheria antitoxin, and arsphenamine were available. Today we have antiinfectious agents, tranquilizing agents, cardiovascular and diuretic agents, steroids, antidiabetic agents, analgesics and anesthetics, antihistamines, antianemics, hormones, vitamins, and biological products (3).

While we may be critical at times of the seemingly high cost of drugs to our patients, we are quick to recall that the cost of medicine consists of only 20% of the total cost of health care in the United States and has risen little, comparatively speaking, in the past 10 years. We also recognize that the drug industry invests approximately one million dollars a day in the search for new and better drugs (7).

How the pharmaceutical industry operates in the eyes of the clinical physician is best described by Chester Keefer (3) in "The Medicated Society."

They work in chemistry—on physical, organic and medicinal chemistry, and today pursue the micromolecular fields of DNA–RNA, polypeptides and enzymes. They seek to relate the changes in the configuration of a chemical compound with its impact on the human organism, in the tradition of—but fortunately much more knowledge than—Erlich seventy years ago as he sought the "magic bullet" for target sites or target diseases.

They work with microorganisms—bacteria, viruses, fungi, and the cyclic existence of parasites; and they seek vaccines, as for polio, influenza, measles, mumps, and rubella.

They work with animals—mice, rats, monkeys, dogs, cats, pigs, chickens, horses—an estimated nine million of them a year. Each plays a role in finding out first whether the drug does anything to the living organism and secondly whether it has toxic effects in the range of amounts necessary to achieve useful effects.

They work with tissues—the sections of organs and samples of blood that, when examined, show microscopically whether damage has been done and how much of the drug may be harmful, and what to look for if humans take too much.

They work in the skills of the apothecary, carried into the modern science of pharmacy, to prepare the chemical in a form the body can and will take, absorb, metabolize, and excrete—the capsule, the tablet, the solution or suspension or ointment.

Their laboratory work done, they turn to the clinics, medical centers, and physician's offices for the study of drugs in humans.

And when all the studies have been completed, they will ask approval of the Federal Food and Drug Administration to market the product for the uses that have been proved out by research.

From the basic chemical industry come raw materials to use in large-scale formulation of the new product. From the vast fermentation vats come antibiotics. In laboratory-like formulation facilities, the mixing, baking, compressing, coating, and other pharmaceutical processes take place, under the watchful eye of quality control inspectors. In the space-age-clean rooms of biological production, virus vaccines are grown, harvested, purified, and endlessly tested. From start to finish, statistical, numerical, procedural, physical, chemical, and analytical control systems attempt to reduce to near-zero the potential error, mixup, distortion, or hazard.

Concurrently, a large group of well-informed men promote useful knowledge about the newly discovered drugs and provide information to doctors, pharmacists, and hospitals.

Communication

What a superb job Dr. Keefer has done in describing the pharmaceutical industry as the physician knows it today. However, the story would not be complete without discussing the methods of communication between the industry and the physician for here is the mechanism by which benefits of the described system reach the patient—the ill and the disabled.

This education and communication mechanism is complex and extremely involved. It takes many paths in an attempt to reach all areas with considerable duplication and overlapping. Included are the detail men, advertisements in medical journals, direct mail advertising, exhibits at medical meetings, scientific articles in medical journals, scientific programs at medical meetings, therapeutic handbooks, U. S. Pharmacopeia, the P.D.R., publications such as the *Medical Letter,* and an obvious source, the medical school with its undergraduate instruction and increasingly active postgraduate schools for practicing physicians. The degree of involvement of the pharmaceutical industry in these educational and communication mechanisms varies considerably in different areas, but certainly its contribution is a major factor.

In all of these endeavors perhaps the best representatives the industry has are the detail men, most of whom the practicing physician has come to respect and enjoy. They bring information concerning new drugs directly to the physician in his office, clinic, and hospital. These men are truly the public relations people for pharmaceutical companies. The wise detail man regards the physician as the intelligent and educated individual that he is and discusses only one or two drugs at each visit. He carefully relates adverse or side effects of the drug as well as its therapeutic effect and advantages. The relatively new and inexperienced man will stress the therapeutic advantages and tend to ignore the adverse effects. The experienced man will present both sides. The physician tolerates the first and welcomes the latter.

An increasing problem to the busy physician is finding the time for postgraduate education. The detail man is no exception. The number of pharamaceutical companies seems to be increasing, and more than 30 representatives now visit my office as well as men from x-ray laboratories, clinical laboratories, supply companies, surgical supply houses, etc. Time simply does not allow for a session with each representative at every visit, and I am sure that most physicians hope that these men realize this.

Equally helpful is the presence of the detail men with their technical exhibits at medical meetings. Here the physician, away from his office, may seek the drug information he needs at his leisure. He is at the meeting intent on postgraduate education and is "tuned in" to the learning process.

Most physicians seek postgraduate education at every opportunity to keep abreast of new knowledge and techniques. The nearer these educational programs are to the busy physicians, the better their attendance since they can continue to serve their patients. Thus, the popularity of postgraduate education has increased in community hospitals. The pharmaceutical industry has performed a great service in contributing so generously to these local seminars.

Mention was made previously to advertisements in medical journals as a means of communication between the drug industry and the clinical physician. This mechanism must rate high on the value scale of effectiveness in postgraduate education, and the observant doctor recognizes a double contribution in this source. First, he has the opportunity to scan quickly for names he does not recognize and which he may wish to pursue further; secondly, he has available the benefits of the scientific articles in a journal made economically possible by the advertising.

Perhaps the least effective means of communications is one we live with daily, one which fills our wastebaskets and increases the load on our janitorial services—the direct mailings. According to Deno and his colleagues in 1959 (4) "An eastern medical journal recently completed a survey which indicated that the practicing physician receives annually by direct mail more than 4,000 pieces of pharmaceutical literature." I have no accurate statistics to offer for I could find none I felt were valid.

Most pharmaceutical companies probably have figures on this subject, but I wonder about their accuracy. My acquaintanceship with physicians span this land, and from personal conversations I conclude that most of the direct mailing is never read. Occasional worthwhile information may be missed, but there are just too many empty oyster shells to find the pearl.

New Drugs

I suppose the physician is a born skeptic or perhaps becomes one in medical school for although he appreciates the benefits of new drugs, he does not turn to them as rapidly and as eagerly as his critics would like to have others believe. He is aware of possible toxicity and adverse side effects of drugs. He knows that most drugs in proper dosage help his patients if his diagnosis is correct and that overdosage produces adverse effects and can be fatal. He is comfortable with the drugs he knows well and can prescribe with confidence to produce the therapeutic and physiologic effect he desires.

The majority of clinical physicians move slowly in using new drugs. They must know, specifically, what advantages a new medication has over a current one and how it will fit into their armament of therapy. They insist on having the important facts relating to physiological action, dosage range, adverse effects, and possible short and long range toxicity. Only then will most change to a new drug or add it to their list for trial.

Often the physician must decide whether the benefits of a certain drug outweigh its possible adverse effects. However, he has been making such decisions since the days of Hippocrates, and there is no indication that he intends to desert this responsibility now. Aristotle expressed it well (5). "It is an easy matter to know the effects of honey, wine, helebone, cautery and cutting. But to know how, for whom, and when we should apply them—is no less an undertaking than being a physician."

The difference today is that there are so many more scientifically valid uses for drugs and so many new drugs to consider. Still the wise physician does not make decisions without facts. "Every year," says pharmacologist Louis Lasagna (6), "300 to 400 new formulations hit the market, each with an average life span of well under five years. Many of these are merely combinations of old remedies—there are 300 antibiotic preparations on the market, but only a dozen or so useful single antibiotics—but in any case the doctor is faced with the overwhelming task of evaluating these new remedies, their claimed effects and side effects, and integrating them into his practice." The young physician today certainly faces a lifetime of learning.

Let us look now at the dispute concerning tradenames and generic names for drugs. The average physician has viewed this tug-of-war with amusement and at times with anger and alarm. Most who advocate the change to generic prescribing and the discarding of tradenames are not in clinical medicine and the "front-line" of patient care. They simply do not understand nor have they experienced daily office practice. They have not faced long office schedules and evenings filled with emergencies. Any factor which would unnecessarily consume more time would place an overwhelming burden on those who carry a major portion of the medical care load—the primary physician. This includes the general practitioner, the general internist, the general pediatrician, and the general surgeon.

I have no argument with the thought that the physician should know the generic name as well as the trade name of the drug he prescribes. Furthermore, he should know the "family" of drugs to which each belongs. However, to require him to write the usually long generic name rather than the usually shorter trade name is to me unreasonable and absurd.

Undoubtedly, the use of generic prescribing, ignoring the quality of the drug involved, would result in some lowering of cost to the consumer. However, the man-hours lost would most certainly result in an increase in total health care costs. To the economist this may seem illogical, but to a busy primary physician it makes a great deal of sense.

I am familiar with all of the pros and cons in this controversy, having followed it with interest the past few years, but the simple saving of time without decreasing quality in the delivery of health care during this era of health manpower shortage is the most salient of all.

Summary

The world of drugs and the world of medical care are revolving in the same direction with amazing synchronization. In the world of medical care the clinical physician has a great deal of respect and gratitude for the industry that has placed at his disposal more drugs for preventing and treating human ills than at any time in history. The system which has been developed to perform this task is complex but follows a definite pattern. It has developed through cooperation between the drug industry, private and public medical institutions, and government. There is no better system in the world. It will change as time dictates, but the physician has every confidence that it will always serve the best interests of the American people.

The methods of communicating drug information to physicians follow many paths to many areas and are improving daily. A chief concern is the shortage of health manpower necessary to deliver the benefits of new therapy to those in need, but this is a problem of the world of medical care and not the world of drugs.

At times the physician is annoyed by too many tradenames for the same or a similar drug, but he is grateful for the tradename for its ease in determining quality and in prescribing. He dislikes information which stresses benefits of therapy without stating clearly adverse effects, but this is changing rapidly.

What does the clinician expect of the drug industry in the future? He confidently expects more miracles for tomorrow. Such ailments as arteriosclerotic cardiovascular disease and cancer which together with highway accidents are today's chief killers offer major challenges. The physician is certain that research scientists in industry and private and public medical institutions will continue to find new methods to diagnose and cure disease and that the system of drug manufacturing and distribution will become even more efficient in making benefits available to all.

Literature Cited

(1) Barber, B., Ed., "Drugs and Society," The Russell Sage Foundation.
(2) Goodman, L., Gilman, A., "The Pharmacologic Basis of Therapeutics," 2nd ed., Macmillan, New York.
(3) Keefer, Chester, "The Contributions of the Pharmaceutical," in "The Medicated Society," S. Proger, Ed., Macmillan, New York.
(4) Deno, R. *et al.*, in "Drugs and Society," B. Barber, Ed., The Russell Sage Foundation.
(5) Lasagna, Louis, "Drugs through the Ages," in "The Medicated Society," S. Proger, Ed., Macmillan, New York.
(6) Lasagna, Louis, "The Doctors Dilemma," in "The Medicated Society."
(7) Garland, J., "Dissemination of Information on Drugs to the Physician," in "Drugs in Our Society," P. Talalay, Ed., The Johns Hopkins Press, 1964.

RECEIVED November 5, 1970.

Discussion

Warren J. Close: To open this discussion, I shall bring up a subject which has important implications in many of the papers presented today —*i.e.*, the cost of research. In dealing with this matter I feel that we are too often confusing "research" with "research and development." Frequently I see published data labeling certain costs "research" when, indeed, the research and development process was being alluded to. We see this in financial analyses, too, and we hear corporation heads using the term "research" when indeed they mean "research and development." Even today, I noted that some of our distinguished panelists referred to "research" when they meant "research and development."

The point I am making is this: the development activity has different dimensions from the research activity. If one were to go to a research man and say, "Discover a new synthesis of Pentothal," that scientist would not be able to predict with any degree of accuracy how long it would take him to do this or how much it would cost. However, if he were to succeed in discovering a new process and were to bring it to a development chemist and say, "I have a new way of making Pentothal; how long is it going to take and how much is it going to cost to install this new process," the development chemist can make predictions with an almost uncanny degree of accuracy. I think we get into a bind when we try to lump these two kinds of activities together. I would like to refer this comment to Mr. Blee; I wonder if he accepts this thesis or disagrees with it.

Frank J. Blee: Dr. Close raises a very interesting question. When I say research, I guess I usually mean research and development, and what I mean is the amount of money that is spent on the people in the organizational chart from director of research and development on down to the lab technician. In other words, I refer to the process which is devoted to discovering and developing a *new* drug product. This is the creative process of coming up with that unique new chemical entity. I feel that this is the major reason for existence of the Research and Development Division—development meaning getting that product ready for the market.

The other situation Dr. Close mentions relates to product X which, let's say, your company has been making for five years and someone thinks that it can be made cheaper. The attempt to determine whether or not it can be made cheaper I would call process improvement. I wouldn't really call this research at all because you are not in search of a new compound; you are attempting to lower costs. Also, I might say quality control—in other words, the process that takes place in the Production Division to insure that the product is up to quality—is not research and development.

What the industry fails to realize is that the figure we talk about when we say 10–11% of sales are spent on R & D is a fairly pure number in the sense that it is devoted to discovering and developing new products. Now the average—and this is why I kept hammering away on the fact that the pharmaceutical industry is unique—the average for all U.S. industry is less than 2%, which means that this industry is spending at least 5 or more times the average amount as a percentage of sales. Another thing is that a good deal of that 2% of other industries is called research but is often nothing more than process improvement or cost reduction. If in a chemical company that is making nylons, for example, someone says, "Let's lower the cost," that's process improvement; it's not research, but it may show up in the R & D budget.

Another point to remember, as Dr. Close said, if you are faced with essentially a production cost accounting problem, which is what process improvement or cost reduction really is, this is much more predictable than the cost of discovering and developing a new compound. Indeed, if the question is asked today, "What is the cost of developing a drug for Parkinson's disease," it would be virtually impossible to answer because the length of time and manpower required are unpredictable.

Harry Yale (to Brian Hoffman): I would question your statement regarding failure to find another drug as useful as quinidine. There is good clinical evidence that procaine amide is a useful and effective medicine. Furthermore, the development of procaine amide was a logical development based on observations concerning procaine in human arrhythmias.

Dr. Hoffman: I don't disagree at all with these statements. I would stick to what I said in my paper, though, that the advent of procaine amide, later diphenylhydantoin and lidocaine and most recently propranolol, as antiarrhythmic agents was not the result of any direct or deliberate attempt by industry to develop useful antiarrhythmic agents. Some chance observations by cardiac surgeons suggested that procaine might be a useful antiarrhythmic agent. The subsequent development of procaine amide is what I would call a good example of goal-oriented research in industry. Procaine was useful but was found to have certain disadvantages, primarily its short biological half-life and the ease with which it penetrated the central nervous system. To overcome these obstacles was not too much of a problem for a good chemist, and so a modification of procaine—procaine amide—was made. It wasn't susceptible to rapid hydrolysis by plasma esterases and didn't penetrate as readily into the CNS and thus became a good antiarrhythmic drug. However, this is simply an improvement of a molecule which did exist and where the necessary manipulation of the molecule was rather minor. What I was talking about this morning was company-sponsored programs which had as a goal the introduction of new antiarrhythmic drugs. I think that useful antiarrhythmic drugs have not come about by searching for them in the laboratory. Dilantin was shown by Merritt and Putnam in 1938 to be useful for epilepsy, and almost by chance it was brought into the treatment of cardiac arrhythmias. Lidocaine was brought in as a local anesthetic. Again almost by chance it was found to be a useful antiarrhythmic, and now it's used very widely. So the additions have been the kind of thing that happens when somebody who knows a little bit about pharmacology and medicine is using drugs and makes observations that clue him in on other diseases or abnormalities where they might be effective. However, development of antiarrhythmics, starting from scratch, I think has not succeeded yet.

I think one could say the same thing for many other classes of drugs. A similar sort of history describes the search for better antianginal agents than nitroglycerine. Many coronary vasodilators have been developed over the years. I think people don't really feel they have made really significant additions to the treatment of angina with them except for changes in duration of action perhaps, and this probably is because the benefit that comes from nitroglycerine is not solely the result of its ability to dilate the coronary arteries. Well this information didn't accumulate until about 10 years ago, so for years and years people tried to develop other coronary dilators because they assumed that this was the only manner by which nitroglycerine was useful. Now I think more companies are beginning to look for antianginal agents that reduce the work of the heart and do other things so it may be successful. So I won't disagree with Dr. Yale, but I will stick by my guns in terms of what I said.

Dr. Yale (to George E. Burket): You have stated that "the physicians do not quickly pick up new drugs until they are convinced of their merits." How then do you explain the phenomenal growth of some of the recent drug entries, some of which have a high incidence of side effects, for example, indomethacin?

Dr. Burket: First, I think you realize that I used the term "majority of physicians." We are all aware that some individuals in the medical profession use drugs quickly and without careful consideration, but you know we like to be comfortable, and I think without knowing exactly the physiological effects of a drug, its adverse effects, its long term—or at least its short term—toxic effects, we just don't sleep well at night when we give such drugs to patients. As an explanation for the specific question I think the physician must decide, as I stated in my presentation, whether the benefits to a particular patient—the benefits that he will receive—outweigh possible adverse effects, and we must do this with an increasing number of drugs now. This is why it is so important that we know the adverse effects so that we can make this decision properly.

Dr. Close: I think we'll turn back to Mr. Blee again since we have a few more questions directed to him. Is the fact that industry promotion and distribution costs are twice those of research sufficient evidence that they are excessive? What is the standard? How do other industries compare in cost and services? Do we know? Shouldn't we know more before we judge?

Mr. Blee: First I didn't say that they were excessive. I raised the question, and I leave it to the industry to ponder this point. I did say that obviously the industry must think they're necessary or they would not spend the money. I would say that in general, given the fact that most other industries spend relatively little on research, it is probably very common to spend a good deal more on advertising and promotion than on research. Even though this industry's research budget is the highest in relationship to sales (10–11%), its advertising is a good deal more. I would say, however, that this is a special kind of industry, and the industry has to realize this. You're not selling automobiles, you're not selling cosmetics, you're not selling cigarettes. There's a special place in the economy for this industry; there are social overtones, and the economics are unique and different. It is not enough to compare it with another industry.

I would also say, as I think we all well know, that there are plans under way which would radically change the distribution system. For example, if drugs are ever included in the out-patient portion of Medicare, in order to process the number of prescriptions that will be involved (which can be 200 or 300 million a year), we are going to have to come up with an automated system to handle them. This would probably involve slave units in every retail pharmacy in the country feeding back to central computers. My feeling is technologically this has to come if everyone is covered in the nation, and indeed you all well know they are talking about a National Health Plan where everybody would be covered. Just multiply that 200 million by 5, and now you have a huge technological problem which will only be solved by automation. When that happens, you can have a radical change in the present distribution system. If the industry isn't ready for it, this can cause substantial consequences. It is incumbent upon industry to work with the problem now because there's no question that it's a very expensive system. Again, I'll not say that it isn't a good system, but I would also say to you that the industry has not convinced the government (and I don't mean the FDA, per se; I'm talking about HEW and I'm talking about HEW economists) that they can justify their advertising and promotion expenditures. They haven't convinced Senator Nelson—not at all. So they've got a lot of work to do.

Dr. Close: I wonder if our industry representative, Dr. Wescoe, has any comments to make in regard to that.

Dr. Wescoe: No, I have no comment at this time.

Dr. Close: I was a little surprised that we received no questions directed to Dr. Jennings. After his presentation, I told Dr. Jennings I thought he gave a very straightforward and frank picture that was at variance with the way some of us viewed research in the drug industry. I would like to be equally frank and straightforward with him and pose a question to him of my own.

Dr. Jennings, you have used the phrase, "molecular manipulation," which, of course, has something of an underhanded connotation. Medicinal chemists use the term "molecular modification"; we feel that this term is more suitable for a process which we consider to be a respectable and necessary form of research. We all know that very small modifications of molecules can result in quite profound changes in biological activity. The steroids are a good example of this; it doesn't take much of a change to get from a female hormone to a male hormone, and yet most of us think the difference is important. I would like to ask Dr. Jennings if he doesn't really believe that molecular modification is a necessary and useful part of the research process?

John J. Jennings: Of course it is. I certainly didn't mean to downgrade it at all. I think one of the questions that has been running through the discussions here is research *vs.* development. Dr. Hoffman pointed out that it took molecular modification or manipulation to make procaine a useful antiarrhythmic drug. Of course, I think this falls somewhere between discovery and development. It is not truly discovery, and yet it is a little bit more than cost-lowering development.

Certainly we need the molecular manipulations that result in improved products in the sense of the example cited here by Dr. Hoffman. Do we need molecular manipulations that allow us to have multiple entries into the same area so that now we give 0.5 mg per dose instead of 50 mg? What benefit is there to increasing the per milligram potency when side effects are as increased per milligram as the therapeutic benefits?

My whole argument, and I offer it simply as a proposal, is that resources be so deployed that we might be in a better position to pick up the leads that have been mentioned over and over today. These leads are truly the origins of innovations. In no way do I downgrade the fine technological apparatus that exists in the drug industry today that allows these innovations once recognized to be brought to the point where they are feasible therapeutic agents.

What I'm trying to say is that since we do accept the studies, the results of scientific studies in other areas, why not in this area? And let's just see if we are not overlooking possibilities for new discoveries. I would hope that the lode has not been mined out. I would sincerely hope that there are many new discoveries waiting to be made, and my whole argument is that we ought to be examining the apparatus to see whether or not there isn't some way of increasing the frequency of these innovative discoveries and recognizing them and then putting them into this mill.

Dr. Close: I wonder if perhaps Dr. Wescoe might have some comments to make on this same subject.

Dr. Wescoe: I think perhaps there is another way to look at it. In part I agree with Dr. Jennings, and in part I disagree. I agree with him in that the reduction in so-called new compounds is not related primarily to the 1962 amendments. I think when we begin to date things from that point we really make a mistake. The fact of the matter is, Dr. Jennings, that discovery has become more difficult, that perhaps the lode has been mined to the point where discovery is going to be less rapid than it used to be. The periodic table of the elements really isn't changing, and many of the molecules that are possible have already been discovered, prepared, or investigated by someone.

This means we're going to have to go back over some of the old ground, and that is research. In fact, Otto Loewi won the Nobel prize on the basis of an experiment with the isolated frog heart. This experiment had been tried a dozen times by others without significant result. The only reason it worked in his hands is that he used the winter frog and not the summer frog. He won the Nobel prize because he was willing to repeat something which someone else had already done. In just the same way we were willing to repeat the work which led to what you called a rejuvenated sulfonamide. For that we make no apology because the compound has saved lives. I think things like that are important; I don't think that research work that goes back over the old fields and brings back something that is really an improvement should be derided.

Nor do I think, as you indicated just in passing, that the people in this room, and you and I, represent factions. We represent the entire system, a system that really can work together now in mutual trust through an understanding of the problems that each of us faces. We can't always be on the same side of the line, but we can be together from the standpoint of integrity and the truth.

Today, discovery is more difficult. Reading the scientific material, having lived in a university for 18 years, I am aware that the great, the monumental discoveries really are not coming through in the way they did in the past. We sometimes need a significant breakthrough in another area before we can make one in a field such as ours. Beyond that I think everyone should know that research institutes and the pharmaceutical industry do not neglect innovative research—that there isn't anybody who would rather have a great breakthrough than we. It is that great breakthrough that we're looking forward to, but it takes a long time to come up with one. When one does come up, I can assure you that there will be some sort of work done by way of molecular rearrangement to find in some way a better product.

Finally, I would like to repeat that I believe the thrust toward one medication for one indication is wrong. I thought maybe Dr. Burket would comment upon that because I think the clinician *needs* the choice of substances that might do nearly the same thing because he might have a patient who responds to one better than he does to another. That is one of the bases of pharmacology and what someone else mentioned this morning, the infinite variation in biologic response.

Dr. Close: Dr. Burket, do you wish to comment on this issue?

Dr. Burket: I hesitate to put a personal interpretation on Dr. Jennings' remark, but I have a feeling that it may stem from the fact that he was at one time in clinical medicine before he assumed his present position. In our offices in medicine the detail men use this at times—this sort of molecular manipulation game. They bring their little books in with them and open them and show how they have switched the molecules and made their product a great deal different from their competitor's. When we study it very carefully, sometimes the actual benefits clinically are not that great, and I just wonder if maybe this didn't affect Dr. Jennings' attitude somewhat. I do agree with Dr. Wescoe, however, that we do appreciate having a choice of valuable drugs that we can use with our patients because many times we run into sensitivities with one drug, and we would like to have one that does not have these adverse effects but still has the same therapeutic benefit.

Question from the floor: I would like to ask a legal or unemotional question of Dr. Jennings. You cited several parts of the mandate from Congress to the FDA. I'd like to ask whether or not included in this mandate is the judgment as to whether a new molecular modification is not desirable even though it is efficacious and safe or relatively so. Do you have the mandate to decide whether the medical profession has too many diuretics or too many compounds in any other class?

Dr. Jennings: I'll answer the question directly, then I'd like to return to some of the discussion that went on here because I think that there's some confusion. We have a few questions mixed in together. First of all, the law does not give us any authority to determine that there are too many of any class of drugs. I was not speaking as a regulator when I asked that we consider, unemotionally and scientifically, the question of whether we are going about our search for new drugs in the most efficient way. Not only are we not allowed to make a determination that there are too many of a particular class of drugs and thus stop approval of further drugs in that class, we are not even allowed to make a determination that one drug is not as effective as other drugs in the same category and, therefore, should not be allowed on the market.

The legislative history of the act is quite clear on this point, the so-called comparative efficacy. This does not enter into the argument. What does enter into it, of course, is the benefit-to-risk ratio of any drug. Let me apologize if I seemed to have spoken slightingly of molecular manipulation. I think it is not only desirable but absolutely necessary in order to render the drug truly useful. However, speaking not as one who must pass an application, but as one who, as Dr. Wescoe pointed out, is a part of this system and is concerned with the ultimate productivity of the system, I am concerned with the utilization of resources to develop another thiazide that now can be given in smaller dosages, another phenothiazine, another corticosteroid with no tremendous increase in therapeutic ratio, no tremendous increase in risk-to-benefit ratio.

My whole question to you was simply this—are we overlooking something? I used a sort of military analogy. We are attacking the problem with a massive frontal assault—a human wave sort of thing—when the enemy is so elusive that perhaps what we need is more patrols out there, more scouts, more probing expeditions.

Maybe we need some way to recognize these serendipitous findings. I think the starting point should be a voyage of discovery but certainly toward the end, or after a certain amount of this type of investigation, we must turn to the heavily financed, well equipped industrial laboratory to bring the product to a point where it will be viable in today's medical and economic situation. That was my whole point. I did not decry the efforts. I applaud the efforts of improving products and lowering costs, and I pointed out that the tremendous, uniquely American technology makes it possible for these discoveries to be brought to a point where they can be useful. But original discoveries have been declining since the early 1950's, and I just suggested that part of the explanation might be that we are not providing the proper climate for this type of discovery.

Another point was brought up, and I must admit that it was the first time that I encountered it, although it came up again and again: the idea of a single entity for a single disease. I know of no policy, I know of no regulation, I know of no authority in our act, I know of no tendency on the part of the agency, to advance that concept.

Glenn Ullyot to Dr. Jennings: I think we're all going in the same direction, but there's a point that's very much missed, although Dr. Hoffman and Dr. Wescoe have alluded to it in some ways. We all would like to get the breakthrough, but what you have to study is how some of the real breakthroughs came about. We work with what we know, and it's like going in an ever-widening circle. Let's just take one real example: in studies on the antihistamines, the phenothiazines came along. It was observed that they produced a sedative effect, and it was decided that this might be an area to pursue. When Largactil, the lytic cocktail, came along, the concept that it would be used to treat mental and emotional disease hadn't developed yet. It just happened that when we eventually became involved (and it would be an interesting story to tell you how that came about) Largactil (as Thorazine) went on the market in this country for treating nausea and vomiting. The tranquilizing effect was then discovered in the clinic. We could not have predicted this. So one works with the tools that we have to proceed from one point to the next, and in this process we make these discoveries. Many other examples of how drugs are truly discovered could be given; these discoveries are not always as reported in the literature.

Question from the floor: We've heard the term "original discoveries" for some time. I would like Dr. Jennings to define "original discoveries" because we all know these do not come as flashes of light. They are often contributions of many people. What is your definition of an "original discovery"?

Dr. Jennings: I'm not sure that I can give one that would satisfy everybody, but the examples that have been cited here would suffice. I would say that it is the putting together of a unique or new or novel chemical entity for treating a clinical disease which heretofore has not been treated with that particular chemical entity. I think it boils down to the original linking of a chemical entity, since we're talking about drugs, with a clinical entity. The finding that isoniazide had the effect on the central nervous system that it did is an example of this. The quinidine and antiarrhythmia story is another example. The effects of the corticosteroids on the inflammatory process is a further example. In contrast to original discovery of that sort would be the further development and refinement of the drug. Where this stops being research and starts being development I'll leave to the economists. I'm not sure that I particularly care about that. My whole modest proposition was that we might not be doing all we can to make sure that we are providing a climate for original discoveries of this sort and then the recognition and development of them.

Dr. Close: Thank you, Dr. Jennings. I believe we have covered essentially all of the questions which were submitted to me. Glenn, do you have final comments before we close?

Dr. Ullyot: I want to thank our speakers and panelists for taking the time to come here and talk to us today. We have reviewed in a very thorough manner the system of drug discovery and development and the problems associated with it.

INDEX

INDEX